THE CONSTRUCTION OF THE SELF

DISTINGUISHED CONTRIBUTIONS IN PSYCHOLOGY
A Guilford Series

Editors: **Kurt W. Fischer**   **E. Tory Higgins**
          Harvard University   *Columbia University*

THE CONSTRUCTION OF THE SELF

A Developmental Perspective

SUSAN HARTER

Foreword by Kurt W. Fischer

THE GUILFORD PRESS
New York   London

Library of Congress Cataloging-in-Publication Data

Harter, Susan, 1939–
  The construction of the self : a developmental perspective / Susan
Harter.
    p.   cm. – (Distinguished contributions in psychology)
  Includes bibliographical references and index.
  ISBN 1-57230-432-4 (hard cover : alk. paper)
  1. Self in children.   2. Self in adolescence.   I. Title.
II. Series.
BF723.S24H37   1999
155.2–dc21   98-56206
                                                                   CIP

To my mother, Alma B. Harter,
whose lifelong commitment to the
education and nurturance of children
inspired me to pursue a career
in developmental psychology

About the Author

Susan Harter, PhD, is Professor of Psychology and Head of the Developmental Psychology Program at the University of Denver. Her research, supported by funds from the National Institutes of Health for over 20 years, has resulted in the construction of a lifespan battery of self-report instruments to tap dimensions of the self-concept. These instruments are currently in use throughout the United States and internationally. In addition, she has received two major faculty awards, University Lecturer of the Year and the John Evans Professorship Award, the highest award to be bestowed upon a faculty member. Both awards are for national and international recognition in one's chosen field of research. Dr. Harter has written numerous journal articles and chapters, including chapters on self-concept, self-esteem, as well as motivational and emotional development in the 1983 and 1998 *Handbook of Child Psychology*. She has also served on National Institute of Mental Health study sections, chaired the Cognition, Emotion, and Personality Committee, and currently is on the editorial boards of a number of journals, including *Developmental Psychology, Child Development, Psychological Bulletin, Development and Psychopathology,* and *American Educational Research Journal.* In two independent citation analyses, published in 1995 and 1997, Dr. Harter has emerged among the top 50 most widely cited developmental psychologists.

Foreword

How do children and adolescents see themselves, and how are their self-perceptions and actions influenced by their relationships with other people? What are the pathways of the development of the self, situated in its natural social context, in relation with others? How do cognitive, social, and emotional processes work together in constructing pathways for the self? These important topics are at the center of this book, and they should be at the center of the study of psychology and child development in general. There has been a lack of strong research on the self in social relationships, and these topics have been relegated to the periphery of the field. Remarkably few scholars have systematically explored the nature of the developing self in relationships and built theories solidly grounded in a broad range of observations. Thus, in this area, very few scholars have succeeded in capturing the natural breadth of human behavior and experience.

This book and the work it represents mark a watershed in the study of the development of the self in relationships. Susan Harter has used her considerable talents to study a wide range of phenomena and bring them together in a coherent portrait of how children and adolescents develop. The field is moving away from overly simple, universalist conceptions of human development toward richly textured, ecological conceptions that depict variable pathways. Harter captures the texture of these variations, showing that self-esteem, for example, reflects a diverse collection of self-evaluations in the distinct, socially defined domains of academics, peer relationships, athletic skills, physical attractiveness, and so on, rather than a single, unified personality characteristic. Gender differences depend on combinations of masculine and feminine characteristics and identifications, with wide variations among girls and among boys. Low evaluations of global self-worth arise along several distinctive pathways, although they lead uniformly to depression and hopelessness. For so many topics, Harter conveys the diversity of developmental pathways. Anyone who reads and connects with this book will come away with a rich view of the natural variations among people in their emotional state, identification, gender, culture, social situation, disability, and trauma. There is no one pathway for development of "*the* child" but instead there are many ways to become human.

A powerful reason for Harter's success in portraying the diversity of these pathways is that she eschews the standard pigeonholing of conventional psychology. Cognition, emotion, and social relations are not separate for children's minds; they are merely arbitrary ways of dividing up psychology. Harter's work is grounded in the assumption that children and adolescents do not stay in social scientists' boxes. She integrates cognitive and social processes in order to capture individuals' development according to their own viewpoints and those of people who live closely with them. Thoughts, feelings, and relationships are all together in the fabric of living.

Another reason for the richness in Harter's work is her skill at building new methods for assessing questions of interest. Besides an ability to raise important issues, she possesses a special ingenuity in constructing methods for eliciting one's conceptions of oneself in important relationships; she has made new assessment tools that have instantly become the best available. Her innovative methods are not esoteric or fancy but go directly to the phenomena of interest, getting to the core of things themselves. Each of her methods is simply the clearest, most straightforward way of assessing a domain, from the viewpoints of both the person being assessed and the researcher. Harter merits a special award for innovative engineering of developmental and social assessment tools.

Harter's work, and this book, are worthwhile and engaging not only for their scientific value, but also because she brings together theory and research with everyday practice. Adults who live and work with children and adolescents—at home, in school, and other institutions in the community—would welcome help from child psychologists in supporting and nurturing the young people in their lives. Yet most psychological research and theory is no more or less successful at improving children's self-worth than anecdotal common sense. Research and theory should try to connect with everyday practice, to enrich our concepts and give us tools to act effectively in our dealings with young people. Harter's approach consistently links her work to practice, especially schooling, clinical intervention, and parenting. These connections are evident on every page of the book.

To bring her book to a fruitful conclusion, Harter takes on the need to link theory to practice and creates an exceptional final chapter. She ties the concepts of research reviewed in the book to diverse interventions that "promote adaptive self-evaluations." Her framework avoids the banal popular belief that everyone should feel wonderful about him- or herself in every way, and instead she outlines how her framework facilitates positive and realistic self-evaluations in people who may be developing quite differently. This creates a much more incisive overview of her arguments and findings than would a simple summary. The book thus ends in a way that reflects its power in depicting the diversity of pathways of development of the self in relationships and in using what we know from that knowledge to enrich and improve children's lives.

KURT W. FISCHER, PhD
Harvard University Graduate School of Education

Acknowledgments

I would first like to express my gratitude to Seymour Weingarten, Editor-in-Chief of The Guilford Press, whose support, encouragement, faith in my mission and message, and patience allowed this volume to come to fruition. I am also indebted to Kurt Fischer for his intellectual contribution to the field. Much of the thinking about development in this book builds upon his own theoretical and empirical efforts. I am also grateful to Kurt for the many hours he spent thoughtfully critiquing earlier drafts of the manuscript. I thank my editor at Guilford, Rochelle Serwator, for her painstaking review of the manuscript and her many suggestions that greatly clarified the points I sought to make. I was greatly assisted by her guidance through the editorial process. I also appreciate the assistance of Anna Nelson who oversaw the production of the book.

Crafting this volume was by no means a solo effort. Many collaborators over the years have enriched my own thinking and have given me insights into the process of self-development. In addition, they have helped steer the course of my research down new and exciting pathways. Donna Marold brought her clinical perspective to bear on the development of a model linking negative self-perceptions to depressive reactions, including suicidal ideation. Moreover, in her expertise in the area of abuse and trauma, she not only increased my understanding of how these experiences negatively impact self-processes but provided me with rich and illustrative case examples. Tricia Waters contributed immensely to the studies we did together of the adolescent voice as well as to the work we did on autonomy and connectedness as dimensions of adult relationship styles. The breadth and depth of her thinking greatly enhanced those efforts.

Over the years, through all the many topics we have addressed together, my colleague Nancy Whitesell has been truly invaluable to me. She has been instrumental in the design and implementation of our studies, and her insights have facilitated the construction of measures and methodological procedures. In addition, her statistical talents have ably guided us through the analysis and interpretation of very complex data. Particularly welcome has been the clarity of her thinking.

Many graduate students and postdoctoral fellows have contributed to the program of research I have been committed to. These trainees have raised intriguing research questions that have moved the thinking of the team in new directions. These individuals include Kauser Ahmed, Kym Baum, Bonnie Buddin, Heather Bouchey, Shelley Bresnick, Cris Chandler, Chris Chao, Jim Connell, Barbara Danis, Jackie Dougherty, Jane Haltiwanger, Brad Jackson, Crystal Johnson, Eric Johnson, Lori Junkin, Jennifer Kofkin, Keven Lancelotta, Wanda Mayberry, Tara Mehta, Bonnie Messer, Ann Monsour, Jennifer Neeman, Kristin Neff, Rosanna Ng, Diana Nikkari, Patty Kowalski, Lisa Pettit, Robin Pike, Mari Jo Renick, Nancy Robinson, Valerie Simon, Clare Stocker, and Ayelet Talmi.

I am grateful as well to the National Institutes of Health for generous financial support of this research program over many years, and I thank the Grant Foundation for its support of the seminal studies I did with Donna Marold on the link between self-evaluations and depression. I wish to thank Principal Steve Cohen, his faculty, and the students at Flood Middle School for their continued collaboration and support of our research over the past 20 years. Additionally, I thank the school administrations and students at Smoky Hill High School, Cherry Creek High School, Rangeview High School, Englewood High School, Bear Creek High School, Laredo Middle School, Indian Hills Elementary School, Steele Elementary School, and the Columbine Psychiatric Center.

Nancy Pleiman deserves special thanks for her tireless typing, and Ayelet Talmi and Tara Mehta for the thankless task of proofreading. I am also grateful to Jennifer Shepard for secretarial assistance.

Very special thanks go to my colleague and friend Cathy Cooper for inspiring me through her own example to create a meaningful vision of the message I wanted to share with readers. Stephen Shirk also served as a supportive role model through the various stages of the evolution of this volume. Finally, I want to thank my family for their continued encouragement, support, and patience with me as well as with the process. Bringing this book to maturity has clearly taken the dedication of a village.

Contents

CHAPTER ONE

Contemporary Issues and Historical Perspectives

Interest in self-processes has burgeoned in the past decade within many branches of psychology. Cognitive-developmentalists, particularly those of a neo-Piagetian persuasion, have addressed normative changes in the emergence of a sense of self (e.g., Case, 1985, 1992; Fischer, 1980; Harter, 1997; Higgins, 1991). Developmentalists interested in memory processes have also described how the self is crafted through the construction of narratives that provide the basis for autobiographical memory (see Fivush, 1987; Nelson, 1986, 1993; Snow, 1990). Contemporary attachment theorists, building upon the earlier efforts of Ainsworth (1973, 1974) and Bowlby (1980), have provided new insights into how interactions with caregivers come to shape the representations of self and others that young children come to construct (see Bretherton, 1991, 1992; Cassidy, 1990; Cicchetti, 1990, 1991; Cicchetti & Beeghly, 1990; Pipp, 1990; Sroufe, 1990). Clinicians within the psychodynamic tradition have also contributed to our understanding of how early socialization experiences come to shape the structure and content of self-evaluations and contribute to psychopathology (Blatt, 1995; Bleiberg, 1984; Kernberg, 1975; Kohut, 1977; Winnicott, 1965). Moreover, social and personality theorists have devoted considerable attention to those processes that produce individual differences in perceptions of self, particularly among adults (see Baumeister, 1987, 1993; Epstein, 1991; Kihlstrom, 1993; Markus & Wurf, 1987; Steele, 1988).

Clearly, there is a "new look" to many of these contemporary formulations. However, the field has also witnessed a return to many of the classic issues that captured the attention of historical scholars of the self. For example, new life has been breathed into James' (1890, 1892) distinction between the I-self—the self as subject, agent, knower—and the Me-self—the self as object, as known. In addition, James' analysis of the antecedents of self-esteem has now been put to an empirical test (see Harter, 1993, 1998a).

1

There has also been a resurgence of interest in the formulations of those symbolic interactionists, namely, Baldwin (1897), Cooley (1902), and Mead (1934), who placed heavy emphasis on how interactive processes with caregivers shape the developing self.

Interest in self-processes has escalated, in part, given increasing emphasis on their *functional* role in development. Thus, far from being an epiphenomenon, the self has taken center stage as a dynamic actor, playing a variety of roles. In fact, it is commonly asserted that the very architecture of the self-theory, by evolutionary design, is extremely functional across the life span. Attachment theorists (e.g., Bretherton, 1991; Cassidy, 1990; Sroufe, 1990) have observed how working models of the self have *organizational* significance, providing infants and young children with a set of expectations that allows them more efficiently to guide their behavior. The development of self-relevant scripts also provides the toddler with predictive structure; moreover, the emergence of autobiographical memories, scaffolded by the narrative co-construction of the self, serves to define the self and cement social bonds (e.g., Crittenden, 1994; Fivush, 1987; Hudson, 1990b; Nelson, 1993; Snow, 1990).

For those focusing on childhood and adolescence, self-structures serve to shape goals (e.g., Dweck, 1991; Ruble & Frey, 1991) and to provide self-guides that aid in appropriate social behaviors and self-regulation (e.g., Higgins, 1991). Positive self-affects, in the form of pride, serve to foster an emotional investment in one's competencies and energize one toward further accomplishments. Negative self-conscious emotions, particularly guilt, have also been afforded very functional, social properties across the life span in that they provoke behaviors directed toward reparation, rebonding, and the maintenance of emotional attachments (see Barrett, 1995; Tangney & Fischer, 1995). Social psychologists who address adult self-processes have also articulated a number of similar functions. Markus and colleagues (e.g., Markus & Kityama, 1991; Markus & Nurius, 1986; Markus & Wurf, 1987; Oyserman & Markus, 1993) have focused on how the self organizes, interprets, and gives meaning to experience, regulates affect, and motivates action by providing incentives, standards, plans, and scripts (see also Carver & Scheier, 1990; Greenwald, 1980). Moreover, the construction of future, possible selves (Markus & Nurius, 1986) further organizes behavior and energizes the individual to pursue selected goals. Discrepancies between real and ideal self-concepts can also motivate the individual to achieve his/her ideals in the service of self-improvement (Banaji & Prentice, 1994; Bandura, 1990; Oosterwegel & Oppenheimer, 1993; Rogers, 1951).

Epstein and colleagues (e.g., Epstein, 1991; Epstein & Morling, 1995) have identified four basic needs that require the construction of a self. The individual needs (1) to maintain a favorable sense of his/her attributes, which in turn will help to (2) maximize pleasure and minimize pain; moreover, one needs to (3) develop and maintain a coherent picture of the world, as well as to (4) maintain relatedness with others. The first self-enhancement function has also been addressed by others (e.g., Beach & Tesser, 1995; Steele, 1988; Tesser, 1988; Tesser & Cornell, 1991). Certain social psychologists have emphasized more specific motives. For example, Greenberg, Pyszczynski, and Solomon (1995) concur that the pursuit of positive self-esteem is a superordinate goal toward which humans aspire. However, they also argue that self-esteem serves as an anxiety buffer against adults' terror over their eventual death. Leary and Downs (1995) have identified a different social function, namely, avoidance of social exclusion. They argue that behaviors that maintain self-esteem decrease the likelihood that one will be ignored or rejected by other people. Clearly, across different theorists addressing different stages of development, the functions of various self-representations have surfaced as an important consideration.

DEFINITIONS OF SELF

Self terminology abounds: self-concept, self-image, self-esteem, self-worth, self-evaluations, self-perceptions, self-representations, self-schemas, self-affects, self-efficacy, and self-monitoring, to name but a few. Certain scholars of the self have argued that the plethora of terminology and contradictory definitions, both conceptual and operational, have rendered much of the literature uninterpretable (see Wylie, 1979, 1989). Given that varying conceptualizations define the landscape of the self literature, leading to potential confusion in how terms are to be interpreted, it is critical to clarify the terminology to be employed in this volume. At the broadest level, I will focus on self-representations, namely, attributes or characteristics of the self that are consciously acknowledged by the individual through language—that is, how one describes oneself. The terms "self-representations," "self-perceptions," and "self-descriptions" will be used interchangeably to denote this general process.

There are those in the field (e.g., Gordon, 1968; McGuire & McGuire, 1980) who have urged that we make a distinction between self-descriptions (namely, "*what* I am") and self-evaluations (namely, "how *good* I am"). This distinction has in part resulted from the use of different methodologies. Many instruments designed to evaluate the self-concept explicitly require that participants react to statements in the form of judgments about whether the self is viewed favorably or unfavorably ("I am scholastically competent," "I am not that popular," etc.). As a methodological alternative, Gordon, McGuire, and colleagues have asked respondents to define themselves in response to the open-ended question "Who am I?" Such a procedure lends itself to a content analysis of spontaneously generated self-descriptions that are then coded into categories that provide a portrait of the dimensions that are most salient to individuals' self-representations. The attributes that individuals produce through such a methodology are viewed by these investigators as self-descriptions rather than self-evaluations. In contrast, those who focus on self-evaluations have employed measures that specifically require individuals to indicate whether they view themselves positively or negatively; that is, the instruments require that individuals attach a valence to self-attributes. Thus, one is forced to report on whether the self is smart or dumb, popular or unpopular, good-looking or unattractive.

However, the distinction between self-descriptions and self-evaluations is rather arbitrary in that it is not very clear-cut. For example, in the "Who am I?" task, a young child may offer descriptions such as "I am strong," "I live in a big house," "I know my ABC's," and "I love pizza." Although this procedure does not require the child to identify the valence of the attributes generated, it is highly likely that if specifically asked to provide this information, being strong and knowing one's alphabet would be judged favorably. It is also likely that self-descriptors such as living in a big house and loving pizza would also represent favorable self-definitions; that is, the self-system is affectively charged in that it represents those characteristics that allow individuals to make *meaning* of their personal transactions with their social and physical environment (see Emde, 1994). Much of this meaning is derived from the construction of self-representations that are judged to be favorable or unfavorable. Building upon Wundt's (1907) observations, Osgood, Suci, and Tannenbaum (1971) convincingly demonstrated, through their use of the semantic differential, that in making meaning out of linguistic concepts, *evaluation* is the most potent dimension; that is, individuals organize concepts, be they about self or others, in terms of judgments that are positive versus negative. Their procedure revealed that this dimension operates across numerous content categories. For example, judgments can be morally evaluative (e.g., good, bad), aesthetically evaluative (e.g., pretty, ugly), socially evaluative (e.g., honest, untrustworthy), and emotionally evaluative (calm, tense). This evaluative dimension was revealed to be primary in human thinking, as evidenced in the responses of adults.

From a developmental perspective, it can be observed that beginning with the first uses of language, young children bifurcate their conceptual world into evaluative judgments of "good" versus "bad." They impose this conceptual framework on self-*attributes* such as nice versus mean (see Fischer, 1980) or smart versus dumb (Harter, 1983, 1986b), as well as on *emotions* experienced by the self, namely, good feelings versus bad feelings (Harter & Whitesell, 1989). Thus, in this volume, it will not be assumed that in studies focusing on self-descriptions, the attributes that children or adolescents generate are valence-free. In all likelihood, since they have affective meaning, they reflect representations that fall somewhere along an evaluative continuum. However, where investigators have not explicitly inquired into the issue of valence, the more general terms, namely, "self-descriptions," "self-perceptions," or "self-representations," will be employed. Where the focus has been the assessment of the valence of self-descriptors, the term "self-evaluations" will be employed.

Global versus Domain-Specific Evaluations

It has become increasingly important to the field to distinguish between self-evaluations that represent global characteristics of the individual (e.g., "I am a worthwhile person") and those that reflect the individual's sense of adequacy across particular domains such as one's cognitive competence (e.g., "I am smart"), social competence (e.g., "I am well liked by peers"), athletic competence (e.g., "I am good at sports"), and so forth (see Epstein, 1990; Harter, 1986a, 1997; Marsh, 1986, 1987; Rosenberg, 1979). Conceptualizations and instruments that aggregate domain-specific self-evaluations into a single score (e.g., Coopersmith, 1967) have been found wanting in that they mask the meaningful distinctions between an individual's sense of adequacy across domains. Moreover, the separation of the evaluation of one's global worth as a person from more domain-specific attributes has allowed investigators to construct hierarchical models of the relationship among these self-constructs, as we shall come to see.

With regard to terminology, global self-evaluations have typically be referred to as "self-esteem" (Rosenberg, 1979), "self-worth" (Harter, 1982a, 1993) or "general self-concept" (Marsh, 1986, 1987). In each case, the focus is on the overall evaluation of one's worth or value as a person. In this volume, I employ the terms "self-esteem" and "self-worth" interchangeably. (I refrain from using the term "general self-concept" except when referring to those few investigators who employ this terminology.) It is important to appreciate the fact that this general evaluation is tapped by its own set of items that explicitly ask about one's perceived worth as a person (e.g., I feel that I am a worthwhile person); that is, it is *not* a summary statement of self-evaluations across different domains.

In this volume, the term "self-concept" is primarily reserved for evaluative judgments of attributes within discrete domains such as cognitive competence, social acceptance, physical appearance, and so forth. Thus, I make reference to "domain-specific self-evaluations." As will become evident, such a focus allows the investigator to construct a *profile* of self-evaluations across domains for individuals or for particular subgroups of interest. Moreover, the separation of global self-esteem or self-worth from domain-specific evaluations allows one to address the issue of whether evaluations in some domains are more predictive of global self-esteem than are others, a topic to which we shall return.

The I-Self versus the Me-Self

This chapter also builds upon another distinction in the literature. The majority of scholars who have devoted thoughtful attention to the self have come to a similar conclusion: Two distinct but intimately intertwined aspects of self can be meaningfully identified, self as *subject* (the I-self) and self as *object* (the Me-self). William James (1890) introduced this distinction, defining the I-self as the actor or *knower*, whereas the Me-self was the object of one's knowledge, "an empirical aggregate of things objectively known" (p. 197). James also identified particular features or components of both the I-self and the Me-self. Components of the I-self included (1) self-*awareness*, an appreciation for one's internal states, needs, thoughts, and emotions; (2) self-*agency*, the sense of the authorship over one's thoughts and actions; (3) self-*continuity*, the sense that one remains the same person over time; and (4) self-*coherence*, a stable sense of the self as a single, coherent, bounded entity. Components of the Me-self included the "material me," the "social me," and the "spiritual me."

The distinction between the I-self and the Me-self has proved amazingly viable and appears as a recurrent theme in most theoretical treatments of the self. While others embellished upon James' formulation, and have employed somewhat different terminology, the essence of the distinction has been retained. Dickstein (1977), for example, contrasted the "dynamic" self that possesses a sense of personal agency and control to the self as the object of one's knowledge and evaluation. Lewis and Brooks-Gunn (1979) initially defined this duality as the *existential* self and the *categorical* self. The task of the developing I-self, the self as *subject*, is to develop the realization that it is "existential" in that it *exists* as separate from others. The Me-self, namely, self as *object*, is referred to as "categorical" in that the developing child must construct categories by which to define himself/herself (e.g., age and gender labels). Wylie (1979) summarized the essence of the distinctions that have been drawn by numerous theorists. The I-self is the active observer, whereas the Me-self is the observed, the product of the observing process when attention is focused on the self.

More recently, Lewis (1991, 1994) has adopted new terminology. He now refers to the I-self as the "machinery of the self," which represents basic biological and perceptual processes that can initially be observed prior to 15–18 months. Lewis describes the Me-self as the "idea of me," namely, cognitive representations of the self that do not emerge until the second half of the second year. The machinery of the self-system is also referred to as "subjective self-awareness," since when attention is directed away from the self to external objects, people, events, one is the *subject* of consciousness. In contrast, the "idea of me" can also be described as "objective self-awareness," which involves focusing on the self as the *object* of consciousness. For Lewis, many of the earliest self-processes do not require the "idea of me" or objective self-awareness; however, other manifestations of self, notably self-conscious emotions, do demand such a representation, as will subsequently be discussed.

Until recently, major empirical attention had been devoted to the Me-self, to the study of the self as an object of one's knowledge and evaluation, as evidenced by the myriad number of studies on self-concept and self-esteem (see Harter, 1983; Wylie, 1979). More recently, the I-self, which James himself regarded as an elusive if not incorrigible construct, has become more prominent in accounts of self-development. As we will come to appreciate in this volume, both the structure and content of the Me-self at any given developmental level necessarily depend upon the particular I-self capabilities, namely, those cognitive processes that define the knower. Thus, the cognitive-developmental changes in I-self processes will directly influence the nature of the self-theory that the child is constructing.

As noted in the introductory section of this chapter, most scholars conceptualize the self as a *theory* that must be cognitively constructed. Those theorists within the tradition of adult personality and social psychology have suggested that the self-theory should possess the characteristics of any formal theory, defined as a hypothetico-deductive system. Such a personal epistemology should, therefore, meet those criteria by which any good theory is evaluated, namely, the degree to which it is parsimonious, empirically valid, internally consistent, coherently organized, testable, and useful. From a developmental perspective, however, the self-theories created by children cannot met these criteria, given numerous cognitive limitations that have been identified in Piagetian (1960) and neo-Piagetian formulations (e.g., Case, 1992; Fischer, 1980); that is, the I-self in its role as constructor of the Me-self does not, in childhood, possess the capacities to create a hierarchically organized system of postulates that are internally consistent, coherently organized, testable, or empirically valid. In fact, it is not until late adolescence, if not early adulthood, that the abilities to construct a self-portrait meeting the criteria of a good formal theory potentially emerge. Therefore, in our developmental analysis of the self as a cognitive construction, it will be essential to examine how the changing characteristics of the I-self processes that define each developmental stage directly impact the Me-self, namely, the self-theory that is being constructed.

ANTECEDENTS OF THE SELF AS A COGNITIVE AND SOCIAL CONSTRUCTION

In examining the development of the self, this volume focuses on the *antecedents* of self-representations as well as on their functional *consequences*. With regard to antecedents, it will become evident that the self is both a *cognitive* and a *social* construction, two major themes around which the material to be presented will be organized. From a cognitive-developmental perspective, the construction of self-representations is inevitable. As neo-Piagetians (e.g., Case, 1992; Fischer, 1980) and self-theorists (e.g., Epstein, 1973, 1981, 1991; Greenwald, 1980; Kelly, 1955; Markus, 1980; Sarbin, 1962) have forcefully argued, our species has been designed to actively create *theories* about one's world, to make *meaning* of one's experiences, including the construction of a theory of self. Thus, the self is, first and foremost, a *cognitive construction*.

As a result, the self will develop over time; that is, as cognitive processes undergo normative-developmental change, so will self-concepts, including their very structure and organization. Thus, because the self is a cognitive construction, the particular cognitive abilities and limitations of each developmental period will represent the template that dictates the features of the self-portrait to be crafted. As will become evident, a cognitive-developmental analysis will focus primarily on changes in the *structure* of the self-system, namely, how self-representations are conceptually organized. As such, primary emphasis will be given to processes responsible for those normative-developmental changes that result in *similarities* in self-representations among individuals at a given developmental level.

Previous ontogenetic accounts highlighted major qualitative differences in the nature of self-descriptions associated with broad stages of development. Within the field of development, observers were initially struck by the most outstanding markers in the psychological landscape, namely, dramatic differences that defined the stage models of the day (e.g., Piaget, 1960). More recent treatments of self-development fill in the gaps by providing a more detailed account of the progression of substages of self-understanding. As a result, we have necessarily had to alter our views about whether the development of self-representations is best viewed as a discontinuous or continuous process. Employing frameworks of the past, self-development was viewed as largely discontinuous, with an emphasis on the saltatory nature of the conceptual leaps from one broadly defined stage to another. From this perspective, theorists highlighted the dramatic *differences* between the self-descriptions and evaluations of young children, older children, and adolescents. However, there has been a shift in emphasis, one that is reflected in this volume. The development of self-representations is now viewed as more continuous, in that investigators specify more ministeps or substages that occur, including how such levels build upon, and transform, one another.

In focusing on normative-developmental changes, we see how cognitive development impacts two general characteristics of the self-structure, the level of differentiation and integration that the individual can bring to bear upon the postulates in his/her self-theory. With regard to differentiation, emerging cognitive abilities allow the individual to create self-evaluations that differ across various domains of experience. Moreover, they permit the older child to distinguish between real and ideal self-concepts, which can then be compared to one another, creating potential discrepancies that have further consequences for the self. During adolescence, newfound cognitive capabilities support the creation of multiple selves in different relational contexts.

With regard to *integration*, cognitive abilities that emerge across the course of development allow the individual to construct higher-order generalizations about the self in the form of trait labels (e.g., demonstrated skills in math, science, and language arts are subsumed under the self-concept of "smart"). Abilities that emerge in middle childhood also permit the individual to construct a concept of his/her worth as a person, namely, an evaluation of one's global self-esteem. Further cognitive advances in adolescence allow one to successfully intercoordinate seemingly contradictory self-attributes (e.g., How can I be both cheerful and depressed?) into meaningful abstractions about the self (e.g., I'm a moody person). Each of these themes will be addressed in subsequent chapters.

In addition to an exploration of the cognitive-developmental antecedents of the self, emphasis is placed upon the self as a social construction. Thus, attention is devoted to an examination of how socialization experiences in children's interactions with caregivers, peers, teachers, and in the wider sociocultural context will influence the particular *content* and *valence* of one's self-representations. Those building upon the symbolic interactionist perspective (Baldwin, 1895; Cooley, 1902; Mead, 1934), as well as those of an attachment theory persuasion, have focused on how socialization experiences with caregivers produce *individual differences* in the content of self-representations, including whether evaluations of the self are favorable or unfavorable. I examine how the reactions of significant others determine whether the child comes to view the self as competent versus incapable, as lovable versus undeserving of others' affection, as worthy of esteem versus lacking in value. Although cognitive-developmentalists emphasize the fact that children are active agents in their own development, including the construction of self, those from the symbolic interactionist and attachment perspectives alert us to the fact that children are also at the mercy of the particular caregiving hand they have been dealt.

To summarize, with regard to antecedents, the self is both a cognitive and a social construction. In examining the self as a cognitive construction, attention focused on those cognitive-developmental processes that result in changes in the *structure* of the self-system, namely, how self-representations are organized. This approach provides an account of normative, developmental change, and emphasizes the *similarities* among individuals at a given stage of development. In treating the self as a social construction, attention turns to those socialization processes that reflect how children are treated by caregivers, interactions that primarily impact the *evaluative content* of self-representations. Although child-rearing practices do impact normative-developmental changes, attention is primarily focused on how they produce *individual differences* in whether judgments about the self are favorable or unfavorable.

CONSEQUENCES OF SELF-DEVELOPMENT

A second major goal of this volume is to examine the consequences of these cognitive and social processes. Why, for example, should we care about self-development? It will be argued that self-representations are of little interest unless it can be demonstrated that they have broader behavioral implications, unless there are ramifications for how individuals adapt to or cope with the developmental tasks that confront them. As observed earlier in this chapter, the self has been afforded many *positive* functions. These can be organized into three general categories. Self-processes perform *organizational* functions in that they provide expectations, predictive structure, and guidelines that allow one to interpret and give meaning to life experiences and to maintain a coherent picture of oneself in relation to one's world. Structures that serve to define the self also cement social bonds and foster appropriate social behavior as well as self-regulation. Self-processes also perform *motivational* functions in that they energize the individual to pursue selected goals, they provide plans and incentives, and they identify standards that allow one to achieve ideals in the service of self-improvement. Finally, self-processes perform *protective* functions toward the goal of maintaining favorable impressions of one's attributes and more generally to maximize pleasure and minimize pain.

The Liabilities of Self-Development

Unfortunately, as will become obvious in this volume, self-processes do not always conform to this functional job description. Rather, there are numerous potential negative correlates and consequences on the path to self-development. Paradoxically, some of these forks in the road are inevitable, given developmental advances; that is, emerging cognitive-developmental structures not only pave the way for a more mature self-structure but also usher in the potential for a variety of negative correlates and consequences. The path to self-development, therefore, represents a veritable minefield. As others have also pointed out, there are costs to development (Leahy, 1985), as new cognitive acquisitions provoke vulnerabilities for the self-system (Higgins, 1991). These liabilities are apparent at every level of development. Thus, attention is devoted to both positive and negative outcomes that result from normative-developmental acquisitions.

For example, during toddlerhood, a positive view of oneself as an active agent, including confidence in one's abilities, will lead to a sense of *self-efficacy*, namely, the perception that one has control over certain outcomes that can be successfully performed (Bandura, 1990). Moreover, there are positive affective consequences, in that such mastery produces feelings of pleasure, if not elation (Case, 1991; Connell & Wellborn, 1991; Deci & Ryan, 1995; Stipek, Recchia, & McClintic, 1992; White, 1959). However, there are also liabilities associated with the new cognitive-developmental acquisitions that emerge during this period. To take one example, the ability to differentiate the self from others, which involves the realization that self and others are each independent agents, dramatically reduces one's sense of omnipotence and control over caregivers; that is, if mother is her own independent agent, she may not share the same agenda, leading the toddler to experience frustration, anger, and distress as the mother engages in actions that are beyond the toddler's control.

Language represents another very potent acquistion for the development of the self. It allows the toddler to craft and to verbalize representations of the self, including the creation of a personal narrative. However, as Stern (1985) argues, language can drive a wedge between two simultaneous forms of interpersonal experience, namely, as it is lived, and as it is verbally represented. The very capacity for objectifying the self through verbal representations allows one to transcend, and therefore potentially distort, one's immediate experience and to create a fantasied construction of the self. Language also provides descriptive labels, for example, "good" versus "bad," that allow the child to evaluate his/her behavior, and these evaluations come to define the self. However, the emergence of cognitive structures that produce all-or-none thinking may lead young children, in the face of failure or censure, to conclude that they are "all bad."

During middle childhood, cognitive acquisitions allow the child to differentiate his/her abilities across domains (e.g., one is better in some arenas than others), and they also allow the child to compare his/her performance to that of others. These advances lead to more realistic evaluations of one's competencies (see Harter, 1998a). However, social comparison also ushers in the likelihood that many who fall short of others will develop perceptions of incompetence and inadequacy. Moreover, the emerging capacity to differentiate the real from the ideal self leads to potential discrepancies that can threaten the self-system. Newfound cognitive abilities also scaffold the construction of a more complex hierarchy of self-evaluations in which there are general self-schemas at the apex (e.g., global self-esteem), under which more specific attributes (e.g., cognitive competence, social skills) are conceptually nested. However, the global self-postulates at the apex are more resistant to change (Epstein, 1991), particularly if they have become highly automatized (Siegler, 1991). If such schemas are negative, the individual will display low self-esteem that may not be responsive to interventions and that may be associated with other liabilities, such as depression.

During adolescence, the emergence of abstract thinking, introspection, and self-reflection moves self-representations to a new level in that the teenager is compelled to differentiate his/her attributes into multiple, role-related selves. Simultaneously, the developing cognitive apparatus compels the individual to attempt to integrate these differing self-attributes into a coherent and consistent self-theory (Fischer, 1980; Harter & Monsour, 1992). However, the adolescent does not yet have the cognitive skills to create such an integrated self-portrait. As a result, given the normative proliferation of multiple selves, he/she will experience conflict over self-attributes in different roles that are seemingly contradictory. This multiplicity, in turn, provokes concern and confusion over which is the real self (Harter, Bresnick, Bouchey, & Whitesell, 1997).

In addition to the contribution of cognitive-developmental processes, the second class of antecedents, *socialization* experiences, can also result in both positive and negative consequences. As the symbolic interactionists observed, the self is primarily a social construction crafted through linguistic exchanges (i.e., symbolic interactions) with significant others (Baldwin, 1897; Cooley, 1902; Mead, 1925, 1934). Thus, the personal self develops in the crucible of interpersonal relationships with caregivers. One outcome is that the child adopts the opinions that significant others are perceived to hold toward the self, reflected appraisals that will define one's sense of self as a person. Through an *internalization* process, the child comes to own these evaluations as his/her personal judgments about the self. Although the symbolic interactionists pointed to critical processes in the normative construction of the self, they did not alert us to the fact that self-development could go awry; that is, there are potential liabilities associated with the construction of a self that is so highly dependent upon social interactions with significant others.

Benevolent socializing agents readily provide the nurturance, approval, and support that is mirrored in self-evaluations that are positive. Approval, in the form of the reflected appraisals of others, is, therefore, internalized as acceptance of self. However, in the search for his/her image in the social mirror, the child may well gaze through a glass darkly. Caregivers lacking in responsiveness, nurturance, encouragement and approval, as well as socializing agents who are rejecting, punitive, or neglectful, will cause their children to develop tarnished images of self. In the extreme, children subjected to severe and chronic abuse create images of the self as despicable. Attachment theorists echo this theme (see Bretherton, 1991; Sroufe, 1990). They observe that the child who experiences parents as emotionally available, loving, and supportive of their mastery efforts will construct a working model of the self as lovable and competent. In contrast, a child who experiences attachment figures as rejecting or emotionally unavailable and nonsupportive will construct a working model of the self as unlovable, incompetent, and generally unworthy.

Moreover, not only do the evaluations of significant others result in representations of self, but also they provoke powerful self-*affects* in the form of pride and shame. Thus, the child who receives praise and support for his/her efforts will develop a sense of pride in his/her accomplishments. However, the child who is chronically criticized for his/her performance will develop a sense of shame that can be psychologically crippling. There are other affective consequences associated with the valence of one's self-representations. Individuals who internalize favorable views of the self are highly likely to be cheerful. Conversely, the most common affective correlate of negative self-perceptions is depression. In the extreme, depressive reactions associated with negative self-perceptions will lead to suicidal behaviors (see Harter, Marold, & Whitesell, 1992).

In addition to the incorporation of the opinions of significant others, children come to internalize the *standards* and *values* of those who are important to them, including the values of the larger society. As will be discussed, perceptions of one's physical attractiveness, in relation to the importance that is attached to meeting cultural standards of appearance, contribute heavily to one's overall sense of worth as a person (see Harter, 1993). Those who feel they have attained the requisite physical attributes will experience relatively high levels of self-esteem. Conversely, those who feel that they fall short of the punishing standards of appearance that represent the cultural ideal will suffer from low self-esteem. Moreover, a related liability can be observed in the eating-disordered behavior of females in particular, many of whom display symptoms (e.g., associated with anorexia) that are life threatening.

Finally, if significant others provide support for who one is as a person, for attributes that the child or adolescent feels truly define the self, then one will experience the self as authentic. However, the construction of a self that is so highly dependent upon the internalization of the opinions of others can, under some circumstances, lead to the creation of a false self that does not mirror one's authentic experience. False-self behavior is particularly likely to emerge if caregivers make their approval contingent upon the child's living up to their own unrealistic standards of behavior, since the child must adopt a socially implanted self; that is, children may come to suppress what they feel are true self-attributes in an attempt to garner the needed approval from caregivers.

In this volume, therefore, the focus not only includes an analysis of the primary antecedents or determinants of self-representations but also an examination of the consequences. The consequences of cognitive-developmental level as well as of the particular socialization experiences at the hands of caregivers is explored. Although the self has been touted for its ability to provide numerous adaptive functions, liabilities associated with each cognitive-developmental level, as well as vulnerabilities stemming from socialization experiences, are examined. As we shall see, self-development is a double-edged sword. In exploring both the antecedents and consequences, the ultimate goal of this volume is to identify pathways to healthy development, including interventions that may enhance the self-evaluations of those who have come to construct an unfavorable self-portrait.

HISTORICAL ROOTS OF CONTEMPORARY ISSUES INVOLVING SELF-DEVELOPMENT

As noted at the outset, the field has witnessed a return to classic issues that captured the attention of historical scholars of the self. Thus, it behooves us to briefly review the scripts of the major actors in this drama as a conceptual backdrop against which more contemporary issues can be examined. The history of interest in the self can be traced back to ancient Greek philosophy, as revealed in the injunction to "know thyself." However, contemporary scholars of the self-concept typically pay major intellectual homage to James (1890, 1892) and to such symbolic interactionists as Cooley (1902), Mead (1934), and Baldwin (1895), scholars in whom there has been a recent resurgence of interest. The reader interested in the history of the self prior to the turn of the century is referred to excellent treatments by Baumeister (1987), Broughton (1987), and Logan (1987). The historical contributions of James and the symbolic interactionists are first presented, followed by a discussion of the shape of self psychology in the 20th century.

The Legacy of William James

The contributions of James (1890, 1892) were legion. As observed in an earlier section, of paramount importance was his distinction between two fundamental aspects of the self, the I-self as subject or knower and the Me-self as object or known. It is the Me-self that came to be labeled the self-concept and took center stage as the major focus of empirical attention. Those interested in individual differences in the self-concept focused primarily on the correlates of favorable versus unfavorable self-evaluations (see Wylie, 1979). Within the field of developmental psychology, earlier attempts to identify age-related changes in self-representations concentrated exclusively on the Me-self (see Harter, 1983, 1997). Thus, the data consisted of the differing self-descriptions produced by children at different age levels, with little analysis of what accounted for such shifts (see Montemayor & Eisen, 1977).

For James, it was essential to posit an I-self, the knower, the active agent responsible for constructing the Me-self, although he became increasingly less invested in this construct, which, he concluded, was best left to the realm of philosophy. However, contemporary developmentalists have afforded the I-self a far greater role as the architect of the Me-self. It has become apparent that an appreciation for developmental changes in I-self processes is critical in order to understand how and why the structure and content of the Me-self changes with age. Thus, James' I-self/Me-self dichotomy has been warmly embraced by many developmentalists (see Damon & Hart, 1988; Harter, 1983, 1997) as a framework for understanding the reciprocal influence of I-self and Me-self processes.

For James (1890), the "Me" self could be subdivided into "constituents": the *material* self, the *social* self, and the *spiritual* self. The material self subsumed the bodily self as well as one's possessions. The social self consisted of those characteristics recognized by others. Given the potential diversity of others' opinions, James concluded that "a man has as many social selves as there are individuals who recognize him and carry an image of him in their mind" (p. 190). The spiritual self was considered to be an inner core comprised of thoughts, dispositions, moral judgments, and so on, that were more enduring aspects of the self. James sought not only to dimensionalize the self but also to impose a hierarchical structure onto its constituents. At the bottom of the hierarchy is the material self. The social self occupies the next position, given James' assumption that we should care more about friends, human ties, and honor among others than about our bodies or wealth. The spiritual self, which James regarded as "supremely precious," occupies the highest tier. Thus, James paved the way for future models in which the self is viewed as multidimensional and hierarchical.

In differentiating various aspects of the self, including the multiplicity of social selves, James (1890) noted that these multiple selves may not all speak with the same voice. For example, James observed that "many a youth who is demure enough before his parents and teachers, swears and swaggers like a pirate among his tough young friends" (p. 169). James further noted that this multiplicity can be harmonious, for example, when an individual is tender to his children but also stern to the soldiers under his command. Alternatively, there may be a "discordant splitting" if one's different selves are experienced as contradictory.

The "conflict of the different Me's" could also be observed in the incompatibility of potential adult roles. James, himself, fantasized about his own desires to be handsome, athletic, rich, witty, a *bon vivant*, ladykiller, philosopher, philanthropist, statesman, warrior, African explorer, as well as a tone-poet and a saint! He knowingly concluded that since all of these roles could not possibly coexist, it was necessary to selectively choose, suppressing the alternatives. Thus, "the seeker of his truest, strongest, deepest self must review the list carefully, and pick out the one on which to stake his salvation" (p. 174).

The repudiation of particular attributes or roles was not, for James, necessarily damaging to the individual's overall sense of worth, the "average tone of self-feeling which each one of us carries about" (p. 171). Thus, his own deficiency at Greek led to no sense of humiliation, since he had no *pretensions* to be proficient at Greek. The role of pretensions became paramount in James' formulation of the causes of self-esteem. Self-esteem could not simply be reduced to the aggregate of perceived successes, but rather represented a ratio of successes to one's *pretensions*. If perceived successes were equal to or greater than one's pretensions or aspirations for success, high self-esteem would result. Conversely, if pretensions exceeded successes, that is, if an individual were unsuccessful in domains deemed important, he/she would experience low self-esteem. Critical to this formulation is the assumption that lack of success in an area in which one does *not* have pretensions (e.g., Greek for James) will not erode self-esteem, since it can be discounted. Thus, both the presence and absence of pretensions figured heavily in James' theorizing. He argued that abandoning certain pretensions can be as much a relief as striving to meet goals: "How pleasant is the day when we give up striving to be young" (p. 201).

In James, therefore, we find many themes that anticipate contemporary issues about the self. First and foremost is the distinction between "I" and "Me" selves, which has become of paramount importance to developmental psychologists. James' multidimensional, hierarchical view of the Me-self has been modernized in recent treatments of the self-structure, where investigators have sought to examine the particular relationships among global and domain-specific self-evaluations. Moreover, the potential conflict between different Me-selves that James observed has served as a springboard to contemporary interest in the construction of multiple selves. In this literature, as we shall come to see, differing attributes across role-related selves that appear contradictory (e.g., depressed with parents but cheerful with friends) usher in the potential for both conflict and concern. Finally, James' formulation concerning the causes of self-esteem has been revived, leading investigators to empirically investigate its viability.

The Contribution of the Symbolic Interactionists

In contrast to James, the symbolic interactionists placed primary emphasis on how social interactions with others profoundly shaped the self. For Cooley (1902), Mead (1934), and Baldwin (1895), the self is viewed as a *social construction*, crafted through linguistic exchanges (symbolic interactions) with others. Several themes can be identified in the writings of the original symbolic interactionists, themes that have found their way into contemporary theorizing. For example, beginning in childhood, (1) one engages in the *imitation* of significant others' behaviors, attitudes, and values or standards; (2) the developing child adjusts his/her behavior to garner the *approval* of salient socializing agents; moreover, (3) one comes to adopt the *opinions* that significant others are perceived to hold toward the self, reflected appraisals that come to define one's sense of self as a person. The fact that these processes occur in multiple social contexts, with different significant others, adds to the complexity of the construction of a self that can be experienced as coherent, as integrated, and as authentic.

Charles Horton Cooley

Cooley's formulation was perhaps the most metaphorical, given his postulation of the "looking glass self." In his now-famous couplet he observed that

> Each to each a looking glass
> Reflects the other that doth pass

For Cooley, significant others constituted a social mirror into which the individual gazes in order to detect their opinions toward the self. These opinions, in turn, are incorporated into one's sense of self. Cooley contended, therefore, that what becomes the self is what we imagine that others think of us, including our appearance, motives, deeds, character, and so on. One comes to own these reflected appraisals. Such a "self-idea" was comprised of three components: (1) the imagination of our appearance to the other person; (2) the imagination of that person's judgment of that appearance; and (3) some sort of self-feeling, namely, an affective reaction to these reflected appraisals. These components gradually become removed from their initial social sources through an implied internalization process.

In describing the affective reactions of the adult self, Cooley singled out the emotions of pride and shame, in particular, and in so doing set the stage for a developmental analysis of how these emotions might emerge. Although pride and shame could clearly be experienced by adults in the absence of others, Cooley noted that "the thing that moves us to pride and shame is not the merely mechanical reflection of ourselves, but an imputed sentiment, the imagined effect of this reflection upon another's mind" (1902, p. 153). Cooley was clear on the point that this sentiment is social in nature, based upon social custom and opinion, although it becomes somewhat removed from these sources through an implied internalization process. Cooley writes that the adult is "not *immediately* dependent upon what others think; he has worked over his reflected self in his mind until it is a steadfast portion of his thought, an idea and conviction apart, in some measure, from its external origin. Hence this sentiment requires time for its development and flourishes in mature age rather than in the open and growing period of youth" (1902, p. 199; emphasis in original).

Thus, Cooley's views on the internalization of others' opinions about the self paved the way for a more developmental perspective on how the attitudes of others are incorporated into the self. Moreover, his looking-glass-self perspective provides an alternative to James' contentions regarding the determinants of global self-esteem. James focused largely on those cognitive processes whereby an individual actively compares particular aspirations to perceived successes in corresponding domains. In contrast, for Cooley, the antecedents were far more social in nature, and less consciously driven, in that children inevitably internalized the opinions that they believed significant others held toward the self. Cooley also spoke more directly to developmental changes, including the consequences of the internalization process for adults. He contended that the more mature sense of self is not buffeted about by potentially transient or disparate views of significant others. As Cooley observed, the person with "balanced self-respect has stable ways of thinking about the image of self that cannot be upset by passing phases of praise or blame" (p. 201). His thesis anticipates contemporary interest in whether self-concepts are malleable versus resistant to change, a topic to which we shall return.

George Herbert Mead

In Mead (1925), we find an elaboration of the themes identified by Cooley, with an even greater insistence on the role of social interaction. For

Mead, "We appear as selves in our conduct insofar as we ourselves take the attitude that others take toward us. We take the role of what may be called the 'generalized' other" (p. 270). Mead also spoke to the origins of these attitudes in childhood. He postulated a two-stage developmental process through which the child adopted the attitudes of others toward the self, labeling these stages as the "play" and the "game." The "play" involved the imitation of adult roles, which Mead documented in his description of the young child "continually acting as a parent, a teacher, a preacher, a grocery man, a policeman, a pirate, or an Indian" (p. 270). In the subsequent stage of "games," there are proscribed procedures and rules.

> The child must not only take the role of the other, as he does in the play, but he must assume the various roles of all the participants in the game and govern his actions accordingly. If he plays first base, it is as the one to whom the ball will be thrown from the field or from the catcher. Their organized reaction becomes what I have called the 'generalized other' that accompanies and controls his conduct. And it is this generalized other in his experience which provides him with a self. (p. 271)

Thus, for Mead, the individual comes to adopt the generalized perspective of a group of significant others that shares a particular societal perspective on the self. In predicting global judgments of self, Mead's formulation implies a process through which the judgments of numerous significant others are somehow psychologically weighted in order to produce an overall sense of self-worth as a person. However, Mead was not explicit on precisely how the judgments of others were combined. Contemporary researchers have begun to address these processes more directly, as will become evident.

James Mark Baldwin

For Baldwin (1897), the construction of the self was a very social, dialectical process between the self and other, whom he labeled the "alter." Baldwin wrote (in what has become the obligatory quote), "My sense of myself grows by my imitation of you, and my sense of yourself grows in terms of my sense of myself. Both ego and alter are thus essentially social; each is a *socius* and each is an imitative creation" (p. 335). In less arcane language, Baldwin (1897) subsequently asserted that "the development of the child's personality could not go on at all without the modification of his sense of himself by suggestions from others. So he himself, at every stage, is really in part someone else, even in his own thought of himself" (p. 30).

From a developmental perspective, the *imitative* process is particularly powerful during childhood where the young child is, for Baldwin, a "veritable copying-machine." In imitating others, one transfers behaviors "to myself by trying to act as if they were true to me, and so coming to find out that they are true of me" (1897, p. 12). Thus, although others are imitated, the behaviors come to be owned as central to one's self-definition. Baldwin also spoke to the issue of how the child adjusts or accommodates his/her behavior to garner the approval of significant others. Thus, the child acts in accord with the wishes of caregivers, initially, for example, by demonstrating the type of obedience that is required by family members. Baldwin contrasted the *accommodating* self to the *habitual* self, which represented the child's more natural inclinations. However, the accommodating self, which represents behaviors that are "modified by the influences outside," leads the individual to "pass the new things learned over to the self of habit" (p. 35). There is a transfer of attributes first encouraged and rewarded by others and later assimilated into the individual's sense of his/her habitual self. Here, as with imitative processes, there is an implicit internalization process through which the developing individual comes to own particular behaviors, initially prompted by others, as central to the self.

For Baldwin, the family provides the initial models to be imitated, the authorities whose standards and opinions were to be respected. However, the spheres of social influence widen as the child moves out of his/her immediate domestic life into the world of school, including teachers and peers. As more spheres become salient, more alters appear on the social horizon, leading to greater complexities in the adoption of attributes that will come to define the self. This perspective has been adopted by contemporary developmentalists who have charted shifts in the impact that different significant others have upon the developing self.

Inherent in Baldwin's explication of these processes are two themes that reappear in contemporary treatments of the self. The first involves his contention that the self during its formative years represents a process of change. In Baldwin's words, an individual undergoes "constant modification of his sense of himself by suggestions from others" leading to "changes in the content of one's sense of self" (1897, p. 30). Baldwin also described the multiplicity of the self-structure, namely, that attributes of the self may differ *across* relational contexts, as well as *within* a given relational context. With regard to differing selves across contexts, Baldwin cites how the child who is aggressive with brothers or sisters is far more docile, obedient, and less aggressive with elders. Moreover, in certain social situations, the child may display generosity and altruism, contrasted to other contexts in which he/she appears quite selfish. *Within* a given context, Baldwin gives examples of how the child might be quite fearful in the presence of his father's wrath, but quite playful if the father, himself, was jovial. For Baldwin, "the growing child is able to think of self in varying terms as varying social situations impress themselves upon him" (p. 37). Thus, we have in Baldwin a model for the development of multiple selves, a theme that has found its way into contemporary theorizing, and one to which we will return.

In Cooley, Mead, and Baldwin, we can identify several themes that have found their way into contemporary treatments of the self. Paramount is the role of the opinions of others in shaping the self-concept, through social interaction. Cooley hinted at a developmental internalization process whereby the reflected appraisals of specific others become incorporated in the form of relatively *enduring* attitudes about the self, a process that has implications for the stability of the self-concept. Baldwin also described how the individual assimilates the self-attributes initially encouraged or identified by others into his/her habitual sense of self. For Mead, a more generalized sense of self was internalized, although just how the opinions of various others are psychologically homogenized into a collective sense of self remained elusive. In Baldwin, we also observe the significance of social imitative processes in fashioning a sense of self and other, founded upon the infant's realization that others have subjective experiences like the self. As such, Baldwin anticipated later contentions concerning the infant's rudimentary "theory of mind." Moreover, Baldwin pointed to the multiplicity of the self-structure, observing that the individual can possess different self-attributes both across and within different relational contexts. He did not, however, posit that the multiple selves may produce intrapsychic conflict, as did James. Finally, Cooley's observation that self-judgments are accompanied by self-*feelings* highlighted the role of affective processes in self-concept development, particularly the self-conscious emotions such as pride and shame.

Self Psychology in the 20th Century

During the early period of introspection, inquiry into topics concerning the self and psyche flourished. However, with the emergence of radical behaviorism, such constructs were excised from the scientific vocabularies of many theorists for whom the writings of James and the symbolic interactionists gathered dust on the shelf. Historically, it is of interest to ask why the self was for so long an unwelcome guest at the behaviorists' table. Why was it that constructs such as self, including self-esteem, ego strength, sense of omnipotence, narcissistic injury, feelings of unconscious rejection, and so on, did little to whet the behaviorists' appetite? Several related reasons appear responsible.

The very origins of the behaviorist movement rested on the identification of *observables*. Thus, hypothetical constructs were both conceptually and methodologically unpalatable. Cognitions, in general, and self-representa-tions, in particular, were deemed unmeasurable, since they could not be operationalized as observable behaviors. Moreover, self-report measures de-signed to tap self-constructs were not included on the methodological menu, since people were assumed to be very inaccurate judges of their own behav-ior. Those more accepting of introspective methodologies found the exist-ing measures of self-concept ungratifying, in large part because their con-tent was overly vague and general. Finally, self-constructs were not satisfying to the behaviorist's palate because their *functions* were not clearly specified. The very cornerstone of behavioral approaches rested upon a functional analysis of behavior. In contrast, approaches to the self did little more than implicate self-representations as *correlates* of behavior, affording them little explanatory power as causes or mediators of behavior.

Several shifts in emphasis, beginning in the second half of the century, have allowed self-constructs to become more palatable. Hypothetical con-structs, in general, gained favor as parsimonious predictors of behavior, of-ten far more economical in theoretical models than a multitude of discrete observables. In addition, we witnessed a cognitive revolution within the fields of both child and adult psychology (Bruner, 1990). For develop-mentalists, Piagetian and neo-Piagetian models came to the forefront. For experimental and social psychologists, numerous cognitive models found favor. With the emergence of this revolution, self theorists jumped on the bandwagon, resurrecting the self as a *cognitive* construction, as mental repre-sentations that constitute a theory of self (e.g., Brim, 1976; Case, 1985; Epstein, 1973, 1981; Fischer, 1980; Greenwald, 1980; Kelly, 1955; Markus, 1977, 1980; Sarbin, 1962). Finally, self-representations gained increased le-gitimacy as behaviorally oriented therapists were forced to acknowledge that the spontaneous self-evaluative statements of their clients seemed power-fully implicated in their pathology.

A more *sociocultural* perspective on the history of the self has been offered by Gergen (1991) who identifies three major periods: Romanticism, Modernism, and Postmodernism. Romantic visions of the self flourished during the late 18th and 19th centuries, during which the vocabulary about the self emphasized such commodities as love, passion, loyalty, intrinsic worth, morality, creative inspiration, and will. Thus, the psychological inte-rior was accented, namely, characteristics that constituted the depths of one's soul. The period of Modernism was ushered in by the scientific and techno-logical advances of the 20th century. Emerging values of reason, objective evidence, and rational utility were incompatible with, and therefore replaced, the romanticist perspective. The machine became the metaphor for the self. Individuals were characterized in computer terminology, for example, as networks of associations, perceptual mechanisms, and cognitive structures, all of which highlighted *rationality* as the essence of humanity. From a developmental perspective, proper molding by one's family and wider societal forces would result in the well-designed person whose behavior would be self-directing, authentic, trustworthy, and consistent. As Gergen observes, "Modernist man is genuine rather than phony, principled, rather than craven, stable, rather than wavering" (p. 44).

Modernism has, for Gergen, more recently given rise to our current period of *Postmodernism*, which he partially traces to further advances in technology (see also Overton, 1994). In developing his portrait of the "saturated" self, Gergen observes that easy access to air travel, electronic and express mail, fax machines, cellular phones, beepers, and answering machines have all dramatically accelerated our social connectedness. As a result, contemporary life has become a dizzying swirl of social relations, where the "social caravan in which we travel through life remains always full" (p. 62). For Gergen, these changes have profound implications for self-development, in that they dictate the creation of multiple selves across a variety of social contexts. As such, they force us to revisit James' (1892) conclusion that the individual must create multiple role-related selves that may not be compatible, leading to the "conflict of the different Me's."

Despite historical precedent for considering the multiplicity of the self, theoreticians in the first half of the century did not embrace James' contentions. As Gergen (1968) has observed, there was historical resistance to such a stance in the form of a "consistency ethic." Thus, many scholars placed major emphasis on the integrated, unified self (Allport, 1961; Horney, 1950; Jung, 1928; Lecky, 1945; Maslow, 1954; Rogers, 1951). For Allport, the self includes all aspects of personality that make for a sense of inward unity. Lecky (1945) fashioned an entire theory around the theme of self-consistency, emphasizing how behavior expresses the effort to maintain the integrity and unity of the self. Epstein (1973, 1981) has argued that among the criteria that one's self-theory must meet is *internal consistency*. Thus, one's self-theory will be threatened by evidence that is inconsistent with the portrait one has constructed of the self, or by postulates within the theory that appear to be contradictory. Epstein (1981) has formalized these observations under the rubric of the "unity principle," emphasizing that one of the most basic needs of the individual is to maintain the unity and coherence of the conceptual system that defines the self.

The pendulum would appear to have swung back to an emphasis on multiplicity, with increasing zeal for models depicting how the self varies across situations (see Ashmore & Ogilvie, 1992; Kihlstrom, 1993; Markus & Cross, 1990; Rosenberg, 1988; Stryker, 1987). In contrast to the emphasis on unity, several social psychologists (Gergen, 1968; Mischel, 1973; Vallacher, 1980) began to argue that the most fruitful theory of self must take into account the multiple roles that people adopt. Thus, Gergen contended that the "popular notion of the self-concept as a unified, consistent, or perceptually whole psychological structure is possibly ill-conceived" (1968, p. 306). Although consistency *within* a relationship was deemed desirable, consistency *across* relationships was viewed as difficult, if not impossible, and in all likelihood damaging, that is, people are compelled to adjust their behavior in accord with the specific nature of the interpersonal relationship and its situational context. In the extreme, high self-monitors (Snyder, 1987) frequently and flexibly alter their self-presentation in the service of creating a positive impression, enacting behaviors that they feel are socially appropriate and will preserve critical relationships. For Gergen, such multiplicity is not only a response to the demand characteristics of different interpersonal contexts, but also rests heavily on social comparison. As Gergen (1977) observes, "In the presence of the devout, we may discover that we are ideologically shallow; in the midst of dedicated hedonists, we may gain awareness of our ideological depths" (1977, p. 154).

In his more recent discussion of the postmodern era, Gergen (1991) has elevated his argument to new heights in his sociocultural treatise on the "saturated" or "populated" self. Gergen observes that in contemporary life, individuals have been forced to contend with a swirling sea of multiple social relationships, which in turn require the construction of numerous, disparate selves. Although the construction of multiple selves may allow the individual to adaptively respond to different relationships, the demands of these relationships can lead to a cacophony of multiple selves, in that their different voices may not necessarily harmonize. Moreover, according to Gergen, the need to craft different selves to conform to the particular relationship at hand leads to doubt about one's true identity; that is, the sense of an obdurate, core self is compromised in playing out one's role as "social chameleon."

Lifton (1993) develops a similar theme in his analysis of the emergence of the postmodern "protean self," named after Proteus, the Greek sea god who possessed many forms. For Lifton, the protean self emerges out of "confusion, from the widespread feeling that we are losing our psychological moorings" (p. 1). He attributes this confusion to unmanageable historical forces, rapid societal and economic changes, and social uncertainties. Lifton is a bit more sanguine than Gergen, however, emphasizing the flexibility and resilience of the protean self, whereas Gergen focuses more on the erosion of the belief in one's essential self. There are those (see Chandler, 1997) who have been critical of this postmodern analysis of the self, arguing that it is nihilistic, contradictory, and does not capture the phenomenological reality of the self for most individuals. Nevertheless, some do experience an erosion of a sense of an immutable, core self, a topic to which we shall return (in Chapter 9) in considering how the authenticity of the self can be compromised.

OVERVIEW OF CHAPTER TOPICS

Against this historical backdrop we turn to an analysis of how the self is both cognitively and socially constructed during childhood and adolescence. Although self-development begins at birth and proceeds through predictable stages during infancy (see Harter, 1997), the present volume focuses on those *verbal* representations of self that begin to emerge toward the end of the second year of life. Attention is first devoted to cognitive-developmental processes that represent I-self changes, which in turn impact developmental differences in the nature of the Me-self, among children (Chapter 2) and adolescents (Chapter 3). The focus is on *normative-developmental* changes that lead to similarities in the self-structure among individuals at a given developmental level. Within this framework, emphasis is placed on how cognitive-developmental advances lead to more mature self-structures while at the same time ushering in potential liabilities that may compromise the functionality of self-system. Chapter 4 pursues the theme of developmental differences, shifting to the emergence of self-*affects* (e.g., pride, shame, and guilt) as both cognitive and social constructions.

In Chapters 5, 6, 7, and 8, the focus shifts to *individual differences* in self-*evaluative* judgments, namely, domain-specific self-concepts as well as global self-esteem or self-worth. In Chapter 5, the content, valence, and organization of self-evaluative judgments are examined, including how such judgments are differentiated and integrated into a hierarchical model of self-representations. These issues are addressed in normative samples, as well as examined in special groups of children and cross-cultural samples. Chapter 6 focuses on the construction of ideal as well as real self-concepts, exploring how the discrepancy or congruence between these two self-concepts will determine the level of one's overall sense of worth. Findings relevant to James' formulation are reviewed within this context.

Attention then shifts, in Chapter 7, to those social sources of self-evaluation initially observed by the symbolic interactionists. Child-rearing practices leading to individual differences in the valence of self-attributes are examined against a backdrop of models specifying how the opinions of others are internalized. Of particular relevance is how the process of internalization emerges and is transformed as a function of development. Here, as in the treatment of developmental changes, both positive and negative outcomes are identified. Chapter 8 presents a broader model of the causes and consequences of self-worth that has emerged in our own work. With regard

to causes, attention focuses on the relative contribution of those antecedents of self-worth identified by James as well as Cooley, and, to a lesser
extent, Mead and Baldwin. A central assumption in our thinking is that
self-processes must have meaningful *consequences* if they are to be considered
worthy of study. One constellation of negative consequences associated with
low self-worth, namely, depressive reactions (depressed affect, hopelessness,
and suicidal thinking) has been central to our work. Although these efforts
have resulted in a general model that has been empirically supported by
group data, we have also documented the fact that there are multiple pathways to these outcomes that need to be considered in understanding how
the pattern of antecedents can differ across individuals.

Chapters 9, 10, and 11 address additional processes through which the
self can become compromised. Chapter 9 focuses on factors leading to the
construction of self-representations that are judged to be *false*, that lack authenticity. Social processes that promote the suppression of one's true self
are examined. One particular form of false-self behavior, the inability to
voice one's opinions, is highlighted. In so doing, I present findings relevant
to Gilligan's (1993) contention that adolescent girls, in particular, are at risk
for loss of voice. Chapter 10 deals with how extremely negative social experiences at the hands of caregivers, in the form of severe and chronic abuse,
compromises the functionality of numerous I-self and Me-self functions,
including one's sense of authenticity, and lead to debilitating dissociative
reactions.

Across the various chapters of this volume, I highlight an important
developmental goal, namely, the cognitive and social construction of a sense
of self that increasingly becomes less dependent upon external evaluations,
and that represents a core set of inner attributes perceived to reflect one's
true self. However, as discussed in Chapter 11, healthy development does
not mean that one retreats into an autonomous, independent, self-focused
orientation, constructing impenetrable boundaries between self and others. Much of what has been cast as self-theory reflects Western models that
have underscored autonomy, independence, separateness, individualism, and
distinctiveness. The perspective advanced in this volume is more in keeping
with the recent emphasis on healthy adaptation as an integration of autonomy and connectedness, a theme that can be observed in literatures
addressing early childhood, adolescence, and adulthood. Our own research
with adults reveals that an orientation that is either overly autonomous or
overly connected will compromise the self, particularly with regard to a sense
of authenticity, self-esteem, and associated feelings of depression.

Finally, the last chapter of this volume, Chapter 12, deals with practical applications. It addresses both conceptual and methodological issues in
considering interventions to promote self-evaluations that involve both cog-

nitive and social processes. In so doing, it is important to wrestle with the issue of whether the self is merely an epiphenomenon, a correlate with little explanatory power, which can therefore be ignored in our intervention efforts. Alternatively, if the self is deeply embedded in the very fabric of maladaptive behaviors, it should be taken quite seriously in our efforts to improve the lives of those plagued by damaging self-images and self-doubt. In Chapter 12, the implications of research on the stability and the accuracy of self-evaluations, as well as on the previous models presented, are reviewed; guidelines to aid in program evaluation efforts and the choice of measuring instruments are offered; and the major themes of this book are summarized, concluding with implications for how to facilitate healthy pathways to self-development.

CHAPTER TWO

The Normative Development of Self-Representations during Childhood

In this chapter, we examine the development of the self as both a cognitive and social construction from early to late childhood. Attention focuses on the development of *verbalized* self-representations, namely, how the child comes to describe the self through the use of language. This chapter first offers a discussion of how the emergence of language paves the way for self-development. Attention then turns to an analysis of developmental differences in self-representations across three age periods during childhood: (1) toddlerhood to early childhood, (2) early to middle childhood, and (3) middle to late childhood.

A major goal is a consideration of how particular cognitive-developmental changes in the I-self, as agent, knower, and constructor, influence the differences observed in the Me-self, the self as known or constructed. A neo-Piagetian approach is adopted, given limitations in purely descriptive approaches as well as in the application of Piagetian stage principles, to be discussed later. Three general influences are highlighted at each age period, namely, how cognitive development affects the (1) actual structure of the self-concept, how it (2) mediates the impact of the reactions of socializing agents to the self, and (3) how the social context, in turn, impacts these cognitive-developmental acquisitions. Against a backdrop of the advances that result in more mature self-structures, consideration is given to how such shifts usher in certain vulnerabilities that influences the child's functioning.

THE LIMITATIONS OF EARLIER
FINDINGS AND FRAMEWORKS

Initial investigations into the development of the self were largely *descriptive* and focused primarily on the *content* of self-representations, namely, how the Me-self evolves across childhood and adolescence (see Harter, 1983). Investigators sought to document developmental differences in self-representations through the coding of spontaneously generated descriptions of the self (Bannister & Agnew, 1977; Guardo & Bohan, 1971; McGuire, 1981; Montemayor & Eisen, 1977; Mullener & Laird, 1971; Rosenberg, 1979). These efforts identified broad, discontinuous, qualitative shifts in how the self was described. However, there was little analysis of the structural organization of self-descriptions.

Given that many theorists (e.g., Epstein, 1973, 1981; Greenwald, 1980; Markus, 1980) began to forcefully argue that the self-theory was a *cognitive construction*, an analysis of how cognitive-developmental shifts might be implicated in the age differences that had been documented thus represented the next conceptual approach. It was suggested (see Harter, 1983) that the broad, developmental changes observed across early childhood, later childhood, and adolescence could be interpreted within a Piagetian framework. Thus, the finding that the young child described the self in terms of concrete, observable characteristics such as physical attributes, material possessions, behaviors, and preferences that were not coherently organized was consistent with the cognitive abilities and limitations of the preoperational period. The earlier studies had reported that in middle to later childhood, the self was described in terms of trait-like constructs (e.g., smart, honest, friendly, shy) that would require the type of hierarchical organizational skills to emerge during Piaget's period of concrete operations. For example, a trait label such as "smart" could be cognitively viewed as a higher-order generalization that subsumed the behavioral manifestations of scholastic competence in several school subjects (e.g., doing well at reading, spelling, and math). For the period of adolescence, earlier findings had documented the emergence of more abstract self-definitions based on psychological processes such as inner thoughts, emotions, attitudes, and motives. This type of self-portrait was consistent with the formal operational advances identified by Piaget, for example, the ability to construct higher-order abstractions and the capacity for introspection. However, it has become apparent that this broad, three-stage Piagetian analysis does not do justice to the complexity of self-development across childhood and adolescence.

Within the general field of cognitive development, numerous critiques of Piagetian theory have emerged (see Case, 1985, 1992; Feldman, 1994;

Fischer, 1980; Fischer & Canfield, 1986; Flavell, 1985; Flavell, Miller, & Miller, 1993; Pascual-Leone, 1988; Siegler, 1991), critiques that have specific implications for our understanding of self-development. As Case (1992) observes, Piagetian theory painted a picture of cognitive development that was "too monolithic, universal, and endogenous" (p. 10). For example, findings documenting the tremendous unevenness or décalage in development across domains argued against some single, underlying set of developing cognitive structures (see also Costanzo, 1991; Graziano & Waschull, 1995). Moreover, the theory has been considered to be primarily descriptive, with insufficient attention to specific underlying processes and transition rules. The broad shifts that Piaget identified have also been viewed as too discontinuous. In addition, there was little emphasis on individual differences in the rate of cognitive development, or on the potential for different pathways of development. Finally, issues involving contextual factors that might affect cognitive development were virtually ignored, for example, specific instructional and socialization experiences as well as broader cultural influences.

The theorists cited here have adopted various neo-Piagetian frameworks that have been infused with new concepts and methodologies, many of which can be applied to an analysis of self-development. Several common principles across these newer frameworks represent contemporary solutions to those problems identified in Piaget's theory. For example, a greater number of structural levels have been identified, with more emphasis on the continuity of development. Higher structures are considered to build upon and incorporate lower structures that become more intercoordinated. Décalage is accepted as the rule, rather than the exception; therefore, it is expected that the particular level of development at which one is functioning will vary across different domains of knowledge. The particular processes and transition rules that govern such development have also become more precise. For example, certain neo-Piagetians focus on memory functions and their development (e.g., Case, 1985, 1992; Pascual-Leone, 1988). Others highlight the role of the automatization of skills (e.g., Case, 1985; Siegler, 1991). Siegler, from an information-processing perspective, also identifies the processes of encoding and strategy construction. Encoding involves the identification of the most important features of objects and events that form the basis for internal representations. Strategy construction refers to those processes through which concepts are combined to form categories or higher-order generalizations.

Such processes may be influenced by social and contextual factors. For example, the child's culture as well as the more proximal family and social milieu will play an important role in dictating what features of events and objects, including the self, are most salient and are therefore to be encoded (see also Rogoff, 1990; Vygotsky, 1978). Moreover, the child's experience will partially determine how particular structures are coordinated (see also Costanzo, 1991). The inclusion of contextual variables also contributes to an understanding of individual differences in the rate and manner in which structures are integrated. Although experience, instruction, and practice may influence the rate of the progression through cognitive levels, most neo-Piagetians acknowledge that there are factors that constrain the upper limit that one may achieve at any given age. For example, brain development, in general, and working memory capacity, in particular, represent such constraints.

In applying many of these principles to self-development, we will see, for example, that a greater number of age-related levels can now be identified. Moreover, there is more emphasis on how a given level of self-understanding builds upon the previous level. Processes through which concepts are combined to form categories or higher-order generalizations can be invoked to explain the developmental emergence of trait labels and abstractions that come to define the self. In addition, socialization experiences and related contextual factors contribute to our understanding of the normative-developmental trajectory of self-representations, as well as the tremendous individual differences that can be found at particular age levels. I begin such an analysis with a discussion of language development.

THE DEVELOPMENT OF LANGUAGE

The emergence of language represents a potent acquisition in the development of the self (Stern, 1985). Language allows for the verbal expression and representation of the Me-self, the categorical self, which Lewis (1991, 1994) has more recently relabeled the "idea of me." Thus, the toddler comes to label the self and others with appropriate personal pronouns—for example, "Look at me," "That's mine" (see Bates, 1990)—as well as by name—for example, "I'm Anna." Those investigators who have employed a visual recognition paradigm, in which infants and toddlers respond to their images in a mirror, report that these labeling processes begin at approximately 18 months of age (Berthenthal & Fischer, 1978; Lewis & Brooks-Gunn, 1979). Language also makes possible what Neisser (1991) refers to as the "extended or remembered self," namely, a representational Me-self based upon memories and narrative conventions. Employing somewhat different terminology to describe these processes, Case (1991) observes that verbal and representational skills permit the shift from an "explicit" self that was sensorimotor in nature (analogous to James' I-self) to an "implicit" self that he terms the "referential Me-self." As others have noted (Hart & Karmel, in press; Lewis, 1991, 1994; Sander, 1975; Sroufe, 1990; Stern, 1985), with the emergence of linguistic and symbolic representational capabilities, toddlers move to a new level of self-awareness; that is, they can now conceptualize the self as an object.

The emergence of language also provides toddlers with the capacity to symbolically represent parental rules and standards and their own ability to meet them (Kagan, 1981; Lewis, 1991, 1994). For Emde (1988; Emde, Birigen, Clymen, & Oppenheim, 1991), these acquisitions form the earliest manifestations of moral behavior and contribute to an elaboration of the "we-self," a shared sense of meaning between the toddler and caregiver. Attention to rules and prohibitions represents a more sophisticated form of social referencing in that the toddler checks with the caregiver about the appropriateness of his/her behavior. In situations where there might be a conflict between the mother's wishes and the toddler's desires, Mahler (1967, 1968) placed emphasis on the battle of wills that might ensue. In contrast, Emde has focused on the fact that the internalization of rules and prohibitions actually *empowers* toddlers, allowing them to regulate their own behavior and to resist temptation in situations where the caregiver is not present. Kagan (1981) speaks to the toddler's adoption of another type of caregiver's standards, namely, expectations about competence and achievement. He reports that toddlers express distress when they cannot succeed on tasks that have been modeled by adults, from which he infers that they have a rudimentary form of self-awareness signaling that they have not measured up to the standards.

Self in Memory and the Role of Narrative in the Co-Construction of the Self

With the emergence of language comes the ability to construct a narrative of one's "life story" and therefore to develop a more enduring portrait of the self. Our understanding of the processes of memory and the construction of narratives has increased dramatically in recent years. Developmentalists (see Crittenden, 1994; Fivush, 1987; Fivush & Hudson, 1990; Nelson, 1986, 1993) now distinguish among a number of types of memories, elaborating on Tulving's (1972, 1983) initial distinction between semantic and episodic memory. *Semantic* memory refers to verbally encoded, context-free or generalized information, which, when applied to the self, represents summary trait knowledge (e.g., "I am a good girl; I am a generous person"). *Episodic* memory refers to the memory of an experience that happened once, at a specific time and place (e.g., "I went to McDonald's and had a hamburger and french fries yesterday"). Episodic memories are initially relegated to a holding pattern. If the episodes are reinstated frequently, they are transformed into generic event memory or *scripts*, namely, schemas derived from experience that sketch the general outline of a familiar event without providing details about the specific time and place. Finally, *autobiographical* memory is another special form of episodic memory that codifies experiences of the self. These memories are very personal and have long-lasting significance for the individual, becoming the basis for one's own life story (e.g., "I go to Grandma's every summer and help her pick apples; she always gives me a hug and says I am her favorite grandchild"). As Nelson (1990, 1993) points out, another initial function of autobiographical memories is that they allow one, through language, to share these recollections with significant others, which serves to cement social bonds. Autobiographical memory (see also Hudson, 1990a, 1990b; Snow, 1990) has also been referred to as *personal narrative memory* (Eisenberg, 1983; Nelson, 1986).

Very young children can construct episodic memories for certain events as well as generic event memory or scripts (e.g., of bedtime rituals). However, there are no *autobiographical* memories before the age of 2, and the average age is 3½ (Pillemer & White, 1989). This infantile amnesia can only be overcome by learning from adults how to formulate their own memories as *narratives*. Thus, parents recount stories about a child's past experiences that are told to the child. With increasing age and language facility, children come to take on a more active role in that parent and child co-construct the memory of a shared experience (Eisenberg, 1983; Hudson, 1990a, 1990b; Nelson, 1986, 1990, 1993; Rogoff, 1990; Snow, 1990). However, for the young child, such narratives are still highly scaffolded by the parents, who reinforce aspects of experience that they feel are important to codify and remember (Fivush, Gray, & Fromhoff, 1987; Fivush & Hudson, 1990; Nelson, 1989). Through these interactions, an autobiographic account of the *self* is created. Of further interest are findings demonstrating individual differences in maternal styles of narrative construction (see Bretherton, 1993; Nelson, 1990, 1993). For example, Tessler (1991) has distinguished between an *elaborative* style (where mothers present an embellished narrative) and a *pragmatic* style (focusing more on useful information). Elaborative mothers were more effective in establishing and eliciting memories with their young children.

For most developmental memory researchers, language is the critical acquisition allowing one to establish a personal narrative and to overcome infantile amnesia (Fivush & Hammond, 1990; Hudson, 1990a; Nelson, 1990; Pillemer & White, 1989). The mastery of language, in general, and of personal pronouns, in particular, enables young children to think and talk about the I-self and to expand their categorical knowledge of the Me-self (Bates, 1990; Miller, Potts, Fung, Hoogstra, & Mintz, 1990). Moreover, representations of the self in language are further facilitated by acquisition of the past tense, which occurs toward the latter half of the third year.

Howe and Courage (1993) argue, however, that the emergence of language is not sufficient to explain the demise of infantile amnesia and the emergence of an ability to create autobiographical memories. They note that *self-knowledge* is also required, that is, an appreciation for the self as an independent entity with actions, attributes, affects, and thoughts that are distinct from those of others is required for the development of autobiographical memory. Without the clear recognition of an independent I-self and Me-self, there can be no referent around which personally experienced events can be organized. Thus, for Howe and Courage, the emergence of the infant's sense of self is the cornerstone in the development of autobiographical memory that further shapes and solidifies one's self definition.

Linguistic interactions with parents also impact the developing child's representation of self in *semantic* memory (Bowlby, 1979; Nelson, 1989, 1993; Snow, 1990). As Bowlby first noted, early semantic memory is conferred by caregivers. Parents convey considerable descriptive and evaluative information about the child, including labels to distinguish one from others (e.g., "You're a big boy"), evaluative descriptors of the self (e.g., "You are so smart;" "You're a good girl"), as well as rules and standards and the extent to which the child has met parental expectations ("Big boys don't cry"). Consistent with Cooley's (1902) model of the looking-glass self, children incorporate these labels and evaluations into their self-definition in the form of general *trait* knowledge (represented in semantic memory). Thus, the linguistic construction of the self is a highly interpersonal process, with caregivers making a major contribution to its representation in both autobiographical and semantic memory.

Language as a Double-Edged Sword

Language clearly promotes heightened levels of relatedness and allows for the creation of a personal narrative. Stern (1985), however, also alerts us to the liabilities of language. He argues that language can drive a wedge between two simultaneous forms of interpersonal experience, as it is lived and as it is verbally represented. The very capacity for objectifying the self through verbal representations allows one to transcend, and therefore potentially distort, one's immediate experience and to create a fantasied construction of the self. In addition, there is the potential for incorporating the biases of caregivers' perspectives on the self, since initially, adults dictate the content of narratives incorporated in autobiographical memory (Bowlby, 1980; Bretherton, 1987; Crittenden, 1994; Pipp, 1990). Children may receive subtle signals that certain episodes should not be retold or are best "forgotten" (Dunn, Brown, & Beardsall, 1991). Bretherton describes another process, namely, "defensive exclusion," in which negative information about the self or other is not incorporated since it is too psychologically threatening (see also Cassidy & Kobak, 1988). Wolf (1990) further describes several mechanisms such as deceit and fantasy, whereby the young child, as author of the self, can select, edit, or change the "facts" in the service of personal goals, hopes, or wishes (see also Dunn, 1988).

Such distortions may well contribute to the formation of a self that is perceived as *unauthentic* if one accepts the falsified version of experience. Winnicott's (1958) observations alert us to the fact that intrusive or overinvolved mothers, in their desire to comply with maternal demands and expectations, lead infants to present a false outer self that does not represent their own inner experiences. Moreover, such parents may reject the infant's "felt self," approving only of the falsely presented self (Crittenden, 1994). As Stern notes, the display of false-self behavior, selected because it meets the needs and wishes of someone else, incurs the risk of alienating oneself from those inner experiences that represent one's true self (see also Main & Solomon, 1990). Thus, linguistic abilities not only allow one to share one's experiences with others but also to withhold them as well.

DEVELOPMENTAL DIFFERENCES IN SELF-REPRESENTATIONS DURING CHILDHOOD

In the following sections, the nature of self-representations at each of three periods of childhood, beginning in toddlerhood and ending in late childhood, are examined. Each period begins with a prototypical self-descriptive cameo reflecting the cardinal features of the content and the self-structure at that developmental level. In addition to an analysis of the defining features of each stage, including both advances and potential liabilities, the practical implications of the nature of self-representations are explored. An appreciation for these normative-developmental changes is especially critical as a backdrop against which one can judge whether a given child's self-representations are age-appropriate or, conversely, immature, with possible clinical implications. The major developmental shifts are summarized in Table 2.1. These shifts represent a general sequence or order through which most children progress. The age categories identified are still rather broad, in large part because there is tremendous variability in the particular ages at which these acquisitions are attained. Moreover, as Fischer and his colleagues have argued (see Fischer & Ayoub, 1994; Fischer & Pipp, 1984), there may be deviations in such developmental patterns, depending upon the child's socialization history. For example, severe and chronic abuse in childhood will lead to distortions in self-development, discussed in Chapter 10.

TABLE 2.1. Normative-Developmental Changes in Self-Representations during Childhood

Age period	Salient content	Structure/ organization	Valence/ accuracy	Nature of comparisons	Sensitivity to others
Very early childhood	Concrete, observable characteristics; simple taxonomic attributes in the form of abilities, activities, possessions, preferences	Isolated representations; lack of coherence, coordination; all-or-none thinking	Unrealistically positive; inability to distinguish real from ideal selves	No direct comparisons	Anticipation of adult reactions (praise, criticism); rudimentary appreciation of whether one is meeting others' external standards
Early to middle childhood	Elaborated taxonomic attributes; focus on specific competencies	Rudimentary links between representations; links typically opposites; all-or-none thinking	Typically positive; inaccuracies persist	Temporal comparisons with self when younger; comparisons with age-mates to determine fairness	Recognition that others are evaluating the self; initial introjection of others' opinions; others' standards becoming self-guides in regulation of behavior
Middle to late childhood	Trait labels that focus on abilities and interpersonal characteristics; comparative assessments with peers; global evaluation of worth	Higher-order generalizations that subsume several behaviors; ability to integrate opposing attributes	Both positive and negative evaluations; greater accuracy	Social comparison for purpose of self-evaluation	Internalization of others' opinions and standards, which come to function as self-guides

VERY EARLY CHILDHOOD

"I'm 3 years old and I live in a big house with my mother and father and my brother, Jason, and my sister, Lisa. I have blue eyes and a kitty that is orange and a television in my own room. I know all of my ABC's, listen: A, B, C, D, E, F, G, H, J, L, K, O, M, P, Q, X, Z. I can run real fast. I like pizza and I have a nice teacher at preschool. I can count up to 100, want to hear me? I love my dog Skipper. I can climb to the top of the jungle gym, I'm not scared! I'm never scared! I'm always happy. I have brown hair and I go to preschool. I'm really strong. I can lift this chair, watch me!"

Such descriptions will typically be observed in 3- to 4-year-olds. Noteworthy in this descriptive cameo is the nature of the attributes selected to portray the self. Theory and evidence (see Fischer, 1980; Fischer & Canfield, 1986; Griffin, 1992; Harter, 1996a, 1998a; Higgins, 1991; Watson, 1990) indicate that the young child can only construct very concrete cognitive representations of observable features of the self (e.g., "I know my ABC's," "I can count," "I live in a big house"). Damon and Hart (1988) label these as categorical identifications, reflecting the fact that the young child understands the self only as separate, taxonomic attributes that may be *physical* (e.g., "I have blue eyes"), *active* (e.g., "I can run real fast, climb to the top"), *social* (e.g., "I have a brother, Jason, and a sister, Lisa") or *psychological* (e.g., "I am happy"). It is noteworthy that particular skills are touted (running, climbing) rather than generalizations about abilities such as being athletic or good at sports. Moreover, often these behavioral descriptions spill over into actual demonstrations of one's abilities ("I'm really strong. I can lift this chair, watch me!"), suggesting that these emerging self-representations are still very directly tied to behavior. From a cognitive-developmental perspective, they do not represent higher-order conceptual categories through which the self is defined. In addition to concrete descriptions of behaviors, the young child defines the self in terms of *preferences* (e.g., "I like pizza; I love my dog Skipper") and well as *possessions* ("I have an orange kitty and a television in my own room"). Thus, as Rosenberg (1979) cogently observes, the young child acts as a demographer or radical behaviorist in that his/her self-descriptions are limited to characteristics that are potentially observable by others.

From the standpoint of organization, the self-representations of this period are highly differentiated or isolated from one another; that is, the young child is incapable of integrating these compartmentalized representations of self, and thus self-descriptive accounts appear quite disjointed. This lack of coherence is a general cognitive characteristic that pervades the young child's thinking across a variety of domains (Fischer, 1980). As Piaget (1960) himself observed, young children's thinking is *transductive*, in that they reason from particular to particular, in no logical order.

Neo-Piagetians have elaborated on these processes. For example, Case (1992) refers to this level as "Interrelational," in that young children can forge rudimentary links in the form of discrete event-sequence structures that are defined in terms of physical dimensions, behavioral events, or habitual activities. However, they cannot coordinate two such structures (see also Griffin, 1992), in part because of working memory constraints that prevent young children from holding several features in mind simultaneously. Fischer's (1980) formulation is very similar. He labels these initial structures "Single Representations." Such structures are highly differentiated from one another, since the cognitive limitations at this stage render the child incapable of integrating single representations into a coherent self-portrait.

Moreover, self-evaluations during this period are likely to be unrealistically positive (e.g., "I know all of my ABC's" [which he/she doesn't!]) since young children have difficulty distinguishing between their desired and their actual competence, a confusion initially observed by both Freud (1952) and Piaget (1932). Thus, young children cannot yet formulate an *ideal* self-concept that is differentiated from a *real* self-concept. Rather, their descriptions represent a litany of talents that may transcend reality (Harter & Pike, 1984). For contemporary cognitive-developmentalists, such overstated virtuosity stems from another cognitive limitation of this period, namely the inability of young children to bring social comparison information to bear meaningfully on their perceived competencies (Frey & Ruble, 1990). The ability to use social comparison toward the goals of self-evaluation requires that the child be able to relate one concept (his/her own performance) to another (someone else's performance), a skill that is not sufficiently developed in the young child. Thus, self-descriptions typically represent an overestimation of personal abilities. It is important to appreciate, however, that these apparent distortions are normative in that they reflect cognitive limitations rather than conscious efforts to deceive the listener.

Another manifestation of the self-structure of very young children is their inability to acknowledge that they can possess attributes of opposing valence, for example, good and bad, or nice and mean (Fischer, Hand, Watson, Van Parys, & Tucker, 1984). This all-or-none thinking can be observed in the cameo, in that all of the attributes appear to be positive. Young children's self-representations may also include emotion descriptors (e.g., "I'm always happy"). However, children at this age do not acknowledge that they can experience both positive and negative emotions, particularly at the same time. The majority will deny that they have negative emotions (e.g., "I'm never scared!") as salient features of their descriptive self-portrait. Other procedures reveal that they do have rudimentary concepts of such single negative emotions as mad, sad, and scared (see Bretherton & Beeghly, 1982;

Dunn, 1988; Harter & Whitesell, 1989). However, a growing body of evidence now reveals that young children are incapable of appreciating the fact that they can experience seemingly opposing emotional reactions simultaneously (Carroll & Steward, 1984; Donaldson & Westerman, 1986; Gnepp, McKee, & Domanic, 1987; Harris, 1983a, 1983b; Harter & Buddin, 1987; Reissland, 1985; Selman, 1980). For Fischer and colleagues (e.g., Fischer & Ayoub, 1994), this dichotomous thinking represents the natural fractionation of the mind. Such "affecting splitting," as they term it, constitutes a normative form of dissociation that is the hallmark of very young children's thinking about both self and others.

It is important to appreciate the normative nature of this all-or-none thinking in understanding young children's reactions to everyday life events, particularly as they apply to the experience of negative affects. For example, one of our young interview participants described a situation in which he was being punished by his mother: "When I'm all bad my mother gets all mad, and when she's all mad, she gets a lot bigger!" In other situations, where the child is consumed with anger toward a parent or sibling, he/she may staunchly deny any feelings of affection or love (e.g., claiming only "I hate you!"). With regard to issues of loss, the young child may be pervasively sad over the death of a loved one, totally unable to acknowledge the positive emotions that were undoubtedly also felt for the individual. Thus, at this particular developmental period, one would not want to conclude that such all-or-none reactions are abnormal or have clinical implications.

Cognitive limitations of this period extend to the inability of young children to create a concept of their overall worth as a person, namely, a representation of their global self-esteem or self-worth (Harter, 1990a). Such a self-representation requires a higher-order integration of domain-specific attributes that have first been differentiated. Young children do begin to describe themselves in terms of concrete cognitive abilities, physical abilities, how they behave, how they look, and friendships they have formed (Harter, 1990a). However, these domains are not clearly differentiated from one another, as revealed through factor-analytic procedures (Harter, 1998a; Harter & Pike, 1984).

The fact that young children cannot cognitively or verbally formulate a general concept of their worth as a person does not dictate that they lack the experience of self-esteem. Rather, our own findings (see Haltiwanger, 1989; Harter, 1990a) reveal that young children manifest self-esteem in their *behavior*. In examining the construct of "behaviorally presented self-esteem," we determined, through Q-sorts given to teachers, that young children exude positive self-esteem through displays of confidence, curiosity, initiative, and independence. Those failing to demonstrate these behaviors are identified by teachers as children with low self-esteem. Of particular interest in the Q-sort data was the finding that competence or skills, per se, was not identified by teachers as a cardinal feature of high self-esteem. Rather, the defining features (e.g., confidence, initiative) focused more on the individual's efforts toward mastery rather than manifest success. However, competence does become an important contributor to self-esteem beginning in middle childhood and beyond. (Our efforts to identify the dimensions of self-esteem in early childhood have resulted in the development of an instrument, the Behaviorally Presented Self-Esteem Scale for Young Children, through which adults, familiar with young children, can evaluate these manifestations in young children.)

The Role of the Socializing Environment

Higgins (1991), building upon the efforts of Case (1985), Fischer (1980), and Selman (1980), focuses more on how self-development during this period involves the interaction between the young child's cognitive capacities and the role of *socializing agents*. He provides evidence for the contention that at Case's stage of Interrelational development and Fischer's stage of Single Representations, the very young child can place himself/herself in the same category as the parent who shares his/her gender, which forms an initial basis for identification with that parent. Thus, the young boy can evaluate his overt behavior with regard to the question: "Am I doing what Daddy is doing?" Attempts to match that behavior, in turn, will have implications for which attributes become incorporated into the young child's self-definition. Thus, these processes represent one way in which socializing agents impact the self.

Higgins observes that at the Interrelational stage, young children can also form structures allowing them to detect the fact that their behavior evokes a reaction in others, notably parents, which in turn causes psychological reactions in the self. These experiences shape the self to the extent that the young child chooses to engage in behaviors designed to please the parents. Stipek et al. (1992), in a recent laboratory study, have provided empirical evidence for this observation, demonstrating that slightly before the age of 2, children begin to anticipate adult reactions, seeking positive responses to their successes and attempting to avoid negative responses to failure. At this age, they also find that young children show a rudimentary appreciation for adult standards, for example, by turning away from adults and hunching their shoulder in the face of failures (see also Kagan, 1984, who reports similar distress reactions). For Mascolo and Fischer (1995), such reactions constitute rudimentary forms of *shame*, an issue discussed in more detail in Chapter 4. Although young children are beginning to recognize that their behavior has an impact on others, their I-self cannot yet directly or realistically evaluate the Me-self (see also Selman, 1980).

Summary

Very young children's self-representations reflect concrete descriptions of behaviors, abilities, emotions, possessions, and preferences that are potentially observable by others. These attributes are highly differentiated or isolated from one another, leading to rather disjointed accounts, because at this age, young children lack the ability to integrate such characteristics. Self-representations are also likely to be unrealistically positive, since young children lack the requisite skills (e.g., social comparison) to allow them to distinguish between ideal and real self-concepts. Young children are also unable to acknowledge that they can possess attributes or emotions of opposing valence (e.g., nice and mean, happy and sad). Rather, they demonstrate all-or-none thinking in which, typically, their descriptions are all positive (unless very negative life experiences lead them to construct attributes that are viewed as all unfavorable). Cognitive limitations also extend to the inability to create a concept of global self-worth or self-esteem, although manifestations of positive or negative self-esteem can be reliably observed in their behavior by others. Some of these limitations continue into the next age period, although others are overcome, as new cognitive-developmental acquisitions lead to the creation of new self-structures.

EARLY TO MIDDLE CHILDHOOD

"I have a lot of friends, in my neighborhood, at school, and at my church. I'm good at schoolwork, I know my words, and letters, and my numbers. I can run fast, and I can climb high, a lot higher than I could when I was little and I can run faster, too. I can also throw a ball real far, I'm going to be on some kind of team when I am older. I can do lots of stuff real good. Lots! If you are good at things you can't be bad at things, at least not at the same time. I know some *other* kids who are bad at things but not me! (Well, maybe sometime later I could be a little bad, but not very often.) My parents are real proud of me when I do good at things. It makes me really happy and excited when they watch me!"

Such self-descriptions are typical of children ages 5 to 7. Some of the features of the previous stage persist in that self-representations are still typically very positive, and the child continues to overestimate his/her virtuosity. References to various competencies, for example, social skills, cognitive abilities, and athletic talents, are common self-descriptors. With regard to the advances of this age period, children begin to display a rudimentary ability to intercoordinate concepts that were previously compartmentalized

(Case, 1985; Fischer, 1980). For example, they can form a category or representational *set* that combines a number of their competencies (e.g., good at running, jumping, schoolwork; having friends in the neighborhood, at school, and at church). However, all-or-none thinking persists. In Case's (1985) model and its application to the self (Griffin, 1992), this stage is labeled "Unidimensional" thinking. At this age, such black-and-white thinking is supported by another new cognitive process that emerges at this stage. The novel acquisition is the child's ability to link or relate representational sets to one another, to "map" representations onto one another, to use Fischer's (1980) terminology. Of particular interest to self-development is one type of representational mapping that is extremely common in the thinking of young children, namely, a link in the form of *opposites*. For example, in the domain of physical concepts, young children can oppose up versus down, tall versus short, thin versus wide or fat, although they cannot yet meaningfully coordinate these representations.

Opposites can also be observed within the realm of the descriptions of self and others, where the child's ability to oppose "good" to "bad" is especially relevant. As observed earlier, the child develops a rudimentary concept of the self as good at a number of skills. Given that good is defined as the opposite of bad, this cognitive construction typically precludes the young child from being "bad," at least at the same time. Thus, the oppositional mapping takes the necessary form of "I'm good and therefore I can't be bad." However, other people may be perceived as bad at these skills, as the cameo description reveals ("I know other kids who are bad at things but not me!"). Children at this age may acknowledge that they could be bad at some earlier or later time ("Well, maybe sometime later I could be a little bad, but not very often"). However, the structure of such mappings typically leads the child to *overdifferentiate* favorable and unfavorable attributes, as demonstrated by findings revealing young children's inability to integrate attributes such as nice and mean (Fischer et al., 1984) or smart and dumb (Harter, 1986b). Moreover, the mapping structure leads to the persistence of self-descriptions laden with virtuosity.

In situations involving chronic harsh discipline for misbehavior, or for a subset of children with very negative socialization histories involving abuse, maltreatment, or neglect, children may at times conclude that they are *all bad* (see Chapter 10). To take another example, one young child in play therapy who had been diagnosed with dyslexia, following a history of marked school failure in the first grade, came to the conclusion that she was "all dumb" (see Harter, 1977). Another of my clients, the third daughter in a family whose parents were desperate to have a son, could only report extreme feelings of hatred when her new baby brother finally arrived. However, in these cases, the underlying structure is the same, namely, a mapping in the form of opposites that results in all-or-none, unidimensional thinking. Nevertheless, for those with very negative life experiences, this particular cognitive structure represents a major liability leading to very negative perceptions of the self.

These principles also apply to children's understanding of their emotions, in that they cannot integrate emotions of opposing valence such as happy and sad (Harter & Buddin, 1987). There is an advance over the previous period in that children come to appreciate the fact that they can have two emotions of the *same* valence (e.g., "I'm happy and excited when my parents watch me"); that is, they can also develop representational sets for feelings of the same valence, but these are separate emotion categories, namely, one for positive emotions (happy, excited, proud) and one for negative emotions (sad, mad, scared). However, children at this stage cannot yet integrate the sets of positive and negative emotions, sets that are viewed as conceptual opposites and therefore incompatible. The inability to acknowledge that one can possess both favorable and unfavorable attributes, or that one can experience both positive *and* negative emotions, represents a cognitive liability that will be marked for those whose experiences lead them to conclude that they are all "bad" or "all mad." Finally, it should be noted that the creation of opposing attributes and emotions is not limited to childhood. As Fischer (1980) has demonstrated, one observes this type of structure in adolescents and adults, where mappings of this form are constructed at a more abstract level (a topic to be addressed in Chapter 3). The tendency to organize concepts along such an evaluative dimension, as previously demonstrated by Wundt (1907) and Osgood et al. (1971), is a very central cognitive strategy that is relatively universal.

The Role of the Socializing Environment

Given his focus on social processes, Higgins moves beyond cognitive-developmental structures per se to examine how the child's increasing cognitive appreciation for the perspective of *others* also influences self-development. The relational processes of this level allow the child to realize that socializing agents have a particular *viewpoint* (not merely a reaction) toward them and their behavior. As Selman (1980) also observes, the improved perspective taking skills at this age permit children to realize that others are actively *evaluating* the self (although children have not yet internalized these evaluations sufficiently to make independent judgments about their attributes.) Nevertheless, as Higgins argues, the viewpoints of others begin to function as "self-guides," as the child comes to further identify with what he/she perceives socializing agents expect of the self. These self-guides function to aid the child in the regulation of his/her behavior. The findings of

Stipek et al. (1992) provide direct evidence that these processes begin to be observed shortly after the age of 3.

One can recognize in these observations mechanisms similar to those identified by Bandura (1991) in his theory of the development of self-regulation. Early in development, children's behavior is more externally controlled by reinforcement, punishment, direct instruction, and modeling. Gradually, children come to anticipate the reactions of others and to internalize the rules of behavior set forth by significant others. As these become more internalized, personal standards, the child's behavior comes more under the control of evaluative self-reactions (self-approval, self-sanctions), aiding in self-regulation and the selection of those behaviors that promote positive self-evaluation. The contribution of cognitive-developmental theory, it should be noted, is to identify more clearly those cognitive structures making such developmental acquisitions possible. Moreover, the structures underlying such a shift represent rudimentary processes required for the emergence of *looking-glass-self* behavior involving the incorporation of the evaluative opinions of significant others. However, at this age level, cognitive-developmental limitations preclude the internalization of others' standards and opinions toward the self. Internalization, in which the child comes personally to "own" these standards and opinions, awaits further developmental advances.

As Higgins (1991) and Selman (1980), among others (see also Gesell & Ilg, 1946), have pointed out, although children at this age do become aware that others are critically evaluating their attributes, they lack the type of self-awareness that would allow them to be critical of their own behavior. In I-self, Me-self terminology, the child's I-self is aware that significant others are making judgments about the Me-self, yet the I-self cannot directly turn the evaluative beacon on the Me-self. These processes will only emerge when the child becomes capable of internalizing the evaluative judgments of others for the purpose of self-evaluation. As a result, children at this age period will show little interest in scrutinizing the self. As Anna Freud (1965) has cogently observed, young children do not naturally take themselves as the object of their own observation. They are much more likely to direct their inquisitiveness toward the outside world of events rather than the inner world of intrapsychic experiences.

With regard to other forms of interaction between cognitive-developmental level and the socializing environment, there are certain advances in the ability to utilize social comparison information, although there are also limitations. Frey and Ruble (1985, 1990) as well as Suls and Sanders (1982) provide evidence that at this stage children first focus on *temporal* comparisons (how I am performing now, compared to when I was younger) and age norms, rather than individual difference comparisons with age-mates. As our prototypical subject tells us, "I can climb a lot higher than when I was little and I can run faster, too." Suls and Sanders observe that such temporal comparisons are particularly gratifying to young children given the rapid skill development at this age level. As a result, such comparisons contribute to the highly positive self-evaluations that typically persist at this age level. Evidence (reviewed in Ruble & Frey, 1991) now reveals that younger children do engage in certain forms of social comparison; however, it is directed toward different goals than for older children. For example, young children use such information to determine if they have received their fair share of rewards, rather than for purposes of self-evaluation. Moreover, findings reveal that young children show an interest in others' performance to obtain information about the task demands that can facilitate their understanding of mastery goals and improve their learning (Frey & Ruble, 1985; Ruble & Dweck, 1995). However, they do not yet utilize such information to assess their competence, in large part due to the cognitive limitations of this period; thus, their evaluations continue to be unrealistic.

Summary

Some of the features of the previous stage persist, in that self-representations are typically very positive, and the child continues to overestimate his/her abilities. Moreover, the child at this period still lacks the ability to develop an overall concept of his/her worth as a person. With regard to advances, children do begin to display a rudimentary ability to intercoordinate self-concepts that were previously compartmentalized; for example, they can construct a representational set that combines a number of their competencies (e.g., good at running, jumping, schoolwork). However, all-or-none thinking persists due to a process in which different valence attributes are viewed as *opposites* (e.g., good vs. bad, nice vs. mean). Typically, this all-or-none structure leads to self-attributes that are all positive; however, for those with negative life experiences, unidimensional thinking may support the conclusions that one's attributes are all negative. Rudimentary processes that allow the child to appreciate the fact that others are *evaluating* the self set the stage for the emergence of looking-glass-self behavior, although cognitive-developmental limitations preclude the child from internalizing these evaluations. Further advances include the ability to make *temporal* comparisons between one's current and one's past performance. Given the rapid skill development during these years, such comparisons contribute to the highly positive self-evaluations that typically persist at this age level. The failure to use social comparison information for the purpose of self-evaluation, however, contributes to the persistence of unrealistically favorable self-attributes.

Clinical Implications

Elsewhere I have described in some detail the clinical implications of these self-processes (see Harter, 1977; 1982b; 1990d). Consider those children over whom there is concern because of difficulties in areas such as school failure, behavioral conduct problems, depression, and so forth. What are the implications for therapeutic intervention? First and foremost, there will be roadblocks if the child is not motivated to change. As was pointed out, young children lack interest in the self and are not yet capable of taking themselves as the object of their own cognitive reflection, in part because they have not yet internalized the standards and opinions of significant others. Thus, they show little penchant for analyzing their attributes and the underlying causes of their behavior or emotions. As Anna Freud (1965) points out, conflicts are more likely to be externalized, and environmental solutions are preferred to internal or intrapsychic change. Moreover, she observes that children do not understand the need to analyze their past experiences; they do not appreciate the need to go "backward" in order to progress "forward." Freud notes that the child will typically pin his/her hopes on the clinician making changes in the external environment, in contrast to many adult clients, who appreciate the importance of attending to self-representations and the need for internal change.

There are also challenges to working therapeutically with young children due to the fact that their self-representations will, in all likelihood, be unrealistic. As pointed out, several processes contribute to their inability to evaluate the self realistically. They lack those social comparison skills that provide an anchor of reality in terms of whether they measure up to the performance of others. The fact that they have not yet internalized the evaluative standards of others also deprives them of information through which the self could be judged. Finally, the penchant for all-or-none thinking reinforces the view for most children that their attributes are quite admirable. Thus, in the case of those children whose characteristics are less than desirable from the standpoint of adults, the therapist may meet with resistance in trying to convince such children otherwise.

Those children with negative life experiences that have led them to view the self in pervasively unfavorable terms will also resist seeming evidence to the contrary, given their unidimensional, all-or-none thinking. For example, in my own clinical work with children, it is very common for young children to view themselves as "all bad" in the case of conduct disordered behavior, as "all dumb" in the case of school learning problems, as all "sad" in the case of the loss of a loved one, or as all "mad" in the case of feeling displaced or rejected (Harter, 1977, 1982b, 1990d). In working with such children, I have developed a modest therapeutic technique in which I create visual depictions of how the child actually possesses both positive and negative attributes.

For example, in one case, with a girl referred for serious learning problems, who felt she was "all dumb," I drew a circle with a line down the middle, placing an S (for smart) in the left half of the drawing and a D (for dumb) in the right half (see Figure 2.1). My interpretation to the child was that she was not "all dumb," but rather that she had both smart parts and dumb parts, which I elaborated on with concrete examples from her own life. Gradually, she not only accepted this revision of her self-portrait, but also began to embellish it in her own set of drawings in which the "smart parts" not only became larger in number but more *central* to her visual representations of self, as can be seen in Figure 2.1. Thus, she was able to use both size and centrality to chart the changes that she was experiencing due to therapy as well as to educational interventions within the school that were meeting with success. It should be noted, however, that such techniques will not be effective unless the child is developmentally ready to move beyond the rigid application of the all-or-none thinking that is the hallmark of

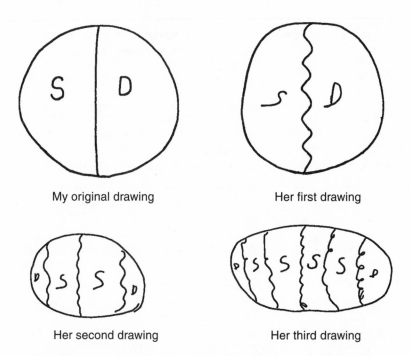

My original drawing   Her first drawing

Her second drawing   Her third drawing

FIGURE 2.1. Child client's representation of smart and dumb representations.

this period. Nor will they lead to changes in the child's self-representations if the socializing environment continues to reinforce the view that the child does indeed possess extremely negative characteristics, as is typically the case with children who are experiencing severe and chronic abuse at the hands of caregivers (see Chapter 10).

MIDDLE TO LATE CHILDHOOD

"I'm in fourth grade this year, and I'm pretty popular, at least with the girls. That's because I'm nice to people and helpful and can keep secrets. Mostly I am nice to my friends, although if I get in a bad mood I sometimes say something that can be a little mean. I try to control my temper, but when I don't, I'm ashamed of myself. I'm usually happy when I'm with my friends, but I get sad if there is no one to do things with. At school, I'm feeling pretty smart in certain subjects like Language Arts and Social Studies. I got A's in these subjects on my last report card and was really proud of myself. But I'm feeling pretty dumb in Math and Science, especially when I see how well a lot of the other kids are doing. Even though I'm not doing well in those subjects, I still like myself as a person, because Math and Science just aren't that important to me. How I look and how popular I am are more important. I also like myself because I know my parents like me and so do other kids. That helps you like yourself."

Such self-descriptions are typically observed in children ages 8 to 11. In contrast to the more concrete self-representations of younger children, older children are much more likely to describe the self in such terms as "popular," "nice," "helpful," "mean," "smart," and "dumb." Children moving into late childhood continue to describe themselves in terms of their competencies (e.g., "smart," "dumb"). However, self-attributes become increasingly interpersonal as relations with others, particularly peers, become an increasingly salient dimension of the self (see also Damon & Hart, 1988; Rosenberg, 1979).

From the standpoint of those emerging cognitive-developmental (I-self) processes that impact the organization of the self-structure, these attributes represent traits in the form of *higher-order generalizations* or concepts, based upon the integration of more specific behavioral features of the self (see Fischer, 1980; Siegler, 1991). Thus, in the preceding cameo, the higher-order generalization that she is "smart" is based upon the integration of scholastic success at both Language Arts and Social Studies. Her conclusion that she is also "dumb" represents a hierarchical construction in which her performance in Math and Science is integrated into a higher-order generalization. Similarly, she has developed the perception that she is "popular" by combining several behaviors, namely, "nice to people," "helpful," and "can keep secrets" into a higher-order concept.

It should be noted that from a developmental perspective, trait labels represent a cognitive construction in which behavioral features are subsumed under a higher-order generalization. One cannot, therefore, merely infer that if a child employs a self-descriptor such as "smart," that it automatically reflects such a construction, since some younger children may also employ these labels. Rather, one must document the underlying *structure* of such self-representations. Thus, the term "trait label" should only be inferred if it can be demonstrated that such a label does indeed represent a hierarchically constructed concept that subsumes specific, relevant behaviors. Too often in the literature, it is simply assumed that if a child describes the self with words such as "smart" or "dumb," this reflects the use of trait labels, an assumption that is unwarranted. For example, if when asked how one knew one was "smart," a younger child replied, "Because I know my numbers" (and said nothing else), this would not reflect a trait-label structure. Rather, the term "smart" in this example is merely a description of a single skill.

Nor should it be assumed that trait labels representing higher-order generalizations are necessarily stable across situations or time, an assumption underlying the use of the term "trait" in the personality literature (see Rosenberg, 1979). Beginning at this age level, children come to the realization that they can be "smart" in some situations and "dumb" in others, as well as "nice" in some situations and "mean" in others, suggesting that they view their attributes as more situation-specific (see also Mischel, 1973); that is, from a cognitive-developmental perspective, one feature of self-representations is that they not only become more integrated into higher-order generalizations, but they also become more differentiated across domains.

The newfound cognitive ability to form higher-order concepts also allows the older child to construct a more global evaluation of the self as a *person*, namely, to formulate a representation of one's overall self-worth. As the cameo child describes herself, "I like myself as a person." This observation is consistent with our own empirical work in which we have demonstrated that the concept of global self-worth, defined as how much one likes the self as a person, does not emerge until middle childhood (Harter, 1990a). Moreover, at this age level, children begin to show some appreciation for those antecedents of self-worth that were identified by James (1892), namely, the role of perceived success in areas where one has aspirations. Our prototypical subject observes that "even though I'm not doing well in Math and Science, I still like myself as a person, because those subjects just aren't that important to me." Her assertion bolsters James' contention that lack of success in domains judged unimportant will not erode global self-worth or self-esteem. Thus, cognitive abilities that now allow the child to simultaneously compare two concepts, in this case judgments of importance with perceptions of success, foster an understanding of the *causes* of one's self-worth.

Another major advance of this period is the ability to coordinate self-representations that were previously differentiated or considered to be opposites. In Case's (1985, 1992) theory, this level is labeled "Bidimensional" thought. In identifying similar structures, Fischer (1980) labels this stage as "Representational Systems." The very hallmark of a representational system is the integration of concepts that were previously isolated. Siegler's (1991) strategy construction processes at this level also include higher-order generalizations of features previously compartmentalized. Thus, concepts viewed as opposing, at the previous level, can now be integrated, leading to both positive and *negative* self-evaluations. For example, as the cameo description has revealed, the older child can acknowledge that he/she can be both smart and dumb, both nice *and* mean. Such self-representations are no longer viewed as opposites but can now cognitively coexist within a more integrated self-system.

There is considerable evidence for the emergence of this more integrated structure (see Case, 1985, 1992; Fischer, 1980; Harter, 1986; Siegler, 1991). In our own work, we have found that the first emergence of an understanding that one can be both smart and dumb typically involves examples in which one is smart in one broadly defined domain (e.g., scholastic competence) but dumb in a very different domain (e.g., social/interpersonal relationships). As one 8-year-old subject put it, "You could say something really smart in school but could be really dumb with your friends, acting like a jerk." Older subjects (ages 9–10) were more likely to provide examples within the same domain (typically, scholastic competence), where they described how they could be smart at one school subject but dumb at a different subject (see also Harter & Jackson, 1992). Among even older subjects (ages 11–12), there were descriptions that reflected an even higher level of differentiation and integration within a given school subject (e.g., "You could understand some parts of science but not others"). An even more differentiated sequence can be found in the work of Fischer and colleagues (see Fischer et al., 1984) for the attributes "nice" and "mean." These concepts are initially highly differentiated for young children and gradually become integrated at higher and higher levels. In each of these bodies of research, it has been demonstrated that by middle to late childhood, the child comes to appreciate that two attributes, previously viewed as contradictory, can now simultaneously exist within the self.

With the emerging ability to integrate positive and negative concepts about the self, the child is much less likely to engage in the type of all-or-none thinking observed in the previous stages, where typically only positive attributes were acknowledged. As a result, self-descriptions begin to represent a more balanced presentation of abilities in conjunction with one's limitations, perceptions that are likely to be more veridical with others' views of the self. These conclusions are consistent with observations (see Gesell & Ilg, 1946; Harter, 1996a; Selman, 1980) revealing that children at this age become much more self-critical, since the I-self can now reflect on one's negative Me-self attributes as well.

For Case, the emergence of these structures will partially depend upon experiences in which two lower-order features, for example, perceptions of smartness and dumbness, are activated *simultaneously* or in rapid sequence. Thus, events that make *each* of these attributes salient will foster such bidimensional structures (e.g., "On my report card I got an A in English, which shows I am smart, but I only got a C in Math, which makes me feel dumb"). Moreover, Case emphasizes the general role of *practice*. Repeated exposure to such events (e.g., discussing one's grades with different individuals such as classmates, close friends, parents, and other relatives, or multiple report cards that were similar) should facilitate the processing of such information and thereby reinforce its intercoordination.

The preceding developmental analysis has focused primarily upon advances in the ability to conceptualize self-*attributes*. However, the processes that emerge during this age period can also be applied to emotion concepts. Thus, the child develops a representational system in which positive emotions (e.g., "I'm usually happy with my friends") are integrated with negative emotional representations (e.g., "I get sad if there is no one to do things with"), as a growing number of empirical studies reveal (Carroll & Steward, 1984; Donaldson & Westerman, 1986; Fischer, Shaver, & Carnochan, 1990; Gnepp et al., 1987; Harris, 1983a, 1983b; Harris, Olthof, & Meerum-Terwogt, 1981; Harter, 1986a; Harter & Buddin, 1987; Reissland, 1985; Selman, 1980).

This represents a major conceptual advance over the previous two age periods during which young children deny that they can have emotions of opposing valences. Our own developmental findings (see Harter & Buddin, 1987) reveal that at this age, the simultaneous experience of positive and negative emotions can initially only be brought to bear on *different targets*. As one child subject observed, "I was sitting in school feeling worried about all of the responsibilities of a new pet but I was happy that I had gotten straight A's on my report card." In Fischerian (1980) terms, the child at this level demonstrates a "shift of focus," directing the positive feeling to a positive target or event and then shifting to the experience of a negative feeling that is attached to a negative event. In middle childhood, the concept that the very *same* target can simultaneously provoke both a positive and a negative emotion is not yet cognitively accessible. However, by late childhood, positive and negative emotions *can* be brought to bear on one target given the emergence of representational systems that better allow the child to integrate emotion concepts that were previously differentiated. Sample responses from our empirical documentation of this progression (Harter & Buddin, 1987) were as follows: "I was happy that I got a present but mad that it wasn't what I wanted"; "If a stranger offered you some candy, you would be eager for the candy but worried about whether it was okay."

In the cameo self-description, the child not only describes the self in terms of basic emotions such as happy and sad, but also makes reference to self-affects or self-conscious emotions such as pride and shame ("I got all A's in Language Arts and Social Studies on my last report card and was really proud of myself"; "I try to control my temper but when I don't, I'm ashamed of myself"). It is not until this age level that self-affects appear in the child's repertoire of self-representations. As will become apparent in Chapter 4, there is an intriguing developmental sequence governing the acquisition of self-affects that requires both cognitive acquisitions and the response of the socializing environment.

Social Processes

A central tenet of neo-Piagetian models is that movement to a new stage of development can be fostered by socializing agents or, alternatively, can be delayed if such environmental support is not forthcoming. One can imagine scenarios in which there would be little environmental support for the integration of positive and negative attributes or positive and negative emotions. For example, in child-rearing situations where children are chronically and severely abused, family members typically reinforce negative evaluations of the child that are then incorporated into the self-portrait (Briere, 1992; Fischer & Ayoub, 1994; Harter, 1998b; Herman, 1992; Terr, 1990; Westen, 1993). As a result, there may be little scaffolding for the kind of self-structure that would allow the child to develop as well as integrate both positive and negative self-evaluations. Moreover, negative self-evaluations that become *automatized* (Siegler, 1991) will be even more resistant to change.

At a more normative level, differential socialization will affect the self-structures of girls versus boys. Laboratory studies reveal that parents give more negative feedback to girls than boys, despite no gender differences in actual performance (Lewis, Alessandri, & Sullivan, 1992). Similar observations are reported in classrooms where girls receive more negative and less positive feedback from teachers (Dweck & Leggett, 1988; Eccles & Blumenfeld, 1985). This differential treatment contributes to the negative self-evaluations of girls and may well interfere with a more balanced sense of self in which both positive and negative attributes are integrated.

A more balanced view of self, in which positive as well as negative attributes of the self are acknowledged, is also fostered by social comparison. As our prototypical subject reports, "I'm feeling pretty dumb in Math and Science, especially when I see how well the other kids are doing." A number of studies conducted in the 1970s and early 1980s presented evidence revealing that it is not until middle childhood that children come to utilize comparisons with others as a barometer of the skills and attributes of the self (see reviews by Frey & Ruble, 1985, 1990). As Damon and Hart's (1988) model and supportive evidence also reveals, it is not until middle childhood that the child can apply comparative assessments with peers in the service of self-evaluation. From a cognitive-developmental perspective, the ability to use social comparison information toward the goal of self-evaluation requires that the child have the ability to relate one concept to another, simultaneously, an ability not sufficiently developed at younger ages. In addition to the contribution of advances in cognitive development (see also Moretti & Higgins, 1990), age stratification in school stimulates greater attention to individual differences between age-mates (Higgins & Bargh, 1987; Mack, 1983). More recent findings reveal that the primary motive for children in this age period to utilize social comparison is for personal competence assessment.

The ability to utilize social comparison information for the purpose of self-evaluation is founded on cognitive-developmental advances, namely, the ability to simultaneously compare representations of self and others. However, it is also supported by the socializing environment. For example, evidence reveals that as children move up the academic ladder, teachers make increasing use of social comparison information (Eccles & Midgley, 1989; Eccles, Midgley, & Adler, 1984) and that students are well aware of these educational practices (Harter, 1996b). Moreover, parents may contribute to the increasing salience of social comparison, to the extent that they make comparative assessments of how their child is performing relative to siblings, friends, or classmates.

However, cognitive-developmental advances in conjunction with the increasing emphasis on social comparison usher in potential liabilities (Maccoby, 1980; Moretti & Higgins, 1990), contributing to individual differences in self-evaluation. With the emergence of the ability to rank-order the performance of other students in the class, all but the most competent children will fall short. Jacobs (1983) notes that this is a major liability for children with learning disabilities. Other research supports this observation in that mainstreamed learning-disabled students have been found to have more negative perceptions of their scholastic competence than those in self-contained classrooms restricted only to learning-disabled students (Renick & Harter, 1989). Thus, the very ability and penchant to compare the self with others makes one's self-concept vulnerable in those domains that are valued (e.g., scholastic competence, athletic prowess, and peer popularity).

Moreover, to the extent that negative self-evaluations are now organized as higher-order *traits* (rather than mere behaviors), they may be more resistant to disconfirmation.

Social processes can also be observed in the older child's appreciation of the attitudes that others hold toward the self, attitudes that come to be internalized in the form of domain-specific self-judgments as well as global self-worth. Thus, children at this age level recognize that if other people approve of them, they will approve of themselves. As the cameo child explains, "I also like myself because I know my parents like me and so do other kids. That helps you like yourself." The ability not only to form the concept of global self-worth, but also to appreciate its antecedents, therefore, is a major developmental acquisition emerging in middle childhood.

As Higgins observes, cognitive acquisitions that facilitate *perspective taking* at this age allow the child to incorporate the expectations as well as attitudes toward the self into self-guides that become even more internalized (see also Selman, 1980). The ability to appreciate the perspective that others have of the self facilitates the incorporation of both their standards and opinions, allowing the I-self to directly evaluate the Me-self. Thus, the advances of this period also have implications for those looking-glass-self processes that require the ability to internalize the opinions of significant others, in the formation of domain-specific self-concepts as well as a more global perception of one's worth as a person.

Summary

There are major cognitive advances at this developmental level that impact the nature of self-representations. The child now describes the self in terms of trait labels (e.g., "smart") that represent higher-order generalizations, based on the integration of more specific behavioral features (e.g., scholastic success in Language Arts and Social Studies). The newfound cognitive ability to form higher-order concepts also allows the older child to construct a more global evaluation of the self as a *person*, namely, to formulate a representation of one's overall self-worth. Another major advance is the ability to coordinate self-representations that were previously differentiated or considered to be opposites (e.g., smart and dumb). Thus, children can acknowledge that they simultaneously possess both positive and negative attributes. These processes apply to emotion labels, as well (e.g., happy and sad), in that the child can now experience opposite valence affects simultaneously. A more balanced view of self, in which both positive and negative self-representations are integrated, is also fostered by social comparison, which not only requires the ability to relate two constructs to each other (i.e., perceptions of self and perceptions of others) but is increasingly made salient by the socializing environment. Moreover, cognitive acquisitions that facilitate perspective taking allow the child to appreciate the opinions that others hold toward the self, opinions that become internalized as domain-specific as well as global self-representations. Thus, the child now has in place those processes required by the looking-glass model of the self (Cooley, 1902). In addition, the ability to compare judgments of importance to perceptions of success allows the child to create the type of discrepancies that are central to James' (1892) formulation. Finally, both cognitive-developmental factors and the response of caregivers to the child's behavior conspire to facilitate the understanding of self-affects (e.g., pride and shame), which will be further explored in Chapter 4.

Clinical Implications

The advances of this period lead to a self-structure that is more mature in that concepts are more highly integrated. However, they also usher in new vulnerabilities that may have mental health implications. For example, it is not until this age period that certain children's presenting problems will involve negative self-evaluations, for example, unfavorable evaluations in particular domains (e.g., scholastic ability, behavioral conduct, lack of peer acceptance) as well as low self-worth. Newfound acquisitions that lead the child to be self-critical, namely, perspective-taking abilities that allow him/her to incorporate the opinions of others, the emergence of social comparison processes, and the skill to compare aspirations to perceptions of success, represent potential liabilities if the child is performing poorly in particular domains. From a clinical perspective, it is critical first to determine whether unfavorable evaluations are *realistic*. If the child is indeed deficient in areas that are eroding his/her sense of competence as well as overall self-worth, then direct interventions to enhance the child's skill level may be appropriate. Alternatively, if it becomes apparent that the child's negative self-evaluations are unrealistically low, then efforts are better directed toward altering the child's self-perceptions, in order to make them more congruent with his/her abilities. For example, we (Shirk & Harter, 1996) report one case in which a 10-year-old boy held unrealistic assumptions about both himself ("I am inferior and will be rejected") and about his peers ("They all think they're better than me; they wouldn't give me the time of day!") that were maladaptive in that they led to rejection by peers. His sense of isolation and alienation, in turn, contributed to low self-worth, including self-punitive behaviors. Cognitive interventions to alter his unrealistic beliefs and assumptions were a major part of the treatment plan.

It is also critical to determine whether the structure of the child's self-representations are age-appropriate with regard to his/her ability to integrate positive and negative self-evaluations. For example, if a child aged 9 or older laments that he/she is "all dumb," one should be concerned about the all-or-none quality of such thinking, as well as the pervasive negative content. Such thinking represents a diagnostic red flag that may signal negative life experiences that lead to the unidimensional thinking characteristic of previous stages of development. For example, in my own clinical work (see Harter, 1977) I encountered a 9-year-old boy with dyslexia, who was convinced that he was totally dumb, that there was not a smart part in his brain or body. An 8-year-old boy with conduct problems, which he displayed both at home and at school, asserted that he was "all bad." In both cases, these self-evaluations were far too harsh. The boy with dyslexia was, in reality, quite intelligent, despite his specific reading deficits. The conduct-disordered child displayed many endearing qualities and under certain circumstances showed considerable self-control. In these, and other clinical cases, the child's manifest difficulties, in combination with socializing agents who did not scaffold perceptions of positive attributes, led to distorted self-perceptions characterized by age-inappropriate, all-or-none thinking. Of particular interest is the observation that in areas where each of these clients was *not* experiencing a problem (positive peer relationships for the dyslexic child and athletic prowess for the conduct-disordered child), their thinking was much more age-appropriate, in that they could integrate favorable and unfavorable self-perceptions. Thus, it is important to be sensitive to this type of unevenness, since invariably the child's thinking will be at lower levels of development in the area of clinical concern, leading to unrealistically negative self-evaluations. (See Harter, 1977, 1982b, 1990d; Shirk & Harter, 1996; Shirk & Russell, 1996, for specific suggestions with regard to potential therapeutic interventions.)

From a clinical perspective, one may also observe in older children what therapists refer to as an "impoverished self." Such children lack a vocabulary to define the self, in that there is little in the way of autobiographical memory and descriptive or evaluative concepts about the self. An impoverished self represents a liability in that the individual has few personal referents or self-concepts around which to organize present experiences. As a result, the behavior of such children will often appear to be disorganized. Moreover, to the extent that a richly defined self promotes motivational functions in terms of guides to regulate behavior and to set future goals, such children may appear aimless, with no clear pursuits. A clinical colleague of mine, Donna Marold, has astutely observed that these children do not have dreams for the future, whereas most children do have future aspirations. For example, the prototypical child in early to midchildhood indicates that he/she is going to be on a team someday. Marold notes that the families of such children typically do not create or construct the type of narratives that provide the basis for autobiographical memory and a sense of self. Nor do such parents provide the type of personal labels or feedback that would lead to the development of semantic memory for self-attributes. Often, these are parents who do not take photographs of the children or the family, nor do they engage in such activities as posting the child's artwork or school papers on the refrigerator door. Marold has also observed that such parents do not have special rituals, such as cooking the child's favorite food or reading (and rereading) cherished bedtime stories.

What type of therapeutic interventions might be applicable, and how can they be guided by developmental theory and research? Therapists (myself included) have learned through trial and error that one cannot, with older children, simply try to instill, teach, or scaffold the self-structures appropriate for their age level, namely, trait labels that represent generalizations that integrate behavioral or taxonomic self-attributes. With such children, there are few attributes to build upon. Thus, one must begin at the beginning, utilizing techniques that help the child create the missing narratives, the autobiographical memory, the self-labels. Marold has successfully employed a number of very basic techniques to achieve this goal, techniques that necessarily enlist the aid of parents. She suggests that the parent and child create a scrapbook in which whatever materials that might be available (the scant photograph, perhaps from the school picture; a child's drawing; anything that may make a memory more salient) are collected and talked about. Where such materials are not available, Marold suggests cutting pictures out of magazines that represent the child's favorite possessions, activities, preferences, the very features that define the young child's sense of self. If there have been no routines that help to solidify the child's sense of self, Marold recommends that parents be counseled to establish routines, for example, establishing some family rituals (e.g., Friday night pizza) around a child's favorite food. Obviously, these techniques require collaboration with the parents and depend upon their ability to recreate their child's past experiences, something that not all parents may be equipped to do. In this regard, the therapist can serve as an important role model. From the standpoint of our developmental analysis, the point is that an impoverished self requires this type of support in order to foster the building blocks on which a firm sense of self is founded.

CONCLUSION

In summary, this chapter has described how changes in the cognitive-developmental structures that have been conceptualized as I-self processes lead to a different pattern of Me-self representations at three different age periods during childhood in interaction with socialization experiences. In addition to describing these developmental differences, attention focused on the particular liabilities that are associated with the self-structures of each period, as well as clinical implications. This type of analysis continues in the next chapter on the development of self-representations during adolescence.

CHAPTER THREE

The Normative Development of Self-Representations during Adolescence

The period of adolescence represents a dramatic developmental transition, given pubertal and related physical changes, cognitive-developmental advances, and changing social expectations. With regard to cognitive-developmental acquisitions, adolescents develop the ability to think *abstractly* (Case, 1985; Fischer, 1980; Flavell, 1985; Harter, 1983; Higgins, 1991). From a Piagetian (1960) perspective, the capacity to form abstractions emerges with the stage of Formal Operations in early adolescence. These newfound acquisitions, according to Piaget, should equip the adolescent with the hypothetico-deductive skills to create a formal theory. This observation is critical to the topic of self-development, given the claims of many (e.g., Epstein, 1973, 1981, 1991; Greenwald, 1980; Kelly, 1955; Markus, 1980; Sarbin, 1962) that the self is a personal epistemology, a cognitive construction, that is, a theory that should possess the characteristics of any formal theory. Therefore, a self-theory should meet those criteria by which any good theory is evaluated, criteria that include the degree to which it is parsimonious, empirically valid, internally consistent, coherently organized, testable, and useful. From a Piagetian perspective, entry into the period of formal operations should make the construction of such a theory possible, be it a theory about elements in the world or a theory about the self.

However, as will become apparent, the self-representations during early and middle adolescence fall far short of these criteria. The self-structure of these periods is not coherently organized, nor are the postulates of the self-portrait internally consistent. Moreover, many self-attributes fail to be subjected to tests of empirical validity; as a result, they can be extremely unrealistic. Nor are self-representations particularly parsimonious. Thus, the Piagetian framework fails to provide an adequate explanation for the dramatic developmental changes in the self-structure that can be observed across the substages of adolescence. Rather, as in our analysis of how self-representations change during childhood, a neo-Piagetian approach is needed to understand how changes in cognitive-developmental I-self processes result in very different Me-self organization and content at each of three age levels: early adolescence, middle adolescence, and late adolescence. As in our examination of self-development during childhood, in addition to describing these changes, the liabilities of each type of self-structure are examined. The major changes are summarized in Table 3.1.

EARLY ADOLESCENCE

"I'm an extrovert with my friends: I'm talkative, pretty rowdy, and funny. I'm fairly good-looking if I do say so. All in all, around people I know pretty well I'm awesome, at least I think my friends think I am. I'm usually cheerful when I'm with my friends, happy and excited to be doing things with them. I like myself a lot when I'm around my friends. With my parents, I'm more likely to be depressed. I feel sad as well as mad and also hopeless about ever pleasing them. They think I spend too much time at the mall with my friends, and that I don't do enough to help out at home. They tell me I'm lazy and not very responsible, and its hard not to believe them. I get real sarcastic when they get on my case. It makes me dislike myself as a person. At school, I'm pretty intelligent. I know that because I'm smart when it comes to how I do in classes, I'm curious about learning new things, and I'm also creative when it comes to solving problems. My teacher says so. I get better grades than most, but I don't brag about it because that's not cool. I can be a real introvert around people I don't know well. I'm shy, uncomfortable, and nervous. Sometimes I'm simply an airhead. I act really dumb and say things that are just plain stupid. Then I worry about what they must think of me, probably that I'm a total dork. I just hate myself when that happens."

With regard to the *content* of the self-portraits of young adolescents, interpersonal attributes and social skills that influence interactions with others or one's social appeal are typically quite salient, as findings by Damon and Hart (1988) reveal. Thus, our prototypical young adolescent admits to being talkative, rowdy, funny, good-looking, and downright awesome. Presumably, these characteristics enhance one's acceptance by peers. In addition to social attributes, self-representations also focus on competencies such as one's scholastic abilities (e.g., "I'm intelligent"), as well as affects (e.g., "I'm cheerful" and "I'm depressed").

TABLE 3.1. Normative-Developmental Changes in Self-Representations during Adolescence

Age period	Salient content	Structure/ organization	Valence/ accuracy	Nature of comparisons	Sensitivity to others
Early adolescence	Social skills, attributes, that influence interactions with others or one's social appeal; differentiation of attributes according to roles	Intercoordination of trait labels into single abstractions; abstractions compartmentalized; all-or-none thinking; opposites; don't detect, oppposing integrate, opposing abstractions	Positive attributes at one point in time; negative attributes at another; leads to inaccurate overgeneralizations	Social comparison continues although less overt	Compartmentalized attention to internalization of different standards and opinions of those in different relational contexts
Middle adolescence	Further differentiation of attributes associated with different roles and relational contexts	Initial links between single abstractions, often opposing attributes; cognitive conflict caused by seemingly contradictory characteristics; concern over which reflect one's true self	Simultaneous recognition of positive and negative attributes; instability, leading to confusion and inaccuracies	Comparisons with significant others in different relational contexts; personal fable	Awareness that the differing standards and opinions of others represent conflicting self-guides, leading to confusion over self-evaluation and vacillation with regard to behavior; imaginary audience
Late adolescence	Normalization of different role-related attributes; attributes reflecting personal beliefs, values, and moral standards; interest in future selves	Higher-order abstractions that meaningfully integrate single abstractions and resolve inconsistencies, conflict	More balanced, stable view of both positive and negative attributes; greater accuracy; acceptance of limitations	Social comparison diminishes as comparisons with one's own ideals increase	Selection among alternative self-guides; construction of one's own self-standards that govern personal choices; creation of one's own ideals toward which the self aspires

From a developmental perspective, there is considerable evidence that the self becomes increasingly differentiated (see Harter, 1998a). During adolescence, there is a proliferation of selves that vary as a function of social context. These include self with father, mother, close friends, romantic partners, peers, as well as the self in the role of student, on the job, and as athlete (Gecas, 1972; Griffin, Chassin, & Young, 1981; Hart, 1988; Harter, Bresnick, et al., 1997; Harter & Monsour, 1992; Smollar & Youniss, 1985). For example, as the cameo reveals, the adolescent may be cheerful and rowdy with friends, depressed and sarcastic with parents, intelligent, curious, and creative as a student, and shy and uncomfortable around people whom one does not know. A critical developmental task, therefore, is the construction of multiple selves that will undoubtedly vary across different roles and relationships, as James (1892) observed over 100 years ago.

In keeping with the major themes of this volume, both cognitive and social processes contribute to this proliferation of selves. Cognitive-developmental advances described earlier promote greater differentiation (see Fischer, 1980; Fischer & Canfield, 1986; Harter, 1990a; Harter & Monsour, 1992; Keating, 1990). Moreover, these advances conspire with socialization pressures to develop different selves in different relational contexts (see Erikson, 1968; Grotevant & Cooper, 1986; Hill & Holmbeck, 1986; Rosenberg, 1986). For example, bids for autonomy from parents make it important to define oneself differently with peers in contrast to parents (see also Steinberg & Silverberg, 1986; White, Speisman, & Costos, 1983). Rosenberg points to another component of the differentiation process in observing that as one moves through adolescence, one is more likely to be treated differently by those in different relational contexts. In studies from our own laboratory (see Harter, Bresnick, et al., 1997; Harter & Monsour, 1992), we have found that the percentage of overlap in self-attributes generated for different social contexts ranges from 25% to 30% among seventh and eighth graders and decreases during adolescence, to a low of approximately 10% among older teenagers.

Many (although not all) of the self-descriptions to emerge in early adolescence represent *abstractions* about the self, based upon the newfound cognitive ability to integrate trait labels into higher-order self-concepts (see Case, 1985; Fischer, 1980; Flavell, 1985; Harter, 1983; Higgins, 1991). For example, as the prototypical cameo reveals, one can construct an abstraction of the self as "intelligent" by combining such traits as smart, curious, and creative. Alternatively, one may create an abstraction that the self is an "airhead" given situations where one feels dumb and "just plain stupid." Similarly, an adolescent could construct abstractions that he/she is an "extrovert" (integrating the traits of rowdy, talkative, and funny) as well as that he/she is also an "introvert" in certain situations (when one is shy, uncomfortable, and nervous). With regard to emotion concepts, one can be depressed in some contexts (combining sad, mad, and hopeless) as well as cheerful in others (combining happy and excited). Thus, abstractions represent more cognitively complex concepts about the self in which various trait labels can now be appropriately integrated into even higher-order generalizations.

Although the ability to construct such abstractions reflects a cognitive advance, these representations are highly compartmentalized; that is, they are quite distinct from one another (Case, 1985; Fischer, 1980; Higgins, 1991). For Fischer, these "single abstractions" are overdifferentiated, and therefore the young adolescent can only think about each of them as isolated self-attributes. According to Fischer, structures that were observed in childhood reappear at the abstract level. Thus, just as single *representations* were compartmentalized during early childhood, Fischer argues that when the adolescent first moves to the level of abstract thought, he/she lacks the ability to integrate the many single abstractions that are constructed to define the self in different relational contexts. As a result, adolescents will engage in all-or-none thinking at an abstract level. For Fischer, movement to a qualitatively new level of thought brings with it lack of "cognitive control" and, as a result, adolescents at the level of single abstractions can only think about isolated self-attributes. Thus, contrary to earlier models of mind (Piaget, 1960), in which formal operations usher in newfound cognitive-developmental abilities that should allow one to create an integrated theory of self, fragmentation of self-representations during early adolescence is more the rule than the exception (Fischer & Ayoub, 1994; Harter & Monsour, 1992).

Another manifestation of the compartmentalization of these abstract attributes can be observed in the tendency for the young adolescent to be unconcerned about the fact that across different roles, certain postulates appear inconsistent, as the prototypical self-description implies. (In contrast, at middle adolescence, there is considerable concern.) However, during early adolescence, the inability to integrate seemingly contradictory characteristics of the self (intelligent vs. airhead, extrovert vs. introvert, depressed vs. cheerful) has the psychological advantage of sparing the adolescent conflict over opposing attributes in his/her self-theory (Harter & Monsour, 1992). Moreover, as Higgins observes, the increased differentiation functions as a cognitive buffer, reducing the possibility that negative attributes in one sphere may spread or generalize to other spheres (see also Linville, 1987; Simmons & Blyth, 1987). Thus, although the construction of multiple selves sets the stage for attributes to be contradictory, as James argued in describing the "conflict of the different Me's," most young adolescents do not identify contradictions or experience conflict, given the compartmentalized structure of their abstract self-representations.

Evidence for these claims comes from our own research (see Harter,

Bresnick, et al., 1997; Harter & Monsour, 1992), in which we asked adolescents at three developmental levels, early adolescence (seventh grade), middle adolescence (ninth grade), and late adolescence (11th grade) to generate self-attributes across several roles and then indicate whether any of these attributes represented *opposites* (e.g., cheerful vs. depressed, rowdy vs. calm, studious vs. lazy, at ease vs. self-conscious). After identifying any such opposites, they were asked whether any such pairs caused them *conflict*, namely, were they perceived as clashing within their personality? Across studies, the specific roles have varied. They have included self with a group of friends, with a close friend, with parents (mother vs. father), in romantic relationships, in the classroom, and on the job. Across a number of converging indices (e.g., number of opposites, number of conflicts, percentage of opposites in conflict) the findings revealed that attributes identified as contradictory and experienced as conflicting were infrequent among young adolescents.

An examination of the protocols of young adolescents reveals that there are *potential* opposites that go undetected. Examples *not* identified as opposites included being talkative as well as shy in romantic relationships, being uptight with family but carefree with friends, being caring and insensitive with friends, being a good student as well as troublemaker in school, being self-conscious in romantic relationships but easygoing with friends, being lazy as a student but hardworking on the job. These observations bolster the interpretation, from Fischer's theory, that young adolescents do not yet have the cognitive ability to simultaneously compare these attributes to one another, and therefore they tend not to detect, or be concerned about, self-representations that are potential opposites. As one young adolescent put it, when confronted with the fact that he had indicated that he was both caring and rude, "Well, you are caring with your friends and rude to people who don't treat you nicely. There's no problem. I guess I just think about one thing about myself at a time and don't think about the other until the next day." When another young adolescent was asked why opposite attributes did not bother her, she succinctly exclaimed, "That's a stupid question. I don't fight with myself!" As will become apparent, this pattern changes dramatically during middle adolescence.

The differentiation of role-related selves, beginning in early adolescence, can also be observed in the tendency to report differing levels of *self-worth* across relational contexts. In the prototypical description, the young adolescent reports that with friends, "I like myself a lot"; however with parents, I "dislike myself as a person." Around "people I don't know well, I just hate myself." Although the concept of self-worth has heretofore been reserved for perceptions of *global* worth or self-esteem, we have recently introduced the construct of *relational self-worth* (Harter, Waters, & Whitesell, 1998).

Beginning in the middle school years, adolescents discriminate their level of perceived self-worth, namely, how much they like themselves as a person, across relational contexts. We have examined these perceptions across a number of such contexts including self-worth with parents, with teachers, with male classmates, and with female classmates. Factor-analyses reveal clear factor patterns with high loadings on the designated factors (i.e., each relational context) with negligible cross-loadings. We have also examined the discrepancy between individuals' highest and lowest relational self-worth scores. While a minority of adolescents (approximately one-fourth) were found to report little variation in self-worth across contexts, the vast majority (the remaining three-fourths) report that their self-worth did vary significantly as a function of the relational context. In the extreme, one female participant reported the lowest possible self-worth score with parents and the highest possible self-worth score with female classmates.

In addition to documenting such variability, our goal has been to identify potential causes of these individual differences. In addressing one determinant, we adopted Cooley's (1902) looking-glass-self perspective, in which the opinions of significant others are incorporated into one's sense of worth. Building upon our previous empirical efforts (see Harter, 1990a), we hypothesized that context-specific support, in the form of validation for who one is as a person, should be highly related to self-worth within the corresponding context. The findings corroborated the more specific prediction that support within a given relationship was more highly associated with relational self-worth in that relationship, compared to self-worth in the other three contexts. Thus, the pattern of results suggests a refinement of the looking-glass-self formulation, in that support in the form of validation from particular significant others will have its strongest impact on how one evaluates one's sense of worth in the context of those particular others.

These findings highlight the fact that with the proliferation of multiple selves across roles, adolescents become very sensitive to the potentially different opinions and standards of the significant others in each context. As the cameo description reveals, the adolescent reports high self-worth around friends who think he/she is "awesome," lower self-worth around parents who think he/she is "lazy" and "irresponsible," and the lowest level of self-worth around strangers who probably think "I'm a total dork." As Rosenberg (1986) observes, adolescents demonstrate a heightened concern with the reflected appraisals of others. He notes that other people's differing views of the self (e.g., the respect of the peer group counterposed to the critical stance of parents) will inevitably lead to variability in the self-concept across contexts.

In addition to their sensitivity to feedback from others, young adolescents continue to make use of social comparison information. However, with increasing age, children shift from more conspicuous to more subtle forms of social comparison as they become more aware of the negative social consequences of overt comparisons; for example, they may be accused of boasting about their superior performance (Pomerantz, Ruble, Frey, & Greulich, 1995). As the prototypical young adolescent describes in the cameo, "I get better grades than most, but I don't brag about it because that's not cool."

Summary and Implications

During early adolescence, interpersonal attributes and social skills that influence one's interactions with others or one's social appeal become quite salient. With regard to the *structure* of self-representations, there is a proliferation of selves that vary as a function of social context. Cognitive-developmental advances promoting greater differentiation conspire with socialization pressures to develop different selves in different relational contexts. Cognitive advances also allow the adolescent to construct self-attributes that represent *abstractions* about the self, based upon the ability to integrate trait labels into higher-order generalizations. However, these abstract representations are highly compartmentalized or overdifferentiated, and therefore the adolescent can only think about each as isolated characteristics of the self. As a result, the young adolescent typically does not detect, nor is he/she concerned about, potential contradictions in his/her self-portrait. The differentiation of role-related selves can also be observed in young adolescents' tendency to report differing levels of *self-worth* across relational contexts. The particular level of self-worth within a given context is highly related to the perceived validation that the adolescent experiences from those significant others. Young adolescents become very sensitive to the potentially different opinions and standards of people in different contexts as sources of reflected appraisals in the formation of the looking-glass self. They are also sensitive to social comparison information, although they are less blatant about its use.

As with the entry into any new developmental level, there are liabilities associated with these emerging self-processes. For example, although abstractions are developmentally advanced cognitive structures, they are removed from concrete, observable behaviors and therefore more susceptible to distortion. The adolescent's self-concept, therefore, becomes more difficult to verify and is often less realistic. As Rosenberg (1986) observes, when the self comes to be viewed as a collection of abstractions, uncertainties are introduced, since there are "few objective and unambiguous facts about one's sensitivity, creativity, morality, dependability, and so on" (p. 129). Moreover, the necessary skills to apply hypothetico-deductive thinking to the postulates of one's self-system are not yet in place. Although the young adolescent may have multiple hypotheses about the self, he/she does not yet possess the ability to correctly deduce which are true, leading to distortions in self-perceptions.

The all-or-none thinking of this period, in the form of overgeneralizations that the young adolescent cannot cognitively control, also contributes to unrealistic self-representations, in that at one point in time, one may feel totally intelligent or awesome, whereas at another point in time, one may feel like a dork. The compartmentalization of abstractions about the self also precludes the construction of an integrated portrait of self. The fact that different significant others may hold differing opinions about the self also makes it difficult to develop the sense that the self is coherent. With movement into middle adolescence, abstract self-descriptors become far less isolated or compartmentalized. However, as will be demonstrated, the emerging structures that follow bring with them new liabilities.

MIDDLE ADOLESCENCE

"What am I like as a person? You're probably not going to understand. I'm complicated! With my really *close* friends, I am very tolerant. I mean I'm understanding and caring. With a *group* of friends, I'm rowdier. I'm also usually friendly and cheerful but I can get pretty obnoxious and intolerant if I don't like how they're acting. I'd *like* to be friendly and tolerant all of the time, that's the kind of person I *want* to be, and I'm disappointed in myself when I'm not. At school, I'm serious, even studious every now and then, but on the other hand, I'm a goof-off too, because if you're *too* studious, you won't be popular. So I go back and forth, which means I don't do all that well in terms of my grades. But that causes problems at home, where I'm pretty anxious when I'm around my parents. They expect me to get all A's, and get pretty annoyed with me when report cards come out. I care what they think about me, and so then I get down on myself, but it's not fair! I mean I worry about how I probably *should* get better grades, but I'd be mortified in the eyes of my friends if I did too well. So I'm usually pretty stressed-out at home, and can even get very sarcastic, especially when my parents get on my case. But I really don't understand how I can switch so fast from being cheerful with my friends, then coming home and feeling anxious, and then getting frustrated and sarcastic with my parents. Which one is the *real* me? I have the same question when I'm around boys. Sometimes I feel phony. Say I think some guy might be interested in asking me out. I try to act different, like Madonna. I'll be a real extrovert, fun-loving and even flirtatious, and think I am really good-looking. And then everybody, I mean *everybody* else is looking at me like they think I am totally weird! *They* don't act like they think I'm attractive so I end up thinking I look terrible. I just hate myself when that happens! Because it gets worse! Then I get self-conscious and embarrassed and become radically introverted, and I don't know who I really am! Am I just acting like an extrovert, am I just trying to impress them, when really I'm an introvert? But I don't really care what they think, anyway. I mean I don't *want* to care, that is. I just want to know what my close friends think. I can be my true self with my close friends. I can't be my real self with my parents. They don't understand me. What do *they* know about what it's like to be a teenager? They treat me like I'm still a kid. At least at school, people treat you more like you're an adult. That gets confusing, though. I mean, which am I? When you're 15, are you a still a kid or an adult? I have a part-time job and the people there treat me like an adult. I want them to approve of me, so I'm very responsible at work, which makes me feel good about myself there. But then I go out with my friends and I get pretty crazy and irresponsible. So which am I, responsible or irresponsible? How can the same person be both? If my parents knew how immature I act sometimes, they would ground me forever, particularly my father. I'm real distant with him. I'm pretty close to my mother though. But its hard being distant with one parent and close to the other, especially if we are all together, like talking at dinner. Even though I am close to my mother, I'm still pretty secretive about some things, particularly the things about myself that confuse me. So I think a lot about who is the real me, and sometimes I try to figure it out when I write in my diary, but I can't resolve it. There are days when I wish I could just become immune to myself!"

Self-descriptions are likely to increase in length during this period, as adolescents become increasingly introspective as well as morbidly preoccupied with what others think of them (Broughton, 1978; Elkind, 1967; Erikson, 1959, 1968; Harter, 1990b; Lapsley & Rice, 1988; Rosenberg, 1979). The unreflective self-acceptance of earlier periods of development vanishes, and, as Rosenberg observes, what were formerly unquestioned self-truths now become problematic self-hypotheses. The tortuous search for the self involves a concern with *what* or *who* am I (Broughton, 1978), a task made more difficult given the multiple Me's that crowd the self-landscape. There is typically a further proliferation of selves as adolescents come to make finer differentiations; in the cameo, the adolescent describes a self with really close friends (e.g., tolerant) versus with a group of friends (e.g., intolerant), and a self with mother (e.g., close) versus father (e.g., distant). The acquisition of new roles, for example, self at a job, may also require the construction of new context-specific attributes (e.g., responsible).

Moreover, additional cognitive I-self processes emerge that give the self-portrait a very new look (Case, 1985; Fischer, 1980). Whereas, in the previous stage, single abstractions were isolated from one another, during middle adolescence one acquires the ability to make *comparisons* between single abstractions, namely, between attributes within the same role-related self or across role-related selves. Fischer labels these new structures "abstract mappings," in that the adolescent can now "map" constructs about the self onto one another. Therefore mappings force the individual to compare and contrast different attributes. It should be noted that abstract mappings have features in common with the "representational" mappings of childhood, in that the cognitive links that are forged often take the form of *opposites*. During adolescence, these opposites can take the form of seemingly contradictory *abstractions* about the self (e.g., tolerant vs. intolerant, extrovert vs. introvert, responsible vs. irresponsible, goodlooking versus unattractive, in the cameo).

However, the abstract mapping structure has limitations as a means of relating two concepts to one another, in that the individual cannot yet truly integrate such self-representations in a manner that would resolve apparent contradictions. Therefore, at the level of abstract mappings, the awareness of these opposites causes considerable intrapsychic conflict, confusion, and distress (Fischer et al., 1984; Harter & Monsour, 1992; Higgins, 1991) given the inability to coordinate these seemingly contradictory self-attributes. For example, our prototypical adolescent agonizes over whether she is an extrovert or an introvert ("Am I just acting like an extrovert, am I just trying to impress them, when really I'm an introvert?" "So which am I, responsible or irresponsible? How can the same person be both?"). Such cognitive-developmental limitations contribute to the emergence of what James (1892) identified as the "conflict of the different Me's."

In addition to such confusion, these seeming contradictions lead to very unstable self-representations, which are also cause for concern (e.g., "I don't really understand how I can switch so fast from being cheerful with my friends, then coming home and feeling anxious, and then getting frustrated and sarcastic with my parents. Which one is the *real* me?"). The creation of multiple selves, coupled with the emerging ability to detect potential contradictions between self-attributes displayed in different roles, naturally ushers in concern over which attributes define the true self (a topic to be covered in Chapter 9, where individual differences in false-self behavior are examined). However, from a normative perspective, the adolescent at this level is not equipped with the cognitive skills to solve fully the dilemma (e.g., "So I think a lot about who is the real me, and sometimes try to figure it out when I write in my diary, but I can't resolve it").

As introduced in the previous section on early adolescence, our own research has been directed toward an examination of the extent to which adolescents at three developmental levels both identify opposing self-attributes and report that they are experienced as conflictual (Harter & Monsour, 1992; Harter, Bresnick, et al., 1997). We have determined, across several studies, that young adolescents infrequently detect opposites within their self-portrait. However, it was predicted, according to the analysis presented earlier, that there would be a dramatic rise in the detection of opposing self-attributes as well as an acknowledgment that such apparent contradictions lead to conflict within the self-system. Our most recent procedure for examining these issues is illustrated in the protocol presented in Figure 3.1. Adolescents are first asked to generate six attributes for each role, writing them on the lines associated with each interpersonal context. These contexts have varied from study to study; however, in the sample protocol, we asked them to generate attributes for six roles: self with mother, with father, with a romantic interest, with their best friend, with a group of friends, and in their role as student, in the classroom. As in our original procedure (Harter & Monsour, 1992), respondents were then asked to identify any pairs of attributes they perceived to reflect *opposites*, by connecting them

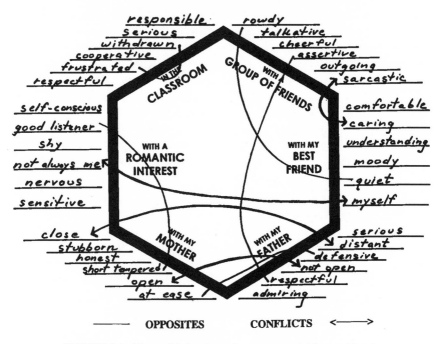

FIGURE 3.1. The multiple selves of a prototypical 15-year-old girl.

with lines. Next, they indicated whether any of these opposites were experienced as clashing or in conflict with each other, by putting arrowheads on the lines connecting those pairs of opposites.

Across three different studies (see Harter, Bresnick, et al., 1997) we have found that the number of opposing self-attribute pairs, as well as the number of opposites in conflict, increases between early and middle adolescence. This pattern of findings supports the hypothesis that the abstract mapping structures that emerge in middle adolescence allow one to detect, but not to meaningfully integrate, these apparent contradictions. Thus, they lead to the phenomenological experience of intrapsychic conflict. We have asked teenagers to verbally elaborate on the opposites and conflicts that they reported on our task. As one 14-year-old put it, "I really think I am a happy person and I want to be that way with everyone, not just my friends; but I get depressed with my family, and it really bugs me because that's not what I want to be like." Another 15-year-old, in describing a conflict between self-attributes within the realm of romantic relationships, exclaimed, "I hate the fact that I get so nervous! I wish I wasn't so inhibited. The real me is talkative. I just want to be natural, but I can't." Another 15-year-old girl explained, "I really think of myself as friendly and open to people, but the way the other girls act, they force me to become an introvert, even though I know I'm not." In exasperation, one ninth grader observed of the self-portrait she had constructed, "It's not right, it should all fit together into one piece!" These comments suggest that at this age level, there is a need for coherence; there is a desire to bring self-attributes into harmony with one another, yet in midadolescence, the cognitive abilities to create such a self-portrait are not yet in place.

An examination of the protocol in Figure 3.1 illustrates the fact that adolescents can identify two types of opposing attributes, those occurring *within* a given role (e.g., frustrated and withdrawn in the classroom) and those occurring *across* relational contexts (e.g., close with mother but distant with father, rowdy with a group of friends but quiet with one's best friend). We became curious about whether there were more opposing attributes and associated conflict *within* particular roles (e.g., rowdy vs. withdrawn with friends) or *across different roles* (e.g., tense with a romantic other vs. relaxed with friends). Among those social psychologists who have focused on the *adult* self, it has been argued that consistency within a particular relationship is critical; therefore, perceived violations of this consistency ethic, where one displays opposing attributes within a role, should be particularly discomforting to the individual (Gergen, 1968; Vallacher, 1980). According to these theorists, the adoption of different behaviors in *different* roles should be less problematic or conflictual for adults, since they represent appropriate adaptation to different relational contexts rather than inconsistency.

From a developmental perspective, we did not expect these processes to be in place during adolescence. Adolescents are actively concerned with creating, defining, and *differentiating* role-related selves, and thus there is relatively little overlap in the self-attributes associated with different roles. Moreover, opposing attributes across relational contexts become more marked or salient in midadolescence, when teenagers develop the cognitive ability to detect seeming contradictions. The very salience of these opposites leads to a greater focus on contraditions *across* roles rather than *within* roles. Perceived conflict caused by opposing attributes should also be greater across roles, particularly with the onset of midadolescence, when teenagers can begin to compare characteristics across such roles but cannot integrate these salient and seemingly contradictory self-attributes. As can be seen in Figure 3.2, the number of opposites identified at midadolescence and beyond is far greater for attributes identified *across* roles than within each role, confirming our expectation. The same pattern was obtained for opposites in conflict.

Figure 3.2 also reveals that for across-role opposites, at every age level, females detect more contradictory attributes than do males. These findings replicate two other studies in which similar gender differences were obtained (see Harter, Bresnick, et al., 1997). Moreover, in one study in which we asked subjects to indicate how upset they were over conflicting attributes,

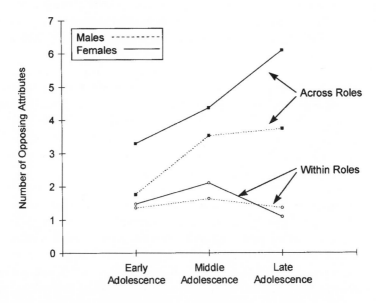

FIGURE 3.2. Mean number of opposing attributes identified *across* versus *within* roles for males and females in early, middle, and late adolescence.

the pattern revealed that females become *more* upset over conflicting attributes across early, middle, and late adolescence, whereas males become *less* upset. Elsewhere, we have offered a general interpretation of this pattern, drawing upon those frameworks that emphasize the greater importance of relationships for females than males (Chodorow, 1989; Eichenbaum & Orbach, 1983; Gilligan, 1982; Jordan, 1991; Miller, 1986; Rubin, 1985). These theorists posit that the socialization of girls involves far more embeddedness within the family, as well as more concern with connectedness to others. Boys, in contrast, forge a path of independence and autonomy in which the logic of moral and social decisions takes precedence over affective responses to significant others.

In extrapolating from these observations, we have suggested that in an effort to maintain the multiple relationships that girls are developing during adolescence, and to create harmony among these necessarily differentiated roles, opposing attributes within the self become particularly salient as well as problematic. Boys, in contrast, can move more facilely among their different roles and multiple selves to the extent that such roles are logically viewed as more independent of one another. However, these general observations require further refinement, including an empirical examination of precisely which facets of the relational worlds of adolescent females and males are specifically relevant to gender differences in opposing attributes displayed across different contexts.

Closer examination of the gender effects reveals that it is a subset of female adolescents who report more opposites and greater conflict compared to males. We have determined that adolescent females who endorse a feminine gender orientation (eschewing masculine traits) may be particularly vulnerable to the experience of opposing attributes and associated conflict. Feminine adolescent females, compared to females who endorse an androgynous orientation, report more conflict, particularly in roles that involve teachers, classmates, and male friends (in contrast to roles involving parents and female friends). Several hypotheses would be worth pursuing in this regard. Is it that feminine girls report more contradictions in those public contexts where they feel they may be acting inappropriately by violating feminine stereotypes of behavior? Given that femininity as assessed by sex-role inventories is largely defined by caring, sensitivity, and attentiveness to the needs and feelings of others, might female adolescents who adopt this orientation be more preoccupied with relationships, making opposing attributes and accompanying conflict more salient? Moreover, might it be more important for feminine girls to be consistent across relationships, a stance that may be difficult to sustain, to the extent that significant others in different roles are encouraging or reinforcing different characteristics? These are all new directions in which attention to gender issues should proceed.

The challenges posed by the need to create different selves are also exacerbated for ethnic minority youth in this country, who must bridge "multiple worlds," as Cooper and her colleagues point out (Cooper, Jackson, Azmitia, Lopez, & Dunbar, 1995). Minority youth must move between multiple contexts, some of which may be with members of their own ethnic group, including family and friends, and some of which may be populated by the majority culture, including teachers, classmates, and other peers who may not share the values of their family of origin. Rather than assume that all ethnic minority youth will react similarly to the need to cope with such multiple worlds, these investigators have highlighted several different patterns of adjustment. Some youth are able to move facilely across the borders of their multiple worlds, in large part because the values of the family, teachers, and peers are relatively similar. Others, for whom there is less congruence in values across contexts, adopt a bicultural stance, adapting to the world of family as well as to that of the larger community. Others find the transition across these psychological borders more difficult, and some find it totally unmanageable. Particularly interesting is the role that certain parents play in helping adolescents navigate these transitions, leading to more successful adaptations for some than others.

The Role of the Socializing Environment

As observed earlier, adolescents during this period become extremely preoccupied with the opinions and expectations of significant others in different roles. As our prototypical respondent indicates, "I care what my parents think about me"; "I want to know what my close friends think"; "I don't care what (everybody else) thinks. I mean I don't *want* to care, that is"; "I want them (adults at work) to approve of me"; that is, adolescents gaze intently into the social mirror for information about what standards and attributes to internalize. However, as the number of roles proliferate, leading to messages from different significant others that are potentially contradictory, adolescents may become confused or distressed about just which characteristics to adopt. We see this in the cameo self-description with regard to scholastic performance, in that the adolescent feels she "should get better grades" to please her parents but confesses that "I'd be mortified in the eyes of my friends if I did too well." As Higgins (1991) observes, in their attempt to incorporate the standards and opinions of others, adolescents at this level develop conflicting "self-guides" across different relational contexts as they attempt to meet the incompatible expectations of parents and peers. He reports evidence indicating that such discrepancies have been found to produce confusion, uncertainty, and indecision with regard to self-evaluation and self-regulation, consistent with our own findings. Moreover, as Rosenberg (1986) notes, the serious efforts at perspective taking that emerge at this stage make one aware that no human being can have direct access to another's mind, leading to inevitable ambiguity about others' attitudes toward the self, producing yet another source of doubt and confusion.

The potential for displaying differing levels of self-worth across relational contexts is also exacerbated during this period, to the extent that the significant others are providing different levels of validation for who one is as a person (see also Rosenberg, 1986). For example, the cameo self-description reveals that the adolescent gets down on herself for not getting the grades her parents expect. She hates herself when she feels peers think she is weird, but she feels good about herself on the job, where supervisors give her more positive feedback. Our own evidence has revealed that not only does self-worth become differentiated by context beginning in early adolescence, but also it becomes further differentiated in middle to late adolescence. For example, individuals come to develop different levels of self-worth with their mothers and their fathers (Buddin, 1998), levels that in turn are directly related to their perceptions of approval from each parent. The contradictory feedback that adolescents may receive from different sources will, therefore, lead to volatility in self-worth across interpersonal contexts.

Contradictory standards and feedback can also contribute to a lowering of global self-worth between early and midadolescence (see findings reviewed by Harter, 1990), to the extent that one cannot meet the expectations of everyone in each relational context. To the extent that the adolescent does not meet the standards of others, he/she is likely to experience less approval, which in turn will lead to lower global self-worth. Moreover, the abstract mapping structure, coupled with the penchant for introspection, may also contribute to lowered self-worth in that it facilitates the comparison of one's ideal and real self-concepts. Such a focus can lead to a heightened awareness of the discrepancy between how one perceives the self to be in reality (e.g., "I can get pretty obnoxious and intolerant") and how one would ideally like to be (e.g., "I'd like to be friendly and tolerant all of the time. That's the kind of person I *want* to be, and I'm disappointed in myself when I'm not").

Cognitive-developmental advances during midadolescence also represent limitations that can lead to distortions in the interpretation of the opinions of significant others. As observed earlier, with the advent of any new cognitive capacities comes difficulty in controlling and applying them effectively. For example, teenagers have difficulty differentiating their own mental preoccupations from what others are thinking, leading to a form of adolescent egocentrism that Elkind (1967) has labeled the "imaginary audience." Adolescents falsely assume that others are as preoccupied with their behavior and appearance as they themselves are. As our prototypical respondent exclaims, "Everybody, I mean *everybody* else is looking at me like they think I am totally weird!" With regard to lack of cognitive control, this phenomenon represents overgeneralization (or failure to differentiate) in that adolescents project their own concerns onto others.

Interestingly, the inability to control and to effectively apply new cognitive structures can result not only in a lack of differentiation between self and others, as in the imaginary audience phenomenon, but also in excessive or unrealistic differentiation. The latter penchant can be observed in another form of egocentrism that Elkind (1967) has identified as the "personal fable." In creating narratives that come to define the self, the adolescent asserts that his/her thoughts and feelings are uniquely experienced. No one else can possible understand or experience the ecstasy of his/her rapture, or the intensity of his/her despair. Adults, particularly parents, are likely to be singled out in this regard. As the prototypical adolescent exclaims, "My parents don't understand me. What do *they* know about what it's like to be a teenager?" Her initial comment to the interviewer when asked to describe what she was like ("You're probably not going to understand") also reflects this type of overdifferentiation between self and other.

Summary

Midadolescence brings with it a preoccupation with what significant others think of the self, a task that is made more challenging given the proliferation of roles that demand the creation of multiple selves. The addition of new role-related selves can be observed in the fact that adolescents make finer discriminations, for example, self with a close friend versus self with a group of friends, and self with mother versus self with father. Moreover, there is relatively little overlap in the personal attributes that define the self in each role. The proliferation of multiple selves ushers in the potential for such attributes to be viewed as contradictory. Moreover, the emergence of new cognitive processes such as abstract *mappings* forces the adolescent to compare and contrast different attributes, exacerbating the likelihood that contradictions will be detected. Mappings, in the form of the identification of *opposites*, are problematic in that the individual cannot yet truly integrate such self-representations in a manner that would resolve the contradictions. Thus, the adolescent is likely to experience conflict, confusion, and distress. Opposites and associated conflict are particularly likely to occur for attributes in *different* roles, rather than in the same role. Females are particularly likely to display these negative outcomes. Opposing self-attributes also lead to unstable self-representations, in addition to concern over which characteristics represent one's true self.

With regard to the impact of the socializing environment, adolescents gaze intently into the social mirror for information about what standards and attributes to internalize. However, contradictory messages from different significant others can lead to confusion about just what characteristics to adopt. Differential support, in the form of approval or validation, will also lead to differing levels of self-worth across relational contexts. Cognitive-developmental advances also represent limitations that can lead to distortions in the interpretation of the opinions of significant others, as in the creation of an "imaginary audience," as well as the perception that one's experiences are uniquely different. The liabilities of this period are legion with regard to potential conflict and confusion over contradictory attributes and messages, concern over which characteristics define the true self, distortions in the perception of self versus others, as well as a preoccupation with discrepancies between the real and ideal self-concepts, which can lead to lowered self-worth. Some of these processes would appear to be problematic for particular subgroups of adolescents, for example, females who adopt a feminine gender orientation, as well as ethnic minority youth who are challenged by the need to create selves that bridge "multiple worlds," for example, with one's own ethnic group as well as groups within the mainstream majority culture.

An appreciation for the ramifications of these normative processes is critical in interpreting the unpredictable behaviors, shifting self-evaluations, and mood swings that are observed in many adolescents during this age period. Such displays are less likely to be viewed as intentional or pathological, and more likely to meet with empathy and understanding to the extent that normative cognitive-developmental changes can be invoked as in part responsible. For many parents, as well as other adults working closely with teenagers, these seemingly inexplicable reactions often lead to perplexity, exasperation, and anger, provoking power struggles and altercations that strain the adolescent–adult relationship. The realization that this is a normative stage of development that should not persist forever may provide temporary comfort to adults who feel beleaguered and ineffectual in dealing with adolescents of this age.

LATE ADOLESCENCE AND EARLY ADULTHOOD

"I'm a pretty conscientious person, particularly when it comes to things like doing my homework. It's important to me because I plan to go to college next year. Eventually I want to go to law school, so developing good study habits and getting top grades are both essential. (My parents don't want me to become a lawyer; they'd rather I go into teaching, but law is what I want to pursue.) Every now and then I get a little lackadaisical and don't complete an assignment as thoroughly or thoughtfully as I could, particularly if our high school has a big football or basketball game that I want to go to with my friends. But that's normal, I mean, you can't just be a total 'grind.' You'd be pretty boring if you were. You have to be flexible. I've also become more religious as I have gotten older, not that I am a saint or anything. Religion gives me a sense of purpose, in the larger scheme of things, and it provides me with personal guidelines for the kind of adult I'd like to be. For example, I'd like to be an ethical person who treats other people fairly. That's the kind of lawyer I'd like to be, too. I don't always live up to that standard; that is, sometimes I do something that doesn't feel that ethical. When that happens, I get a little depressed because I don't like myself as a person. But I tell myself that its natural to make mistakes, so I don't really question the fact that deep down inside, the real me is a moral person. Basically, I like who I am, so I don't stay depressed for long. Usually, I am pretty upbeat and optimistic. I guess you could say that I'm a moody person. I'm not as popular as a lot of other kids. At our school, its the jocks who are looked up to. I've never been very athletic, but you can't be good at everything, let's face it. Being athletic isn't that high on my own list of what is important, even though it is for a lot of the kids in our school. But I don't really care what they think anymore. I *used* to, but now what *I* think is what counts. After all, I have to live with myself as a person and to respect that person, which I do now, more than a few years ago. I'm pretty much being the kind of person I want to be. I'm doing well at things that are important to me like getting good grades. That's what is probably *most* important to me right now. Having a lot of friends isn't that important to me. I wouldn't say I was unpopular, though. While I am basically an introvert, especially on a date when I get pretty self-conscious, in the right social situation, like watching a ball game with my friends, I can be pretty extroverted. You have to be adaptive around other people. It would be weird to be the same kind of person on a date and with my friends at a football game! For example, when our team has a winning season and goes to the playoffs, everyone in the whole school is proud; what the team does reflects on all of us. On a date, the feelings are much more intimate, just between you and the other person. As much as I enjoy my high school friends and activities, I'm looking forward to leaving home and going to college, where I can be more independent, although I'm a little ambivalent. I love my parents, and really want to stay connected to them, plus, what they think about me is still important to how I feel about myself as a person. So leaving home will be bittersweet. But sometimes it's hard to be mature around them, particularly around my mom. I feel a lot more grown-up around my dad; he treats me more like an adult. I like that part of me because it feels more like my true self. My mom wants me to grow up, but another part of her wants me to remain 'her little baby.' I'll probably always be somewhat dependent on my parents. How can you escape it? But I'm also looking forward to being on my own."

With regard to the *content* of the self-representations that begin to emerge in late adolescence and early adulthood, typically, many of the attributes reflect personal beliefs, values, and moral standards that have become internalized or, alternatively, constructed from their own experiences (see findings by Damon & Hart, 1988). These characteristics are exemplified in the prototypical cameo, in that the adolescent expresses the personal desire to go to college, which requires good grades and discipline in the form of study habits. Although classmates tout athletics as the route to popularity, there is less concern at this age with what others think ("I used to care but now what *I* think is important"). In addition, there is a focus on one's *future* selves, for example, not only becoming a lawyer, but also an *ethical* lawyer, as a personal goal. Noteworthy in this narrative is the absence of an explicit reference to the potential origins of these goals, for example, parental encouragement or expectations that one pursue such a career. Moreover, this adolescent's career choice does not conform to the parents' occupational goals for their child.

The failure to acknowledge the socialization influences that might have led to these choices does not necessarily indicate that significant others such as peers and parents had no impact. In fact, findings (see Steinberg, 1990) reveal that the attitudes of adolescents and their parents are quite congruent when it comes to occupational, political, and religious decisions or convictions. Rather, the fact that the impact of significant others is not acknowledged suggests that older adolescents and young adults have come to "own" various values as personal choices, rather than attribute them to the sources from which they may have been derived (Damon & Hart, 1988). In Higgins' (1991) terminology, older adolescents have gone through a process in which they have actively selected among alternative "self-guides" and are no longer merely buffeted about by the expectations of significant others; that is, self-guides become increasingly internalized, namely, less tied to their social origins. Moreover, there is a greater sense of direction as the older adolescent comes to envisage future or "possible" selves (Markus & Nurius, 1986) that function as ideals toward which one aspires.

Another feature of the self-portrait of the older adolescent can be contrasted with the period before, in that many potentially contradictory attributes are no longer described as characteristics in opposition to one another. Thus, being conscientious as a student does not appear to conflict with one's lackadaisical attitude toward schoolwork: "That's normal, I mean, you can't just be a total 'grind.' You'd be pretty boring if you were. You have to be flexible." Similarly, one's perception of the self as ethical does not conflict with the acknowledgment that one also has engaged in some un-ethical behaviors ("It's natural to make mistakes"). Nor does introversion conflict with extroverted behaviors: "You have to be adaptive around other people. It would be weird to be the same kind of person on a date and with my friends at a football game!"

There are cognitive acquisitions that allow the older adolescent to over-come some of the liabilities of the previous period, where potentially oppos-ing attributes were viewed as contradictory and as a cause of internal con-flict. The general cognitive advances during this period involve the construction of higher-order abstractions that involve the meaningful intercoordination of single abstractions (see Case, 1985; Fischer, 1980; Fischer & Canfield, 1986). For example, the fact that one is both introverted and extroverted can be integrated through the construction of a higher-order abstraction that defines the self as "adaptive." The observation that one is both depressed and cheerful or optimistic can be integrated under the per-sonal rubric of "moody." Similarly, "flexible" can allow one to coordinate conscientiousness with the tendency to be lackadaisical. The higher-order concept of "ambivalence" integrates the desire to be independent yet still remain connected to parents. Moreover, "bittersweet" reflects a higher-order abstraction combining both excitement over going to college with sadness over leaving one's parents. Such higher-order abstractions provide self-labels that bring meaning and therefore legitimacy to what formerly appeared to be troublesome contradictions within the self.

Neo-Piagetians such as Case (1985), Fischer (1980), and colleagues, observe that developmental acquisitions at these higher levels typically re-quire greater scaffolding by the social environment in the form of support, experiences, instruction, and so on, in order for individuals to function at their optimal level. If these new skills are fostered, they will help the adoles-cent to integrate opposing attributes in a manner that does not produce conflict or distress. Thus, efforts to assist the adolescent in realizing that it is normal to display seemingly contradictory traits, and perhaps quite appro-priate, may alleviate perceptions of conflict. Moreover, helping teenagers to provide higher-order labels that integrate opposing attributes (e.g., flexible, adaptive, moody, inconsistent) may avert some of the distress that was sa-lient during middle adolescence. These suggestions derive from the obser-vations of Fischer, Case, and others to the effect that these cognitive solu-tions will not necessarily emerge automatically with development. Nor will the potential benefits derived from movement to late adolescence and early adulthood necessarily accrue; that is, the levels described in this chapter represent a normative *sequence* of development. However, the age levels are somewhat arbitrary in that certain individuals may not attain a given level at the designated age period. Development may be delayed or even arrested if there is not sufficient support for the transition to a new level of conceptualization, particularly for the higher stages.

The assertions about how the changing cognitive structures emerge—ideally, in late adolescence to early adulthood—will allow for a potential reduction in the number of contradictory attributes identified in one's self-portrait, as well as diminished conflict, have found partial support in our own findings. For example, in one study (Harter & Monsour, 1992) in which adolescents described their attributes in four roles—with parents, with friends, with romantic others, and as a student—there was a dramatic rise in the number of opposites and conflicts identified at midadolescence, followed by a slight decline among older adolescents. Evidence that older adolescents become better able to consolidate or integrate seeming contradictions within the self-theory come from the comments they made in response to a follow-up interview. As one older adolescent explained, "Sometimes I am really happy, and sometimes I get depressed. I'm just a moody person." Another commented, "I can be talkative, and I can be quiet. I'm flexible, plus they complement each other. It's good to be both ways."

The tendency to *normalize* or find value in seeming inconsistency can also observed in the comments of other older adolescents, for example, "You wouldn't be the same person on a date as you are with your parents, and you shouldn't be. That would be weird." Another asserted, "It wouldn't be normal to act the same way with everyone. You act one way with your friends and a different way with your parents. That's the way it should be." Others made similar comments, for example, "It's good to be able to be different with different people in your life. You'd be pretty strange and also pretty boring if you weren't." "You can be outgoing with friends and then shy on a date because you are just different with different people; you can't always be the same person and probably shouldn't be." Yet another indicated, "There are situations where you are a good listener and others where you are talkative. Its good to be both." Thus, older adolescents come to the conclusion that it is desirable to be different across relational contexts, and in so doing, they would appear to be cultivating the stance that social psychologists (see Gergen, 1968; Mischel, 1973; Vallacher, 1980) identify as more the rule than the exception for adults.

The Role of the Socializing Environment

More recent evidence (see Harter, Bresnick, et al., 1997) indicates that the ability to resolve potentially contradictory attributes may be more difficult for some role-pair combinations than for others, particularly for females. For example, as Figure 3.1 reveals, when all role pairs are combined, there is no decline in the number of opposing attributes identified *across* roles. In fact, for older adolescent females, there is actually a further increase. The fact that six roles were included in the study generating the data in Figure 3.1 (compared to only four in the original Harter and Monsour study) may have been partly responsible, since the inclusion of additional roles increased the probability that opposing attributes might be detected; that is, there were 15 possible role pairs that might contain contradictions compared to only six role pairs in the original study. In increasing the number of roles, we also separated the reports of self-attributes with mother and with father (whereas in the earlier study, we merely inquired about self with parents).

The separation of self-attributes with each parent potentially enhances the likelihood that characteristics with each may contradict attributes in roles with peers. Examples generated by adolescent respondents in mid- to late adolescence included being short-tempered with mother versus a good listener in romantic relationships; respectful with father versus assertive with friends; distant from father but attentive with a romantic interest. Adolescent bids for autonomy from parents (Cooper, Grotevant, & Condon, 1983; Hill & Holmbeck, 1986; Steinberg, 1990), coupled with the increasing importance of the peer group (Brown, 1990; Savin-Williams & Berndt, 1990), would lead to the expectation that attributes expressed with mother and father might well differ from those displayed with *peers* (namely, friends and romantic partners), leading to a greater potential for contradictions.

However, the separation of self with mother and self with father also creates the potential for attributes with mother to be in opposition to attributes with father. The potential for attributes with each parent to appear contradictory can be observed in the cameo, where the prototypical older adolescent feels much more mature with father than with mother. Moreover, such conflicts begin to be observed in midadolescence, where the prototypical teenager indicated that she was "close" with her mother but "distant" with her father, a difference that became problematic if they were all together, such as talking at dinner.

When the findings in Figure 3.1 are broken down by relationship pairs, opposing attributes and associated conflict were most frequent for the combination of self with mother versus self with father, beginning in midadolescence, and increasing in late adolescence, a pattern that we have since replicated in a subsequent study. Examples have included being close with mother versus distant with father; stubborn with mother versus respectful with father; open with mother but not with father; at ease with mother but defensive with father; hostile with mother but cheerful with father. Moreover, such opposites between self with mother versus self with father, as well as associated conflict, increased dramatically for the older girls in particular.

The fact that older female adolescents reported increasing contradictions, whereas male adolescents did not, suggests that cognitive-developmental explanations are incomplete. The separation of attributes with mother and with father, in particular, would appear to make it more difficult for certain adolescents to cognitively resolve or normalize the contradictions that are provoked by these roles, contradictions produced by the opposing attributes with mother *versus* father, as well as those attributes with each parent that contradict the characteristics that one displays with peers. Contradictions between self with parents and self with peers is more understandable, given developmental bids for autonomy. However, why should adolescents (particularly adolescent females) report increasingly different characteristics with mother and father?

Here, we can only speculate. Family therapists observe that children and adolescents typically develop different relationships with each parent, which in turn may cause the salient attributes in each relationship to vary considerably. Contributing to these dynamics is the fact that each parent may have a different set of expectations about those characteristics that he/she values and therefore attempts to foster. First, the adolescent may become caught in a struggle between two parents who are encouraging and reinforcing different facets of his/her personality, provoking opposing attributes and resulting conflict. Second, both of these roles, self with mother and self with father, occur within the *same* general context, namely, the family, whereas other multiple roles are not as likely to be called upon simultaneously. These particular conditions may exacerbate the contradictions and conflicts that adolescents experience in their respective roles with mother versus father. These family dynamics appear to be relevant to the increase in across-role opposing attributes for *female* adolescents in particular, who may be more likely to be sensitive to the fact that they are behaving differently with mother versus father. As observed in the previous section on the period of midadolescence, females display more concern over relationship issues, which may make opposing attributes more salient. Adolescent females may also feel that in order to remain connected to both mother and father, it is important to be *consistent* across these relationships, a task that can be problematic for the reasons cited earlier.

Although the gender literature suggests that connectedness is more critical to females than to males (Chodorow, 1989; Eichenbaum & Orbach, 1983; Gilligan, 1982; Gilligan, Lyons, & Hanmer, 1989; Jordan, 1991; Miller, 1986; Rubin, 1985), the adolescent literature reveals that it is important for teenagers of both genders to remain connected to parents in the process of individuation and the establishment of autonomy (Cooper et al., 1983; Hill & Holmbeck, 1986; Steinberg, 1990). As our prototypical subject reveals, while it is important to go to college where he/she can be more independent, it is also important to stay connected to parents.

Contextual factors such as the family, therefore, will conspire with cognitive development to impact the extent to which opposites and conflicts are experienced. Another example of the role of context can be observed in cross-cultural research by Kennedy (1994). Kennedy has adapted our procedure in comparing the self-understanding of American and Korean youth. He finds that there are different age-related peaks in conflict among adolescents in the two cultures. Korean youth report increased conflict between opposing attributes in 10th and 12th grades, findings that he interprets in terms of the demands of the school context at those particular grade levels. In Korea, 10th grade is the first year of high school, and the new students are required to be deferential to the juniors and seniors, a relationship that many 10th graders find oppressive. Kennedy argues that these demands exert a strain on the self-system and destablize students' sense of self as they struggle to find a niche within the peer hierarchy of high school. During 12th grade, there are different demands, for example, intense preparation for the college entrance exams. This pressure leads to challenges in balancing the demands of academics, peer relationships, and family commitments, resulting in greater conflict.

Future research should attend to such contextual factors and attempt to assess the underlying processes more directly. To return to our own findings in this regard, it would be of interest to determine whether the conflict between self-attributes with mother versus father is more intense if the adolescent is living in a two-parent family where both mother and father are in the same household, or if the parents are divorced and living apart. One hypothesis is that living under the same roof with both parents makes it difficult to avoid conflict if different attributes in each relationship are demanded simultaneously. Alternatively, conflict may be exacerbated in the situation of divorce to the extent that in an acrimonious separation, each parent intensifies his or her differential expectations for the attributes they want the adolescent to display as part of a power struggle in which the adolescent becomes a pawn. Such processes would be intriguing to investigate.

Finally, with regard to developmental changes in the self, evidence from longitudinal studies reveals that self-esteem or global self-worth improves in later adolescence (see Engel, 1959; O'Malley & Bachman, 1983; Rosenberg, 1986; Simmons, Rosenberg, & Rosenberg, 1973). Several interpretations of these gains have been suggested (see Harter, 1990a; McCarthy & Hoge, 1982). Reductions in the discrepancy between one's ideal self and one's real self, between one's aspirations and one's successes, according to James' (1892) formulation, may be in part responsible. As the prototypical adolescent indicates, he/she has more self-respect now, compared to a few years ago and observes that "I'm pretty much being the kind of person I want to be. I'm doing well at things that are important to me like getting good grades and being ethical." Gains in personal autonomy and freedom of choice may also play a role, in that the older adolescent may have more opportunity to select performance domains in which he/she is successful. Such freedom may also provide one with more opportunity to select those support groups that will provide the positive regard necessary to promote or enhance self-worth, consistent with the looking-glass-self formulation. Increased role-taking ability may also lead older teenagers to behave in more socially acceptable ways that enhance the evaluation of the self by others, such that the favorable attitudes of others toward the self are internalized as positive self-worth.

These others include parents. Although it has been common in treatments of adolescent development to suggest that the influence of peers increases, whereas the impact of parental opinion declines, findings do not support the latter contention. As our cameo subject indicates, "What my parents think about me is still important to how I feel about myself as a person." Our own findings reveal that the correlation between classmate approval and global self-worth does increase during childhood and adolescence; however, the correlation between parental approval and global self-worth, which is high in childhood, does *not* decline during adolescence (Harter, 1990a). The latter correlation does decline, however, during the college years among students who are away from home.

More specific evaluations of self-worth continue to vary by relationship context (Harter, Waters, & Whitesell, 1998), throughout the high school years as adolescents make finer distinctions (e.g., between their self-worth with mother and with father). However, we did not anticipate the fact that for the vast majority of individuals, self-worth in one *particular* relational domain is much more highly related to *global* self-worth than is relational self-worth in all other contexts. The specific domain occupying this position varies from adolescent to adolescent. For example, with our prototypical adolescent, self as student in the academic domain is most important ("Getting good grades is what is *most* important to me now") and his/her self-worth in that particular context is higher than in other domains. Thus, focusing on that particular context would appear to be very adaptive in that it should promote more positive feelings of global self-worth.

Summary

Many of the limitations of the preceding period of midadolescence would appear to be overcome as a result of changes during late adolescence. Attributes reflecting personal beliefs, values, and standards become more internalized, and the older adolescent would appear to have more opportunity to meet these standards, thereby leading to enhanced self-worth. The focus on future selves also gives the older adolescent a sense of direction. A critical *cognitive* advance can be observed in the ability to construct higher-order abstractions that involve the meaningful integration of single abstractions that represent potential contradictions in the self-portrait (e.g., depressed and cheerful do not conflict because they are both part of being moody). The older adolescent can also resolve potentially contradictory attributes by asserting that he/she is flexible or adaptive, thereby subsuming apparent inconsistencies under more generalized abstractions about the self. Moreover, older adolescents are more likely to normalize potential contradictions, asserting that it is desirable to be different across relational contexts and that it would be weird or strange to be the same with different people.

Nevertheless, conflict between role-related attributes does not totally abate in later adolescence. Conflict will be more likely to occur if the new skills that allow for an integration of seeming contradictions are not fostered by the socializing environment. Furthermore, opposing attributes across particular role combinations, notably self with mother versus self with father, continue to be problematic in late adolescence, especially for girls. To the extent that one's mother and father elicit or reinforce opposing attributes, cognitive solutions for integrating seeming contradictions would appear to be more difficult to invoke.

Last, although the internalization of standards and opinions that the adolescent comes to own as personal choices and attitudes toward the self represents a developmental advance, there are liabilities as well, associated with this process. As Rosenberg (1986) observes, the shift in the locus of self-knowledge from an external to internal source can introduce uncertainty. As long as major truths about the self derive from omniscient and omnipotent adults, then there is little doubt about their veracity. However, when the locus of self-knowledge shifts inward and adolescents must rely on their own autonomous judgment and insight to reach conclusions about the self, then the sense of certainty can be compromised.

CONCLUSION

The developmental progression of stages identified across the three periods of adolescence allows for an appreciation of what are normative self-representations at each level. Moreover, an understanding of the self-structure at midadolescence helps to demystify the often strange and volatile conceptualizations that teenagers in this stage bring to bear upon the self, conceptualizations that can spill over into erratic and inexplicable behavior patterns. Such an understanding prevents us from overinterpreting certain self-descriptions as potentially pathological, when in fact, they may be quite age-appropriate. For example, the all-or-none thinking that emerges during midadolescence does not constitute the incipient characteristics of a borderline personality or signal the onset of a manic–depressive disorder. Rather, it reflects age-appropriate limitations related to lack of cognitive control over self-attributes, in the form of single abstractions, that cannot be meaningfully integrated. Thus, it leads to "normative distortions" given the cognitive limitations of this developmental period. Appreciating the fact that self-representations undergo major normative, age-related change provides a backkdrop against which one can assess the developmental level of the self-portrait of a given individual.

The more differentiated series of substages that define the changing self-representations across adolescence represents an advance over the earlier Piagetian view that formal operational thought ushered in the potential for a mature self-theory that would meet such criteria as coherence and internal consistency. Rather, the adolescent must move through substages that recapitulate certain structural features of earlier stages, albeit at the more advanced level of abstractions. Thus, the emergence of single abstractions that are highly compartmentalized represents the normative fragmentation of self-representations that characterize early adolescent thought (Fischer & Canfield, 1986). In the stage to follow, the fact that the adolescent can now detect but not *resolve* contradictory attributes in the self-portrait leads to confusion, vacillation, conflict, and distress. This contemporary analysis of adolescent self-development provides a more sympathetic perspective in illuminating the cognitive-developmental liabilities of this period. Moreover, it allows us to appreciate seemingly perplexing features of teenage behavior that have long been observed by parents and educators but have heretofore escaped explanations by those wedded to a more traditional Piagetian model of development.

Such an analysis also underscores the importance of scaffolding adolescent self-development such that they move beyond the all-or-none thinking that resurfaces at the abstract level during the period of midadolescence. Neo-Piagetians (e.g., Case, 1992; Fischer, 1980) have emphasized the fact that at higher levels of development, more support from the socializing environment is required to foster movement toward a new level. Those within the field of education, examining levels of reflective judgment that build upon this framework, concur (see Kitchner, 1986), indicating how instructional techniques and opportunities can aid in helping adolescents and young adults to move beyond these levels of thinking.

Finally, it has become apparent that the ability to construct a self-theory that would meet the criteria of a formal hypothetico-deductive system of postulates represents a much later acquisition than was previously imagined. Most neo-Piagetians place the abilities to construct such a self-system at subsequent levels in adulthood, if at all; that is, further cognitive advances are necessary in order to integrate high-order abstractions into a larger system of abstractions that comes to define a self-theory that is perceived as psychologically unified. A major challenge is the construction of a self-structure that is experienced as coherent, yet can tolerate attributes that appear, on the surface, to be contradictory. I return to potential solutions in the last chapter, which addresses the promotion of healthy self-development.

The Developmental Emergence of Self-Conscious Emotions

The preceding two chapters have emphasized how the development of self-representations is a function of both cognitive and social processes, a theme that continues in the present treatment of self-conscious emotions. In addition to the construction of concepts of self (e.g., nice, mean, smart, dumb), children also develop *affective* reactions to the self in the form of what have been labeled self-affects or self-conscious emotions, terms that are here employed interchangeably. These include pride, shame, guilt, and embarrassment, emotions that emerge within the crucible of interpersonal relationships. With regard to the topic of this volume, namely, self-representations, shame and pride are the most appropriate prototypes in that they represent cognitive-emotional as well as social constructions in which, over the course of childhood development, the I-self eventually becomes "conscious" of the Me-self in that it takes the Me-self as the object of reflection and affective evaluation. Thus, the I-self is proud of the Me-self, or, alternatively, the I-self is ashamed of the Me-self.

Theoretically, such self-conscious emotions can be experienced in the *absence* of an observing other; that is, the individual should be able to reflect upon his/her accomplishments or transgressions and experience pride or shame, despite the fact that other people may initially be unaware that these personal events have occurred (Harter & Whitesell, 1989). However, the ability to verbally acknowledge that one is either proud or ashamed of the self represents a developmental acquisition that is very dependent upon socialization experiences. In fact, it does not emerge until middle to late childhood. From a historical perspective, Cooley (1902) first observed that the ability to experience pride or shame in the absence of an observing other emerges from particular social interactions with significant others, namely, experiences that promote the internalization of these affective, evaluative judgments. For Cooley, to develop a sense of shame, the child must first be caught at something the parent has forbidden. To the extent that the parent expresses shame in the child, gradually this reaction will become internalized, such that the child can experience shame in the absence of the overt reactions of others. The capacity to experience self-affects is not only dependent upon the acquisition of particular cognitive structures, but also is deeply embedded in the matrix of interactions with caregivers and only gradually emerges during childhood. Moreover, the salience and manifestations of self-affects are highly influenced by societal factors that differ across cultures.

Before examining these processes, it is necessary to identify the cardinal features of self-conscious emotions, a topic about which there is considerable agreement across numerous theorists (see Tangney & Fischer, 1995). Attention then turns to the cognitive-developmental prerequisites necessary for the behavioral display of self-affects. This is followed by an analysis of those child-rearing practices critical to the expression of guilt and shame in particular. The behavioral expression of self-affects is to be distinguished from an *understanding* of these emotion concepts, as revealed through language. The focus of this chapter then shifts to the development of such an understanding, first examining cognitive-developmental influences, followed by a discussion of child-rearing antecedents. Finally, in keeping with a major theme of this volume, the functional role of self-conscious emotions is then explored. The focus is on the positive and negative functions of both guilt and shame, noting that these functions vary across cultures.

DIMENSIONS OF PRIDE, SHAME, AND GUILT

It is instructive to consider the following dimensions along which self-affects can vary. These include (1) the particular cause of the emotion, (2) associated attributions and implications for the self, (3) the role of the other, as well as (4) behavioral and other emotional correlates. In this chapter, these dimensions are applied to pride, shame, and guilt. This analysis is summarized in Table 4.1. In the literature on self-affects, a major focus has been the differentiation of the features of shame and guilt. Most writers build upon the seminal distinctions identified by H. B. Lewis (1971). In a recent edited volume on self-conscious emotions (Tangney & Fischer, 1995), numerous chapters describe and elaborate upon these distinctions (see chapters by Barrett; Emde & Oppenheim; Ferguson & Stegge; Lewis; Lindsay-Hartz, De Rivera, & Mascolo; Mascolo & Fischer; Stipek; Tangney).

With regard to pride, the prototypical cause is a personal accomplishment, typically a specific success or achievement in which one has met or exceeded one's goals or ideals. Older children give such examples as "I was

TABLE 4.1. Features of Self-Conscious Emotions

Emotion	Cause	Attribution/implications for the self	Role of the other	Behavioral/emotional correlates
Pride	Specific successful achievements; meeting or exceeding one's ideals	Personal ability and effort; I-self as competent agent; positive Me-self evaluations	Other as proud of the self, reinforcing positive evaluations	Desire to approach evaluating others to communicate the successful event; emotions of happiness, excitement, feelings of hopefulness
Shame	Transgressions, wrong-doings that violate one's own ideals or others' ideals for the self; incompetence or achievement failures	Global (trait-like) evaluation of the self as a bad person; low self-worth; negative Me-self evaluations; actions relatively uncontrollable; lack of ability; self is inadequate, fundamentally flawed	Other as potential shamer, one with power as active agent of scorn; loss of esteem in eyes of others who serve as "social mirrors," negatively evaluating one's behaviors	Desire to hide, avoid others, distance oneself from evaluative others; self is passive, immobilized; dejection-based emotions (disappointment in Me-self, depression, hopelessness)
Guilt	Violations of standards or moral rules for how one *ought* to behave toward others; violations directly affect such others	Evaluation of a specific *behavior* that was wrong; negative evaluation of I-self as agent responsible; actions viewed as controllable; lack of effort	Other as person who was hurt by actions of self; other as passive victim; focus of guilty thoughts	I-self is mobilized to engage in acts of confession, reparation, to approach the other; agitation-type emotions (anxiety, tension, uneasiness) about threat to relationship

proud that I got all A's on my report card," "Getting the lead in the school play made me feel proud," "I made a bathroom shelf all by myself and was so proud." The *attributions* associated with pride are internal in that the individual takes personal responsibility for the accomplishment in the form of ability and/or effort (see Weiner, 1986). In I-self, Me-self terminology, there is a focus on how the I-self, as active agent, is responsible for the accomplishment that in turn leads to a favorable evaluation of the Me-self as competent. Others may also be afforded a role in the experience of pride. To the extent that significant others become aware of one's role in producing the successful outcomes, they will express their pride in the individual. This is likely to occur, given that one is motivated to communicate the event to such others, in anticipation of a positive evaluative reaction. As one older child subject put it, "I couldn't wait to tell my parents because I knew they would be very proud of me for jumping off the high dive." Pride is also accompanied by the emotions of happiness, excitement, and feelings of hopefulness.

Lewis (1994) makes the distinction between pride and "hubris," another positive self-affect. Pride is experienced in reaction to successful achievements that are more specific, whereas hubris is expressed as a more global attribution about the self that has elements of grandiosity, if not narcissism. (Muhammed Ali's frequent self-aggrandizing statements to the public, for example, "I am the greatest!," come to mind.) However, pride itself is not viewed as necessarily a desirable emotion in all cultures. For example, in collectivist or interdependent cultures (as opposed to individualistic societies), pride signals separateness from others, social comparison, and the sense that one feels superior to others (Kitayama, Markus, & Matsumoto, 1995).

Although guilt and shame were initially treated as somewhat indistinguishable in the older emotion literature, more contemporary theorists have articulated a number of differences between these two negative affects, differences that that have interesting implications for the self. With regard to the *causes* of these two emotions, shame is typically experienced when one commits transgressions or wrongdoings that violate one's own ideals or others' ideals for the self ("I'm ashamed of myself for writing all over the family room wall"). Shame is also commonly provoked by incompetence or achievement failures in which the self does not measure up to personal or social standards. As one of our 10-year-old interview subjects explained, "I lost the baseball game for the whole team, I made a really stupid move and felt ashamed of myself for doing such a dumb thing, especially in front of all those people." Guilt, in contrast, is driven by the violation of standards or moral rules for how one *ought* to behave toward others, violations that directly impact particular others. The same subject also provided an example of what would make him guilty: "If I stole something from a friend and then

I thought about it later, I would feel guilty that I took something from another person."

The *attributions* for these two emotions, including their implications for the self, differ (in addition, see Dweck & Leggett, 1988; Weiner, 1986). Shame involves a *global*, trait-like evaluation of the self ("I am a bad person for what I did"). These more general negative evaluations are also associated with feelings of low self-worth. Shame over displays of incompetence are associated with attributions involving inherent lack of ability. In describing his feelings of shame, one respondent exclaimed, "I felt totally stupid when I failed the test. I just don't know what happened." Moreover, shameful acts are perceived to be relatively *uncontrollable*; that is, they could not be prevented or ameliorated. As one of our older child subjects explained, "I felt like a bad person. I was ashamed of myself, and there was nothing I could do to fix it." With shame, therefore, the focus is on the inadequacy and worthlessness of the Me-self, which is judged to be fundamentally defective. Guilt, on the other hand, is linked to attributions involving an evaluation of a *specific behavior* judged to be wrong. The particular act is viewed as potentially controllable through personal effort. With guilt, therefore, the focus is on the I-self as the agent of negative actions against another for which one assumes responsibility.

The role of significant others also varies for each of these negative self-affects. With regard to shame, others are potential shamers if they either witness or later learn about the transgression or achievement failure. Thus, they possess power as active agents of scorn. As such, they serve as "social mirrors" whose negative evaluations of the shameful act provoke loss of esteem in the eyes of others. In contrast, for guilt, the role of the other is as the person who was hurt by the actions of the self. Therefore, the other is the passive victim and becomes the focus of one's guilty thoughts.

These features in turn have implications for the behaviors that one displays, as well as their emotional concomitants. For example, in the case of shame, there is the desire to escape, to hide, to distance oneself from the evaluative gaze of others. The self becomes passive, if not immobilized, in an attempt to avoid further humiliation. As one older child interviewee put it, "I felt terrible. I just wanted to hide my feelings. I didn't want to talk about it. I didn't want to hear what they thought about me." One is also likely to experience *dejection*-based emotions, such as depression and feelings of hopelessness (see Higgins, 1987), in part due to the loss of esteem in the eyes of others (Harter, 1997). For a minority, shame evolves into defensive anger or rage described as the fury of humiliation (Kohut, 1977; Lewis, 1971; Morrison, 1989). In contrast, with guilt, the I-self is typically mobilized to engage in acts of control in the form of confession and/or reparation for the interpersonal damage caused. Emotions involve more agitation; for example, one experiences anxiety, tension, and uneasiness over the potential threat to the relationship (Higgins, 1987). As one interviewee described it, "It grabs you. It sticks to you, and you can't get over it unless you do something about it. I feel guilty about what I did to her and try to fix it so she will still be my friend."

The features described here define the dimensions of these particular self-affects as they typically appear in the emotional repertoire of older children, adolescents, and adults. However, from a developmental perspective, self-conscious emotions are of particular interest since their emergence is gradual and depends upon both cognitive advances and specific socialization experiences. In the remainder of this chapter, attention focuses primarily on those factors responsible for the normative-developmental emergence of these emotions, primarily addressing pride and shame. What becomes apparent is that the capacity to *experience* these emotions, as inferred from *behavioral displays*, developmentally precedes the ability to *verbalize* an understanding of these emotions.

With regard to the displays of young children, overt manifestations of pride include an open stance in which the chest is literally "puffed up," with shoulders back, typically accompanied by eye contact and a wide grin. As Stipek (1983, 1995) observes, there is no unique facial expression for pride, only an accompanying expression of happiness. Shame, on the other hand, is manifested by a slumping posture, with head down, to facilitate gaze aversion, as well as efforts to hide from others. In the next section, I review the cognitive and social prerequisites leading to the *display* of pride and shame in children. Subsequently, I turn to those factors that facilitate the verbal understanding of the *concepts* of pride and shame.

COGNITIVE-DEVELOPMENTAL PREREQUISITES FOR THE DISPLAY OF SELF-CONSCIOUS EMOTIONS

Lewis (1991, 1994) has been the most explicit in identifying what he considers the critical developmental acquisitions necessary for the emergence of self-conscious emotions. For Lewis, the expression of pride, shame, and guilt requires the development of *objective self-awareness*, namely, the toddler's budding ability to become the object of his/her own consciousness and self-evaluation. This rudimentary manifestation of the Me-self (the "idea of me") emerges during the middle of the second year of life, when toddlers can first recognize and label themselves in the mirror, and realize that others are labeling them as well. The identifying characteristics that they begin to acquire include an initial sense of their competence (see Stipek et al., 1992) as well as their conduct. As Lewis (1994) also observes, the emergence of the Me-self allows for the representation of self and other, and helps to transform the behaviors or interactions into an appreciation for standards, goals, and rules. For Lewis, the experience of self-conscious emotions requires some knowledge of the standards of achievement as well as conduct that have been established by primary caregivers; that is, the toddler must take responsibility for violating such standards in order to experience guilt and shame. Taking responsibility, in turn, implies that the toddler can engage in some rudimentary form of self-evaluation, based upon a judgment about whether he/she has performed according to the standards set by caregivers.

Stipek et al. (1992) provide evidence for a three-stage sequence representing the acquisition of these prerequisites of self-conscious emotions, as observed in American samples of children. At the first stage, prior to age 2, infants and toddlers experience joy in mastery, reflecting their sense of agency of causality. Thus, they will display gleeful behavior if they make a block tower or complete a simple puzzle. However, they lack the cognitive-representational skills to evaluate their performance. In addition, they do not call their successful mastery efforts to the attention of adults, nor do they anticipate adults' reactions.

At the second stage, slightly before 2 years of age, children begin to anticipate adult reactions, seeking positive responses to their successes while attempting to avoid negative responses to their failures. This stage corresponds to the age at which "social referencing" is observed, namely, that toddlers turn to caregivers and rely on their signals for feedback that may "disambiguate" uncertain events (Barrett & Campos, 1987; Campos & Stenberg, 1980). Stipek et al. (1992) report that toddlers show evidence of their appreciation of adult standards, for example, by turning away from adults and hunching their shoulders in the face of failures. Kagan (1984) describes similar phenomena in describing toddlers' distress reactions when they watch an adult model perform a set of acts that they could not successfully imitate, implying that they were aware of their lack of competence to achieve the implicit performance standard.

During the third stage, after age 3, there is further evidence that children begin to incorporate adult standards, in that they appear to evaluate their performance and react emotionally to success and failure, independent of adult reactions. For example, frowns and verbal displays of frustration (e.g., "I can't do it!") that are not directed to adults typically accompany failure experiences, suggesting to Stipek and colleagues that the young child is experiencing "dissatisfaction with the *self*, not just the task" (p. 75).

The emergence of the capacity for this rudimentary form of self-awareness, in Lewis' (1991, 1994) terminology, or self-evaluation, according to Stipek et al. (1992), serves to pave the way for the initial experience of self-conscious emotions during the second and third year of life, as argued by Lewis. However, others have taken issue with the age at which Lewis feels that self-conscious emotions can be experienced. For example, Buss (1980) suggests that the behavioral manifestations in toddlers reflect "pseudoshame" in the form of fear of punishment, and that self-conscious emotions such as shame do not emerge until the age of 5, when the cognitive sense of self is sufficiently complex. Moreover, Kagan (1984) contends that guilt is not experienced until the age of 4, at which time children have the cognitive abilities to understand that they caused the transgression and, in so doing, that they had a conscious choice.

Barrett (1995) also challenges the analysis as put forth by Lewis and colleagues, questioning whether toddlers actually experience self-conscious emotions. She makes the logical argument that the cognitive prerequisites postulated to be necessary (e.g., objective self-awareness) are somewhat arbitrarily assigned to a given age; that is, one could always find rudimentary forms of a given cognitive process in early childhood, in keeping with the contemporary trend to identify skills at younger and younger ages. Barrett, herself, considers it unlikely that self-conscious emotions are manifest in toddlers. The approach of Mascolo and Fischer (1995) would appear to circumvent these caveats. They argue that rather than ask at what single point in development do self-conscious emotions emerge, we should ask what forms these affects assume at different points in development. They perform such a developmental analysis for pride, shame, and guilt, utilizing Fischer's (1980) skill theory. Eight levels, covering the age-span of 7 months to 17 years, identify the different skills and behaviors defining the developmental emergence of increasingly complex structures that underlie self-conscious emotions and their precursors.

For example, for the emotion of shame, the earliest precursors (Step 1 in the sequence ages 7–8 months) include distress over failures of outcomes that older infants have tried to produce through sensorimotor actions. Consistent with the Stipek et al. (1992) findings, at Step 2, approximately 11–13 months, distress is also associated with caregivers' reactions of disappointment in their child. At Step 3, approximately 18–24 months, the toddler begins to anticipate the negative reaction of the caregiver, showing rudimentary displays of shame-like behavior, including avoidant posture and gaze aversion. At Step 4, approximately 2–3 years, behaviors suggest that the child is experiencing shame caused by the self performing poorly, as revealed in statements such as "I'm bad at throwing," "Mommy doesn't like what I did."

Their analysis continues beyond this sensorimotor tier into what Fischer (1980) labels the "representational tier" and the "abstract tier." During the intermediate stages (at the representational tier), children exhibit behaviors from which shame over one's comparative performance and valued traits is inferred. At the abstract tier, beginning in adolescence, shame about a general (negative) personality characteristic is experienced, followed by shame over a characteristic or sentiment shared with others possessing a similar identity (e.g., others of the same ethnicity or cultural group). Through such a sequential analysis, one can appreciate the building blocks upon which more mature displays and understandings of self-conscious emotions rest, rather than identifying a particular age at which such emotions "truly emerge."

SOCIALIZATION FACTORS

There is more agreement on those child-rearing practices critical to the establishment of self-conscious emotions, where particular attention has been directed toward the social prerequisites for the display of guilt and shame. Caregivers must convey the *standards* of behavior they expect of their toddler through modeling and instruction, imbuing these goals with significance through social interaction (Barrett, 1995; Emde & Oppenheim, 1995; Ferguson & Stegge, 1995; Lewis, 1991; Stipek, 1995; Zahn-Waxler & Robinson, 1995). Standards concerning expectations regarding age-appropriate achievement behavior as well as conduct are among the most common. In addition, as these authors point out, parents must overtly evaluate their child's ability to meet such standards. Through such practices, young children begin to develop a rudimentary sense of their competence as well as their behavioral conduct or morality (see also Bretherton, Fritz, Zahn-Waxler, & Ridgeway, 1986; Dunn, 1987; Kagan & Lamb, 1987) that should support the experience of self-conscious emotions. These processes are more likely to occur if parents are nurturant (see Barrett, 1995) and if caregivers employ "induction techniques" in which they provide children with explanations that promote insight and understanding into their behaviors and their consequences (Hoffman, 1982, 1991).

Investigators have also illuminated those parental practices that differentially lead to guilt versus shame. Guilt is more likely to be produced if parents focus on the consequences of harm inflicted on others, placing emphasis on the child's obligations and the need for personal responsibility. Those parenting techniques most likely to produce internalized standards and guilt that is associated with toddler reparations for a wrongdoing include emotion-laden explanations that also clarify standards of behavior (see also Zahn-Waxler, Radke-Yarrow, & King, 1979). Shame is more likely to be induced if parents highlight their child's failure to meet high standards. Shame will be particularly intense if parents communicate that failures reflect the fact that the child is fundamentally deficient and will never be good enough or lovable (Barrett, 1995; Lewis, 1991; Potter-Efron, 1989).

Discrepancies between the child's behavior and particular types of expectations also differentially predict the strength of guilt and shame reactions. Guilt is more likely to ensue if parents emphasize the discrepancy between the child's behavior and how the parents feel he/she *ought* to behave (Higgins, 1987). Shame, on the other hand, is more likely if parents underscore how the child is falling short of parental *ideals,* namely, how they *want* the child to behave (Higgins, 1987; Moretti & Higgins, 1990). Barrett also hypothesizes that the precursors of shame will have more of an effect if there is a strong bond between parent and child, such that parental values and associated feedback about performance matter a great deal to the child.

There is also some evidence for gender differences, with girls expressing more guilt as well as shame. Zahn-Waxler and Robinson (1995) review studies demonstrating that girls are more likely to experience empathy and guilt, and to engage in prosocial and reparative behaviors than are boys (see other reviews by Brody, 1985; Eisenberg & Lennon, 1983; Hoffman, 1977; Zahn-Waxler, Cole, & Barrett, 1991). These investigators suggest that greater empathy and guilt among females may reflect biological causes linked to potential childbearing and child rearing, since responsive parenting requires empathy, sensitivity to infant distress, and control of one's anger. However, they also point to socialization factors. For example, aggression is more readily tolerated in boys (Condry & Ross, 1985), and females are judged more harshly than males for failure to engage in the same altruistic act (Barnett, McMinimy, Flouer, & Masbad, 1987).

Alessandri and Lewis (1993) report that girls also experience more *shame* than do boys, consistent with gender differences reported in the adult literature (H. B. Lewis, 1987; Tangney, 1995). Their studies with preschoolers and their parents reveal that in performing achievement tasks in a laboratory setting, girls expressed more shame over failures than boys, despite no gender differences in actual performance (see also Lewis, Alessandri, & Sullivan, 1992). The parents of girls were observed to use more negative comments than parents of boys. These investigators infer, therefore, that negative parental feedback promotes unfavorable self-evaluations in girls, since it focuses attention on their failures, which in turn predisposes girls to experience shame. They relate their findings to the attribution literature (see Dweck & Leggett, 1988), where it has been found that girls are more likely to assume personal responsibility for failure and focus on global, internal attributions than are boys. Girls are also observed to have lower expectations for success and decreased achievement striving in the face of failure or evaluative pressure. Consistent with the laboratory findings reported earlier, girls receive more negative feedback and less positive feedback from teachers than do boys (see also Eccles & Blumenfeld, 1985). Thus, differential treatment of girls and boys both at home and in the classroom would appear to contribute to the experience of more negative self-conscious emotions in girls.

THE EMERGENCE OF AN UNDERSTANDING OF SELF-CONSCIOUS EMOTION CONCEPTS

The preceding discussion has focused on those cognitive and social prerequisites responsible for the emergence of the first behavioral *expressions* of pride, shame, and guilt during toddlerhood and early childhood. At these young ages, verbal references to such emotions do not appear in the child's self-representations among American children. During middle childhood and adolescence, the focus shifts to the emergence of children's *verbal* understanding of self-conscious emotion *concepts*, particularly as they become part of the network of representations that define the self. For example, in the protoypical cameos presented in Chapter 2, there was no mention of pride or shame in the self-descriptive statements of the child in the period of toddlerhood to early childhood. However, at the next stage, early to middle childhood, the prototypical subject described how "my parents are real proud of me when I do good at things"; that is, the child comes to appreciate that significant others can express their pride (or shame) for the self, although the child does not acknowledge that his/her I-self could be proud or ashamed of the Me-self. The latter realization represents an advance that was illustrated for the period of middle to late childhood, where the cameo child described how "when I don't control my temper, I'm ashamed of myself," and "I got A's on my last report and was really proud of myself." As was demonstrated for self-*attributes*, the gradual emergence of an understanding of self-affects requires both cognitive-developmental acquisitions as well as particular child-rearing experiences, which are next explored.

Cognitive-Developmental Factors

There has been relatively little work that specifically addresses developmental changes in the child's *understanding* of self-affects. In one of the few such efforts, Griffin (1995) has examined certain cognitive-developmental prerequisites that underlie an understanding of pride, shame, and embarrassment, employing Case's theory as a framework (Case, 1985; Case & Griffin, 1990). She found support for the prediction that children do not demonstrate an understanding of self-conscious emotion terms until approximately 7 or 8 years of age, when they become capable of "bidimensional" thought. Such thinking allows them cognitively to coordinate two dimensions of social reality—for example, with shame, (1) one's failure to meet standards (2) in the presence of an audience that witnesses and acknowledges one's failure.

In our own laboratory, we have adopted a somewhat different cognitive-developmental framework for exploring the prerequisites of an understanding of two self-affects: pride and shame. We built upon earlier work documenting an age-related sequence in which children come to be able to coordinate the simultaneous representation of two different emotions (Harter & Buddin, 1987). Whereas young children develop *single representations* for discrete emotions (e.g., happy, sad, mad, scared), they cannot combine these representations into more complex emotion blends. As described in Chapter 2, the recognition that a given event can evoke more than one emotion gradually emerges in middle to late childhood through a predictable sequence of stages. An appreciation for the meaning of self-conscious emotions such as pride and shame would also appear to require an understanding of how more than one emotion can be experienced simultaneously. More specifically, an understanding of pride or shame requires the differentiation and integration of several features of single emotions. Both pride and shame involve the integration of features that involve feelings directed toward the *self* as well as toward the *other*. For example, the self-component of pride represents joy over the personal mastery of a particular skill that is combined with a feeling involving a significant other, namely, happiness because the accomplishment was (will be, or hypothetically would be) appreciated by others. If shame is experienced over a failure, then it will combine anger toward the self for personally deficiencies as well as a sense of sadness that one has disappointed another. If shame is experienced in regard to a transgression, it will appear more similar to guilt in that it will combine anger toward the *self* for committing a transgression with some sense of regret for hurting or violating *another*.

In an interview study (see Harter & Whitesell, 1989), we asked children between the ages of 4 and 9 to tell us the meaning of the terms "proud" and "ashamed," giving examples of something that would lead them to feel each emotion. We performed a content analysis to determine at what age children's definitions and examples would meet the criteria described here, namely, that their descriptions exemplified the components in which emotions are explicitly directed toward both self and other. The youngest children (ages 4 and 5) did not have a conceptual understanding of either pride or shame; that is, they could not define these terms, nor did their examples contain the components built into the criteria. However, their responses did indicate that they had some rudimentary appreciation for the *valence* of each feeling. Examples for pride were "You feel good"; "It makes you feel happy." Examples for shame were "It's a bad feeling when you did something wrong"; "Your mom gets mad at you for doing something you shouldn't do."

Six- and 7-year-olds typically showed a greater understanding of these terms, although their responses did not meet the stringent criteria adopted. For example, such children may have acknowledged that they were ashamed or proud, but these affects were not directed toward the self, nor were both self and other components present. Typical responses were "You're proud when something good happens like you ran a race"; "You did something good and you were happy about it." The typical shame responses involved some type of transgression; however, children were usually more concerned about the parental reaction than they were about the harm to others or their own regret. Examples included "You're ashamed of what you did, and scared about what your mom might do"; "Your parents are ashamed of you for doing something bad." Thus, these responses had elements of the proto-type for pride and shame, although they did not successfully integrate each of the components.

Many (although not all) 8- and 9-year-olds provided definitions that did meet the criteria. For pride, examples were "I was proud of myself for getting straight A's on my report card; I was real happy and my parents were happy for me, too"; "I was happy for myself that I did something right, and I knew my mother would be glad too, when I told her." For shame, one 8-year-old told us, "I'd be ashamed of myself if I hit my brother; I'd feel sorry that I hurt him and I'd be mad at myself for hitting him." Another explained, "You feel sad for the other person when you do something bad, and you are ashamed of yourself, mad at yourself that you did it."

Child-Rearing Antecedents

A comprehensive analysis of the development of an understanding of the concepts of pride and shame must not only identify the elements to be cognitively integrated but should also take into account those socialization experiences necessary for their emergence. Pride and shame have been described as "self-affects" in that the I-self is proud or ashamed of the Me-self. An important feature is that in their most mature form, these affects are provoked by events that have not been directly witnessed by other people. It was Cooley (1902), as described in the introductory chapter, who first alerted us to the fact that these emotions do not emerge in an experiential vacuum. Rather, the ability to experience these self-affects is highly dependent upon the individual's socialization history; that is, significant others must first express their pride or shame for the individual; then gradually, the external affective reactions of others come to be internalized.

The themes identified by Cooley have been echoed in more contemporary treatments of shame and pride, in which the initial role of external evaluation by socializing agents appears paramount (Erikson, 1968; Griffin, 1995; Harter & Whitesell, 1989; Lewis, 1994; Stipek, 1995). These authors have argued that the ability to initially experience the emotions of pride and shame, and subsequently to *understand* these emotion concepts, requires the internalization of parental values in the form of an ego ideal, a standard, against which one comes to compare one's performance. Thus, pride and shame are socially derived emotions that also have direct implications for one's feelings of worth, given their origins in parental evaluations of the self. As theorists have suggested, this type of analysis leads to the expectation that the young child would require an actual audience that witnesses, and reacts to, behaviors that are shameful, or alternatively, are worthy of pride. However, the need for such a social audience would decline developmentally as the values or standards of significant others are internalized, since children could then apply these standards themselves in order to feel either proud or ashamed of themselves in the absence of observation.

Until recently, this kind of analysis, while very plausible, has been largely speculative. In our work, we have begun to document the emergence of the understanding of the emotions of pride and shame empirically, utilizing a socialization framework. The first findings were rather serendipitous, resulting from an open-ended interview in which we simply asked children ages 4–11 to describe the feelings of pride and shame, and to provide a cause for each. We discovered that our youngest subjects, 4–5 years old, typically could not provide a compelling description or a very plausible cause, although as described earlier, most were aware of the valence of the two feelings, namely, that pride is a good feeling and shame is a bad feeling.

Interestingly, among our 6- and 7-year-olds, who had some intuitions about these feelings, many of their descriptions included accounts of how parents would be proud or ashamed of *them* for their actions; that is, significant *others* were proud or ashamed of the *self*. Examples of pride included "Dad would be proud of me if I took out the trash"; "Mom would be proud if I cleaned my room"; "My parents would be proud if I won something"; "Dad was proud of me when I made a goal." Examples of shame included: "Mom would be ashamed of me if I did something bad or got into trouble"; "Dad was really ashamed of me when I broke the window"; "Mom was ashamed of me when I got into her stuff after she had told me not to"; "My parents get ashamed when I do something naughty." However, at this age, children did not describe how they could be proud or ashamed of *themselves*.

Typically, it was not until about the age of 8 that children gave examples of how they could be ashamed or proud of *themselves*. In these spontaneous accounts, children would report such examples as "I was really ashamed that I broke my friend's bike and didn't tell him"; "I hit my brother for no real reason and felt ashamed of myself"; "I was ashamed that I took something of my sister's without asking"; "I hurt my friend's feelings and really felt ashamed." For pride, typical examples were "I kicked a goal at our soccer match"; "I got the best grade on a test"; "I did a good deed and got a medal"; "When I did something the best."

Since these latter responses did not *specify* whether an audience was or was not present, nor had we probed for this information, we became curious about this issue; that is, these open-ended examples did not allow us to determine whether the experience of being proud of oneself or ashamed of oneself required the observation of another, or whether one could experience these self-affects in the absence of others. We had some clues, however, from the responses of certain subjects. For example, in pursuing one child's description of an experience in which he had felt ashamed of himself, we asked whether he could feel ashamed when he was all alone, or whether someone had to watch what he had done. His thoughtful reply was quite illuminating: "Well I *might* be able to be ashamed of myself if my parents didn't know, but it would sure help me to be ashamed if they were there to see what I did!"

The Empirical Documentation of a Developmental Sequence

These preliminary findings suggested the fruitfulness of studying the developmental course of the concepts of pride and shame more systematically, particularly with regard to the role of the audience. In so doing, our focus was on the development of children's *understanding* of pride and shame, on their ability to *conceptualize the causes* of these emotions. In particular, we were interested in the substages that appeared to be precursors of the child's emerging ability to appreciate the fact that one could be proud or ashamed of the self in the absence of any observation by others.

Given our framework, focusing on the *socialization* component of both pride and shame, we devised a procedure that would be sensitive to the role of the observing parent; that is, we sought to determine whether parents were required to "support" the reported experience of pride and shame. Toward this end, we designed two sets of vignettes. To assess shame, we constructed a pictorial vignette with several frames and a brief story line to accompany the pictures. The story concerned a situation in which the parents have forbidden the child to take any money from a very large jar of coins in the parents' bedroom. However, the child transgresses and takes a few coins.

There are two separate story sequences. In one sequence, no one observes the act, and no one ever finds out (an outcome we attempted to ensure by describing the money jar as very large, whereas the child only took a few coins). In the second sequence, the parent catches the child in the act. The primary dependent measures included the subject's description of the emotions that the story child would feel in the first sequence (where the act is not detected) and a description of the emotions that both child and parent would feel in the second situation, where the parent catches the child in the act.

To assess an understanding of *pride*, we selected a gymnastic feat as the demonstration of competence. In the first sequence, the child goes to the playground on a Saturday when no one else is there and tries out a flip on the bars, one that he/she has been working on at school. The child attempts this maneuver, which he/she has never been able to perform successfully before, and does it really well. In the first sequence the child leaves the bars knowing that he/she was the only one at the playground and thus no one else observed the flip. The child is then asked what feeling he/she would have at that time.

In the second pride sequence, the parent accompanies the child to the playground and observes the child successfully performing the flip for the first time. The child is asked how he/she would feel, as well as how the observing parent would feel having watched the child doing the flip. In all conditions, pictorial aids in the form of photographs of facial expressions of a series of emotions by a child, for the first sequence, and by a child as well as by a parent, for the second sequence, are presented to the children to facilitate their identification of relevant affects.

The results for both pride and shame revealed a highly age-related, parallel, four-stage sequence that is interpretable within our socialization framework (see Table 4.2 and Figure 4.1). Moreover, the stages that have emerged are consistent with Selman's (1980) developmental model of self-awareness, in which children gradually begin to observe and critically evaluate the self. At our *first level*, ages 4 to 5, there is no mention of either pride or shame on the part of story child or parent in either sequence, whether the child is observed or not observed. Participants give very clear responses about their potential emotional reactions to these situations, reactions that are quite

TABLE 4.2. Emotions Reported by Child Subject for Parent and Child

Age	Transgression		Successful feat	
	Parent	Child	Parent	Child
4–5	Mad at child	Scared	Happy for child	Excited
5–6	Ashamed of child	Scared	Proud of child	Excited
6–7	Ashamed of child when observe child	Ashamed of self when observed	Proud of child when observe child	Proud of self when observed
7–8	(Parent does not observe act)	Ashamed of self when not observed	(Parent does not observe act)	Proud of self when not observed

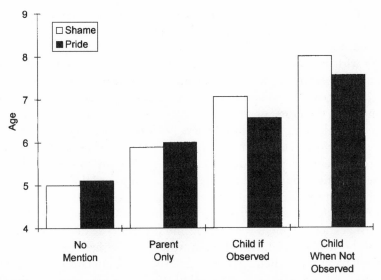

FIGURE 4.1. Ages of subjects at each of the four stages of understanding for shame and pride.

telling. In the transgression situation where the story child is not observed by the parents, participants report that the child character (with whom they are encouraged to identify) would feel scared or worried about the possibility of detection. When they are caught by the parent, they also feel extremely scared or worried about the likelihood of punishment. However, there is no acknowledgment of pride or shame.

In the *pride* sequences of stories, these youngest subjects report that they would feel happy, glad, and excited in the situation where their gymnastic feat is not observed by the parent. In the story where the parent *witnesses* their performance, they report that both they and the parent would feel happy, glad, and excited; that is, there is no mention of pride, either on the part of the parent or the story child. Thus, children at this first level *are* aware that their parents have reactions to their behavior. However, consistent with Selman's (1980) first level of self-awareness and with Higgins' (1991) analysis, the child is not yet aware that others are *evaluating* the self, nor can the I-self critically evaluate or affectively react to the Me-self.

Our *second level*, at ages 5 to 6, represents a very interesting transition period. Children now demonstrate their first use of the terms "ashamed" and "proud." However, their usage is restricted to reactions of the *parents*. Thus, the parental response to the child's transgression is to be ashamed of the child. However, the child does not yet acknowledge that he/she is ashamed of the self. Rather, the child is still scared or worried about the parents' reaction. Similarly, in the case of the gymnastic feat, the subjects describe how the parent is proud of the child. However, the child is not yet proud of the self. Rather, he/she is excited, happy, glad.

This level parallels Selman's second stage of self-awareness and is consistent with Higgins' (1991) analysis; that is, the child's I-self is aware that others are observing and evaluating and affectively reacting to his/her Me-self ("I observe you evaluating and being proud or ashamed of me"). This second level, therefore, provides the necessary building blocks for the emergence of the looking-glass self (Cooley, 1902), in which one comes to internalize the attitudes, opinions, and affective sentiments of significant others toward the self; that is, children must first be sensitive to the fact that they are being evaluated in order to direct their attention to the specific content of others' approval, criticism, and emotional reactions.

At our *third level*, children (between the ages of 6 and 7) demonstrate the first acknowledgment that shame and pride can be directed *by* the self, *toward* the self. Thus, in the situation where the act has been *observed*, not only will parents be ashamed or proud of the child, but children report that they, too, will feel ashamed or proud of themselves, seemingly in response to the parental reaction. However, what also places children at this level is the fact that they do *not* report any feelings of shame or pride in the story sequence specifying the *absence* of parental observation. This seems to be another critical transitional level in our socialization sequence, in that the act must be observed in the case of both a transgression (in order to experience shame) and the demonstration of competence (in order to experience pride). In the absence of parental observation, no such potential self-affects are acknowledged. This level parallels Selman's third stage of self-awareness in that the child begins to incorporate the observations of others into his/her own self-perceptions, such that one can directly evaluate the self. Thus, the I-self can now adopt an attitude toward the Me-self that parallels the attitude of significant others, although these self-attitudes and self-affects must still be scaffolded by the reactions of others.

The hallmark of the *fourth level* (beginning at ages 7 to 8), is that in the absence of parental observation, children spontaneously acknowledge that the story children will feel ashamed of themselves or proud of themselves. (It should be noted that the stories in which the child was *not* observed were always presented first, so that any response of shame or pride on the part of the child was not simply a generalization from the sequence in which they were observed.) Therefore, at this level, children appear to have internalized the standards by which shame and pride can be experienced in the absence of direct, parental observation. Interestingly, the large majority of children at this level do not merely report the emotions of shame and pride, but specifically indicate that "I would feel ashamed, or proud, of *myself*." Thus, they appear to be at the stage where these emotions do function as self-affects in the sense that one is truly ashamed or proud of the self. This final level in our sequence is consistent with Selman's fourth stage, in which the I-self can now observe and critically evaluate the Me-self in the absence of the direct presence or reactions of significant others.

In summary, this sequence not only reveals the gradual nature of the normative, developmental emergence of self-affects, but also suggests that the critical, underlying processes involve parental socialization. Thus, we have inferred that children must first experience others as models who are proud or ashamed of them in order to internalize these functions themselves. Even when they first develop the ability to acknowledge that they are proud or ashamed of themselves, children still need the scaffolding of parental surveillance or observation. The final stage in the internalization process occurs when these self-affects are experienced in the absence of observations by others, when the I-self can be directly ashamed of the Me-self, when one is all by oneself.

Although this empirical effort was designed to illuminate the normative trajectory of the development of self-affects, there are obvious implications for individual differences in their emergence. For this sequence to emerge, it would appear that parental figures must directly express their pride and shame for child behaviors. In the absence of such external affective reactions children will not experience external emotional sentiments that they can internalize. Earlier in this chapter, other conditions fostering the emergence of self-conscious emotions were described. For example, parents must be clear about their standards and their evaluations of whether children are meeting these standards. Moreover, children will be more likely to incorporate parental evaluations and affects if there is a strong bond between parent and child, leading the child to value and want to adopt such parental standards. For children experiencing neglect, or for those who do not experience a close bond, these conditions may not be met. Alternatively, for parents who are abusing, punitive, and excessively harsh in their criticism, where the child nevertheless wants to please the parents, there may be excessive shame but little pride given an absence of parental reactions signalling that they are proud of their child.

It is also critical to appreciate the fact that this developmental sequence, and the ages at which each stage emerged, were documented for an American, middle-class sample. However, there is evidence (Shaver, Wu, & Schwartz, 1992) to reveal that in the Chinese culture, shame emerges in the behavior and the vocabulary of children at much early ages than in the United States. Moreover, the centrality of shame to Chinese socialization practices and to the fabric of interpersonal relationships can be observed in the fact that there are many more shame-related words in the Chinese vocabulary. In addition, Shaver et al. have demonstrated that shame represents a basic emotion category in the hierarchy of emotion concepts for the Chinese (at the same level of anger, sadness, fear, and happiness), further underscoring its salience, whereas in the United States, shame is a subcategory under sadness. It would be of interest to determine in future research how the sequence we have documented for American children may vary as a function of culture.

It should be noted that the developmental trajectories identified in the American sequence of self-affects and discussed by Selman, Higgins, and others represent *acquisition*, rather than acquisition/deletion, sequences; that is, although new stages emerge, the former stages do not drop out of one's repertoire. Thus, a child who has developed the ability to function at the highest stage in the sequence may, under certain circumstances, display behavior characterized by lower levels in the sequence. For example, during environmental transitions (e.g., the shift to junior high school), one is faced with the scrutiny of new significant others whose standards must be identified, as well as new social reference groups to whom one will compare the self. These conditions may necessitate a shift to lower levels in the sequence initially, during which time one comes to observe the standards of others, their attitudes and affects toward the self, as well as the characteristics of others to whom one is comparing the self before the internalization process can proceed. The general point, therefore, is that the ability to observe, evaluate, and critically react to the self, cognitively as well as affectively, must gradually develop through a series of stages that begin with an awareness of how others are evaluating the self and with the ability to compare oneself to an appropriate social reference group.

The particular sequence that we have identified in our own empirical work extends from early to late childhood. We have not yet explored the potential further understanding of pride and shame during adolescence. However, there are some suggestions in the literature. Piaget (1960) was among the first to describe the type of *collective* pride that emerges in adolescence, wherein the individual is proud of a group or members of a group to which he/she belongs, pride that reflects on the self. As the prototypical older adolescent (in Chapter 3) described, "When our team has a winning season and goes to the playoffs, everyone in the whole school is proud. What the team does reflects on all of us." A spontaneous example for collective shame emerged in one of our adolescent interviews in which participants were asked to describe situations in which they would experience shame. This 17-year-old lamented how ashamed he felt as a member of the human race when he saw the movie *Day of the Dolphins*.

Mascolo and Fischer (1995), in applying Fischer's skill theory to the sequence of steps governing the emergence of pride and shame, provide a more detailed structural analysis that includes an account of this type of collective pride or shame. They observe that general identity-related abstractions can be constructed from identifying with the admired (or devalued) traits of others. Such an abstraction involves the integration of traits perceived to be similar in the self and others. In coordinating the identity characteristics of self and other, one can react to others' achievements (or failures) almost as if they were one's own. Mascolo and Fischer provide an example in which an African American individual described how proud he was of Marian Anderson for singing at the Lincoln Memorial after having been denied an opportunity to perform at Constitution Hall. Through this type of identification, he could experience reflected glory or pride. Thus, self-affects continue to undergo development, a topic that requires much needed empirical attention.

THE FUNCTIONAL ROLE OF SELF-CONSCIOUS EMOTIONS

An important theme of this volume is that self-representations, be they domain-specific self-evaluations, global perceptions of self-worth, or self-conscious emotions, should only command our attention if they produce consequences that impact everyday behavior. In many instances, self-representations may be very functional in that they perform a positive role in promoting adaptation. In other situations, self-representations may have negative consequences, as revealed by the liabilities described in the two preceding chapters.

The positive functions associated with pride are perhaps the most obvious. These include an enhanced sense of competence and self-worth, as well as the motivation to perform similar activities in the future, perhaps challenging oneself to perform at a higher level of difficulty. Moreover, the experience of pride may cement social bonds to the extent that the successful behavior is shared with others. As Barrett (1995) notes, pride serves to decrease the distance from socializing agents who are likely to evaluate the self, since the sharing of one's accomplishments with significant others should serve to provoke their expressions of pride for the individual. Our own data, described in this chapter, indicate that among older children, personal pride can be experienced in the absence of an observing other. However, when we specifically asked subjects whether they would tell anyone about the successful gymnastic feat or keep it to themselves, fully 85% indicated that they would relate their triumphs to others, particularly their parents. Moreover, many of the older children specifically indicated that telling someone about their accomplishments would enhance their own positive affective response to the event.

Collective pride, as in the example of how the entire school felt proud of the football team's success, leads to shared, positive affective experiences that also serve to support social relationships. Although pride is generally associated with favorable outcomes, in its extreme form, which Lewis (1991) labels "hubris," it can have negative consequences, alienating others who feel that one's reactions are excessive or narcissistic. From a developmental perspective, such reactions would appear to intensify in early adolescence where, as the prototypical cameo revealed, bragging was identified as not cool, since it would diminish one's popularity. From a cross-cultural perspective, excessive pride may threaten interpersonal harmony in collectivist cultures (e.g., China), to the extent that its expression signals separateness from others as well as superiority (Kityama et al., 1995).

The negative self-conscious emotions, namely, shame and guilt, require a more complex analysis. It is more apparent that they would be associated with *unfavorable* outcomes such as loss of esteem in the eyes of others, lowered self-worth, debilitating self-awareness, and feelings of depression, particularly in the case of shame. To the extent that one is exposed to the negative evaluations of others, shame can cause the individual to shrink in relation to previous images of self, contributing to feelings of worthlessness (Lindsay-Hartz, De Rivera, & Mascolo, 1995). Guilt is also associated with negative self-evaluations about more specific wrongdoings, including emotions such as anxiety.

Of the two self-affects, shame is judged to be less socially functional than guilt, since shame motivates the person to avoid others and to hide the self, signaling greater concern over one's own distress than empathic concern for others. Shame is also much more personally debilitating. In Chapter 10, it becomes evident that shame is particularly crippling for those who have been victims of severe and chronic abuse. Ferguson and Stegge (1995) make the distinction between "trait" and "state" shame and guilt. In the extreme, those for whom shame becomes a trait will develop a shame-prone personality in which daily life is pervaded by feelings of incompetence, fundamental worthlessness, and a sense of helplessness (see also Kaufman, 1985). Analogously, a guilt-prone person would be plagued by agitation-related emotions such as anxiety and restlessness.

Although there clearly are debilitating comcomitants, contemporary theorists have pointed to the positive functions that seemingly negative self-affects can play, particularly guilt, which is viewed as more functional than shame. For example, guilt enhances one's awareness of standards and their importance, and aids in the acquisition of knowledge of the self as *agent*, since it increases one's awareness that the I-self can hurt others but can also engage in reparation (see Barrett, 1995; Ferguson & Stegge, 1995). Furthermore, guilt promotes prosocial behaviors by inhibiting aggressive behavior, as well as communicating contrition and future good intentions to others.

Overall, guilt would appear to be more socially adaptive than shame, since it involves remorse and typically provokes behaviors directed toward reparation, rebonding, and the maintenance of emotional attachments beginning in childhood (see Tangney & Fischer, 1995). Zahn-Waxler and Robinson (1995), building upon Hoffman's (1975, 1982) theorizing, link guilt to *empathy* in that there is empathic concern for the distressed other, coupled with an awareness that one was responsible. These investigators review studies revealing that even very young children show prosocial and reparative behaviors such as helping, sharing, sympathizing, and comforting victims.

Baumeister, Stillwell, and Heatherton (1995) build upon the role of guilt as an interpersonal phenomenon that has particular functions in strengthening more developmentally advanced close relationships. They identify three particular functions. First, they present evidence revealing that guilt stimulates the avoidance of patterns of behavior that threaten the relationship in that people learn lessons and change certain behaviors to avoid hurting, distressing, or upsetting relational partners. Second, partners would appear to contribute to these processes in that they may exaggerate their suffering or distress in order to increase the partner's guilt, toward the goal of altering his/her future behavior. Third, guilt acts to redistribute the emotional distress within the dyad. Guilt makes the transgressor feel worse and the victim feel better, thus effectively transferring negative affect from the victim to the transgressor, which in turn may trigger acts of reparation. However, despite these positive functions, it should be noted that in certain guilt-ridden individuals, the obsession with perceived transgressions and accompanying self-hatred may preclude these positive functions (see Barrett, 1995).

Although shame in U.S. and other Western cultures has been identified as less adaptive than guilt, there are nevertheless interpersonal functions that shame can perform. Shame as a *state* (as contrasted to a trait) can inhibit arrogance, promote humility, and foster deference to standards of conduct valued by significant others (see H. B. Lewis, 1971). These functions are paramount in more collectivist cultures (e.g., China), where shame signals social standards of conduct that ensure appropriate interpersonal interactions within the family as well as society (see Wallbott & Scherer, 1995). In highlighting the importance of standards, the experience of shame can also provide more knowledge about the self as *object*; that is, it illuminates the looking-glass self, the self as others see it, causing the individual to evaluate or modify his/her view of the Me-self. Thus, shame can enhance self-awareness. Moreover, in signaling a discrepancy between one's actual behavior and one's ideal self, shame may, if not excessive, represent a motivation for self-improvement.

Much of the current literature on self-awareness focuses on its negative outcomes, namely, that preoccupation with one's failures can heighten and prolong depressive reactions (Duvall & Wicklund, 1972; Nolen-Hoeksema, 1990; Pyszczynski & Greenberg, 1986). Less attention has been devoted to the potentially enabling functions that self-awareness may perform. For example, in our own research with adolescents, we have examined individual differences in the extent to which preoccupied individuals can employ enabling versus debilitating forms of self-awareness as they think about their failures (Simon & Harter, 1998). This distinction is important, since those who feel that thinking about their problems makes them worse report greater levels of depression, including low self-worth and hopelessness. However, those who can use such self-reflection to their advantage, who think about potential solutions to their failures as springboards to change, report lower levels of depression and self-depreciation. Thus, certain individuals make better use of the self-awareness that can accompany emotions such as shame, leading to more adaptive outcomes.

In the prototypical analysis of shame, summarized in Table 4.1, shame has typically been associated with attempts to hide oneself, to escape the potential evaluative gaze of significant others who may find the self less than admirable, contributing to feelings of low self-worth. However, our own findings (Harter & Whitesell, 1989) reveal that not all older children adopt such a stance. Most *young* children (90%) indicate that in instances of acts that are potentially shameful, they would not want to tell anyone, particularly parents, for fear of punishment (e.g., "I'd be too scared about what mom would do"; "They'd be really mad, so I wouldn't tell them"; "I'd be afraid that I'd get in trouble"). However, among older children, many indicate that they would want to tell parents or relevant others about shameful acts, since such confessions would help them alleviate the negative affective reactions they initially experience when committing an unobserved transgression. Their responses suggest that although they have internalized the capacity to feel ashamed of themselves, relief from the experience of shame could come if they confessed to the external sources (the parents) initially responsible for instilling the standards to be internalized.

Typical examples were "If I confess, then the awful feeling wouldn't be inside of me. I'd be relieved to get rid of it"; "It would make me feel better to get it off my mind"; "You would get if off your conscience"; "Its better to tell the truth and get it off your mind"; "I'd feel a lot better being honest and just telling them." The confessions to others, therefore, seem to play a powerful role in alleviating the internal feeling associated with shame, which would appear more psychologically adaptive than reactions in which one chooses not to tell significant others what he/she had done (particularly if the fear that they will find out persists). Confession, in turn, should serve to reestablish relationships that may have been marred by the actions that produced shame in children and anger in socializing agents. Thus, for those who are able to adopt this stance, shame should be less debilitating than for those who seek to avoid others in an attempt to hide the self.

In addition to generalizations that shame is associated with the need to take oneself into hiding, shame has also been associated with *self-blame*, where it is typically assumed that blaming the self, a negative internal attribution, has debilitating consequences for the individual. For children, items tapping this construct can be found on perceptions of control measures (e.g., Connell, 1985), where children can indicate that their failures are their fault, as well as on depression measures (e.g., Harter, Nowakowski, & Marold, 1988), where children can indicate that they blame themselves for things that go wrong. However, it is not a foregone conclusion that internal attributions for failure are necessarily debilitating. We sought to examine this issue in one Master's thesis (Johnson, 1993), where we made the distinction between *self-blame*, namely, the attribution of failure to a deficit in the self, and *responsibility*, namely, the recognition that one has played a role in failures without attributing it to a deficit in the self. A sample statement tapping self-blame in the achievement domain is "When I don't do well at my schoolwork, I usually blame myself and feel that I am *stupid.*" An example of a responsibility item in this same domain is "When I don't do well at my schoolwork, I take *responsibility* for what I did, since it was my fault, but I *don't* feel that I am stupid."

We found support for the hypothesis that these two orientations to internal attributions for failure would be associated with different motivational patterns, as well as self-representations. Those endorsing the self-blaming attribution, which involved perceived deficiencies in the self, were much more likely to avoid dealing with schoolwork because of the conclusion that they could not do better. Moreover, they reported lower perceptions of scholastic competence, as well as global self-worth. Conversely, those who opted for the responsibility orientation were more likely to display increased effort ("I want to try harder to do better the next time") and to report more positive perceptions of their scholastic competence and global self-worth.

To the extent that internal attributions for failure are associated with shame, these findings suggest that outcomes will differ depending upon the particular nature of such attributions; that is, shame associated with failure attributions that imply deficiencies in the self will be the most debilitating. However, shame linked to failure attributions that imply a sense of responsibility for one's actions, without the perception that one is fundamentally deficient, can have positive, motivational benefits, leading to renewed effort in the face of favorable self-evaluations. The practical implications of this distinction are obvious in that parents, educators, and mental health professionals should, if the conclusion is realistic, support the responsibility orientation, since it should be associated with the most favorable outcomes, even in the face of accompanying feelings of shame; that is, shame in such situations can be functional in the service of enhanced motivation, as well as the maintenance of positive self-evaluations.

CONCLUSION

Self-conscious emotions such as pride, shame, and guilt are important constructs in the repertoire of individuals' self-representations. They represent a constellation of perceptions with regard to their causes, personal attributions, implications for the self, as well as the role of the other, and associated behavioral and emotional reactions. The prototypes that have been identified in the literature, and which were summarized in Table 4.1, characterize relatively mature manifestations of these self-affects. However, these features are only gradually acquired through cognitive-developmental advances and particular socialization experiences. One can identify those prerequisites for the initial *display* of these emotions beginning in early childhood, for example, the emergence of an I-self that has the rudimentary capacity to observe the standards of others in comparison to the performance of the self. Specific child-rearing practices also enhance the experience and display of self-conscious emotions.

With regard to self-representations, the primary topic of this volume, there are also cognitive and social prerequisites governing the emergence in childhood of an *understanding* of the causes of self-affects such as pride and shame, as demonstrated in our own research. Thus, there are predictable developmental sequences revealing that to understand the concepts of pride and shame, children must be able to coordinate representations that involve the impact on the self as well as upon another, an ability that does not emerge until middle childhood. Socialization experiences that facilitate the internalization of the standards of socializing agents, allowing the child to ultimately develop the capacity to be proud or ashamed of the self in the absence of an observing other, are also critical. Moreover, there are cross-cultural differences in these processes, in that in collectivistic cultures, shame is more salient and appears at earlier ages.

The importance of these developmental trajectories hinges upon the *function* of self-conscious emotions. While the positive functions of pride are most obvious, there are also potential positive functions for those self-affects that have typically been described as more negative, namely, guilt and shame. Guilt would appear to have more positive consequences to the extent that the individual engages in confessional and reparative efforts that may serve to restore relational bonds. However, shame, if not excessive, can also lead to self-corrective consequences and thereby serve a motivational function. The ultimate importance of these observations lies in the fact that self-representations are not simply defined as cognitive concepts about the self but include affective reactions that also become codified and integrated into one's self-portrait.

The Content, Valence, and Organization of Self-Evaluative Judgments

The developmental analysis presented in Chapters 2 and 3 made the case for how the structure of the self-system, broadly defined, undergoes change as self-representations first become differentiated and then, at a subsequent stage, are integrated into higher-order generalizations that define the self. In the present chapter, attention focuses more explicitly on those self-representations that represent self-*evaluations*, namely, judgments of self-attributes that range from favorable to unfavorable. Specifically, how do individuals personally evaluate their sense of adequacy across the multiple domains of their lives, as well as construct a more global judgment concerning their overall worth as a person? From a historical perspective, James (1892) set the stage for a *multidimensional* model of the self in distinguishing between three constituents of the self-system, namely, material, social, and spiritual selves. However, James also ushered in the concept of *global self-esteem*, postulating that there is a certain average tone of self-feeling that individuals possess. Cooley voiced a similar sentiment in postulating an overall sense of self-respect.

This chapter begins with a discussion of the shift away from purely unidimensional models of self to multidimensional models that more adequately capture the complexity of the network of self-evaluative judgments. These models, which identify domain-specific self-concepts, as well as preserve the construct of global self-esteem or self-worth, have dictated the development of a variety of self-report instruments to tap these constructs at different points in the life span. An appreciation for both domain-specific and global self-evaluations naturally led theorists to speculate on the relationship between these two types of self-judgments. This focus, in turn, has produced a number of *hierarchical* models in which global self-esteem is placed at the apex and particular domains and subdomains are nested underneath. Multidimensional models also invite an analysis of a *profile* of self-evaluative judgments, where individuals or subgroups report different levels of adequacy or competence across the domains included. Within this context, there is an exploration of gender differences in the profiles for males and females, where the pattern is quite robust across numerous countries. It is also instructive to examine the profiles of special groups of children, such as those with medical conditions (e.g., asthma, diabetes, cancer), since the interpretation of their pattern of scores presents very real challenges. Finally, there may be particular pitfalls in administering instruments designed for Western samples to children and adolescents in Eastern cultures such as China and Japan.

UNIDIMENSIONAL VERSUS MULTIDIMENSIONAL MODELS OF SELF-EVALUATION

The 1960s represented an era in which unidimensional models were fervently embraced (see Coopersmith, 1967; Piers & Harris, 1964). Although the instruments developed by these investigators tapped self-evaluative judgments in a variety of life arenas (e.g., performance at school, peer relationships, family relationships), the underlying additive model dictated that the judgments be averaged into a single score. It was this score that represented an individual's level of self-esteem. Coopersmith (1967) was a major proponent of the view that self-esteem is global in nature. He argued that children do not make self-evaluative differentiations among the various domains of their lives. Unfortunately, inadequacies in his methodology, including selection of item content, the question format, and small sample size, led to this erroneous conclusion (see Harter, 1983). Other investigators, for example, Piers and Harris (1964), began with the assumption that self-esteem is relatively unidimensional and therefore adopted the single-score approach. However, their own empirical work has revealed that children actually do make different evaluative judgments across the different domains they sampled, thereby leading them to alter their conceptualization and to conclude that the self-system of children is indeed multifaceted.

Within recent years, there has been a dramatic shift away from the earlier unidimensional models of self. Such models have been challenged on the grounds that they mask important evaluative distinctions that individuals, including children, make about their adequacy in different domains of their lives. The *zeitgeist*, supported by extensive data, clearly reflects the view that multidimensional models of self far more adequately describe the phenomenology of self-evaluations than do unidimensional models (see Bracken, 1996; Damon & Hart, 1988; Harter, 1982a, 1985b, 1990a, 1993; Hattie, 1992; Hattie & Marsh, 1996; Marsh, 1986, 1987, 1989; Mullener & Laird, 1971; Oosterwegel & Oppenheimer, 1993; Shavelson & Marsh, 1986). Much of the evidence for the multidimensional structure of self-evaluative judgments comes from the administration of instruments that tap a number of different domains of the self-concept, followed by both exploratory and confirmatory factor-analytic procedures revealing that each of the domains defines a discrete factor.

Although there has been a shift to a multidimensional focus, investigators have retained global self-esteem (or self-worth; these terms are used interchangeably) in their models and measures (that are appropriate for middle childhood and beyond). Rosenberg (1979) was one of the first to offer a compelling argument for why we should both retain the notion of global self-esteem and focus on the constituent parts of this whole. "Both exist within the individual's phenomenal field as separate and distinguishable entities, and each can and should be studied in its own right" (p. 20). The findings clearly reveal that beginning in middle childhood, individuals have the cognitive capacity to make global judgments of their worth as a person, in addition to their ability to provide specific self-evaluations across a variety of domains. Young children, however, do not possess a conscious, verbalizable concept of their overall self-worth (Harter & Pike, 1984). As mentioned in Chapter 2, younger children do *exude* a sense of their self-worth or esteem, and these behavioral manifestations (e.g., displays of confidence) can be reliably rated by observers (Haltiwanger, 1989; Harter, 1990a). Thus, the prevailing models do not pit multidimensional models against unidimensional models but recognize that domain-specific judgments as well as global evaluations of worth are represented in an individual's repertoire of self-evaluations beginning in middle childhood.

One cardinal feature of most cognitive-developmental theories is that there is increasing *differentiation* with development. This principle can be applied to the domains of self-evaluation in that the number of domains that can be differentiated increases with development. We have addressed this issue in the construction of a life-span battery of separate instruments that assess self-evaluations across the following periods of development: (1) early childhood, (2) middle to late childhood, (3) adolescence, (4) the college years, (5) the adult years (early through midlife), and (6) late adulthood. Table 5.1 presents the domains that are tapped at each age period. As this table indicates, the number of domains increases across the first four age periods. Moreover, although the absolute number of domains does not differ dramatically across the three periods of adulthood, there are differences in the *content* of the subscales, which are necessary to capture age-appropriate changes in the relevance of particular issues that define the self.

TABLE 5.1. Domains of the Self-Concept Tapped by Our Instruments at Each Period of the Life Span

Early childhood	Middle to late childhood	Adolescence	College years	Early through middle adulthood	Late adulthood
Cognitive competence	Scholastic competence	Scholastic competence	Scholastic competence Intellectual ability Creativity	Intelligence	Cognitive abilities
		Job competence	Job competence	Job competence	Job competence
Physical competence	Athletic competence	Athletic competence	Athletic competence	Athletic competence	
Physical appearance	Physical appearance	Physical appearance	Physical appearance	Physical appearance	Physical appearance
Peer acceptance	Peer acceptance	Peer acceptance Close friendship Romantic relationships	Peer acceptance Close friendship Romantic relationships Relationships with parents	Sociability Close friendship Intimate relationships	Relationships with friends Family relationships
Behavioral conduct	Behavioral conduct	Conduct/morality	Morality Sense of humor	Morality Sense of humor Nurturance Household management	Morality Nurturance Personal, household management
				Adequacy as a provider	Adequacy as a provider Leisure activities Health status Life satisfaction Reminiscence
Global self-worth	Global self-worth	Global self-worth	Global self-worth	Global self-worth	Global self-worth

It should be noted that the domains listed in Table 5.1 represent arenas that to date have been included at each level. One can well imagine other self-concept domains (e.g., mechanical ability, musical aptitude). Moreover, one could further differentiate domains of academic competence, as Marsh and his colleagues have done, and as we have done on our Self-Perception Profile for Learning Disabled Students (Renick & Harter, 1988). The justification for the domains we have included is that they are relatively important to most individuals at a given age. However, if investigators are interested in other domains, they may well want to add these domains by crafting relevant items in the format of our instruments and including them along with the original subscales.

Early Childhood

With regard to the structure and content appropriate during early childhood, findings from 4- to 7-year-olds employing a recent revision of our Pictorial Scale of Perceived Competence and Social Acceptance for Young Children (Harter & Pike, 1984) reveal a factor structure in which judgments in the domains of Cognitive and Physical Competence define one factor, whereas perceptions of Physical Appearance, Social Acceptance, and Behavioral Conduct define a second factor (Nikkari & Harter, 1993). Thus, although young children are able to make evaluative judgments in all five domains, these would appear to reduce to two broad evaluative dimensions, namely, judgments that refer specifically to *competence* versus judgments in other domains that capture *personal* and *social adequacy*. To assess these self-evaluations, we have employed a pictorial format in which the child is presented with two pictures: one of a child demonstrating competence or adequacy, and one in which the child lacks competence or adequacy (see Figure 5.1). The young respondent first selects which of the two children depicted is most life himself/herself. Under each picture are two circles, one small and one large. This child is told that the small circle should be chosen if he or she is just "a little like that," whereas the large circle should be chosen if he or she is "a lot like that." Items are scored on a 4-point scale, where a score of 1 (representing the choice of the large circle under the less than competent child) reflects the lowest perceptions of competence or adequacy and a score of 4 (representing the choice of the large circle for the competent child) reflects the highest perceptions of competence or adequacy.

Middle to Late Childhood

At the next general developmental level of middle to late childhood, we shift to a questionnaire format. The Self-Perception Profile for Children

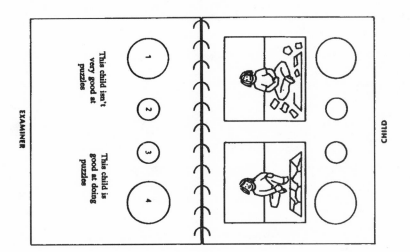

FIGURE 5.1. Sample item from the Pictorial Scale of Perceived Competence and Social Acceptance for Young Children.

(Harter, 1985b) contains five domain-specific subscales tapping Scholastic Competence, Athletic Competence, Peer Likability, Physical Appearance, and Behavioral Conduct, as well as a separate subscale that assesses Global Self-Worth. It should be noted that the index of Global Self-Worth is *not* the sum of the domain-specific subscale scores. Rather, Global Self-Worth is tapped by its own set of items that assesses how much the individual evaluates his/her overall worth as a person.

In shifting to a questionnaire, we sought to develop a question format that would parallel the type of choices that were built into our pictorial scale for younger children, and that could be scored according to a 4-point scale. This principle has guided the construction of each of our instruments such that for purposes of age comparisons, either in cross-sectional or longitudinal research, the potential range of scores is identical, namely, 1 (low) to 4 (high). The structured-alternative question format we developed was also designed to offset tendencies to give socially desirable responses (see Harter, 1982a). Thus, children are presented with items such as the following, below where the first item taps Global Self-Worth and the second taps Scholastic Competence. Respondents are first asked to select the type of kids they are most like, those described in the first part of the statement, or those described in the second part of the statement. Having made this choice, they then indicate whether that description is *Really True for Me* or *Sort of True for Me*. Items are scored from 1 to 4 as the sample items indicate (however, these values are *not* included on the actual questionnaire presented to respondents).

Really True for Me	Sort of True for Me				Sort of True for Me	Really True for Me
☐	☐	Some kids are often *unhappy* with themselves.	BUT	Other kids are pretty *pleased* with themselves.	☐	☐
☐	☐	Some kids feel like they are *just as smart* as other kids their age.	BUT	Other kids aren't so sure and *wonder* if they are as smart.	☐	☐

Several principles guided the development of this question format. The Some kids/Other kids format was designed to reflect more natural statements in the vernacular, contrasting others with whom one could *identify* rather than requiring that subjects endorse the typical bald "I" statements, particularly those that make reference to their limitations (e.g., "I do poorly at schoolwork") that appear on earlier instruments (e.g., Coopersmith, 1967; Piers & Harris, 1964). Evidence (see Harter, 1982a) reveals that this format reduces the tendency to give socially desirable responses. Moreover, we wanted to broaden the range of possible choices from two (as on the previous scales) to four, since we felt that respondents could make these discriminations. Finally, it was desirable to construct a format in which respondents would not have to deal with decisions about statements that were *false*, as in previous instruments that have utilized a true/false or like me/unlike me response choice. The double negatives that such decisions require on certain items (e.g., negating a negative statement about the self) are often confusing to children, as well as to some adolescents and adults.

Factor-analyses across numerous samples reveal that each of the five specific self-concept domains defines its own discrete factor, unlike the factor pattern obtained for younger children, where the five domains collapsed into two factors, as described earlier. Thus, the evidence reveals that the structure of self-evaluations becomes more differentiated as one moves into middle childhood, consistent with what one would expect from a developmental perspective. It should be noted that at this developmental level, as well as at subsequent ages, the Global Self-Worth, subscale is not included in the factoring analysis. Rather, it is a qualitatively different judgment of one's overall worth that is differentially related to particular domains across individual subjects or subgroups of children, in part determined by the importance of success attached to each domain. For example, with children heavily engaged in sports, Athletic Competence may be more closely related to Global Self-Worth, whereas for children in a program for the intellectually gifted, Scholastic Competence may be more predictive of Global Self-Worth. The purpose of factoring the domain-specific subscales is to determine whether children discriminate the domains included, providing evidence for the utility of multidimensional models of self-evaluative judgments. Which domains best *predict* Global Self-Worth is a separate and critical issue to which we shall return later in this chapter.

Adolescence

The Self-Perception Profile for Adolescents (Harter, 1988b) adds three new arenas, Close Friendship, Romantic Appeal, and Job Competence, to the domains included at the previous ages (Scholastic Competence, Athletic Competence, Peer Likability, Physical Appearance, and Behavioral Conduct). The particular issues underlying the new subscales become more salient as one moves into adolescence. This instrument also contains a Global Self-Worth subscale. Factoring of the eight domain-specific subscale scores reveals a very clear factor pattern in which each of the domains defines its own independent factor.

College Years

At the next level, we developed the Self-Perception Profile for College Students (Neemann & Harter, 1987) to tap domains relevant to young adults who were pursuing a college education. The eight domains included on the adolescent version were carried into this instrument, although where needed, there were wording changes designed to make the language more age-appropriate. The content of what was labeled Behavioral Conduct underwent the greatest transformation in that we altered the content, and subscale title, to make reference to Morality. Moreover, additional domains were needed to capture the complexity at the college level. Noteworthy was the fact that in addition to the domain of Scholastic Competence, college students can differentiate the domains of Intellectual Ability and Creativity, each of which define its own factor. For example, a student may work hard to earn good grades but feel that he/she lacks a certain level of intellectual ability or creativity. Another student may judge the self to be extremely creative, or, alternatively, highly intelligent, but is not applying these talents to their academic pursuits. Pilot interviews by Neemann with college students revealed the need to add two new domains that were deemed salient to students' self-representations, Sense of Humor and Ability to Relate to Parents.

Thus, the overall structure at this level includes 12 specific domains, each of which defines its own discrete factor. The instrument also includes a Global Self-Worth subscale.

Early through Middle Adulthood

To assess the self-evaluations of adults in the world of work and family, we developed the Self-Perception Profile for Adults (Messer & Harter, 1989). Subscales tap certain content that is comparable to the college version in that we have included Intelligence, Job Competence, Athletic Competence, Physical Appearance, Sociability, Close Friendships, Intimate Relationships, Morality, and Sense of Humor. Three new subscales were added to tap issues that become salient for adults in the world of work and family. These include Nurturance, Household Management, and Adequacy as a Provider. Employing factor-analytic procedures, each of the 12 domains has been found to define its own discrete factor. As with the other instruments, a Global Self-Worth subscale is included.

Late Adulthood

The most recent instrument to be added to our life-span battery is the Self-Perception Profile for Those in Late Adulthood (Harter & Kreinik, 1998). As can be seen in Table 5.1, a number of the subscale titles are similar. However, the content is somewhat different in that individuals are asked to reflect back on their life. For example, relationships with friends taps satisfaction with the friendships they have formed, including their ability to stay in touch with close friends. A new subscale, Family Relationships, asked them to evaluate how pleased they are with the relationships they have established and maintained with family members. The Nurturance subscale has the same flavor, namely, it taps whether they have been sufficiently nurturant to the important people in their lives. Similarly, Job Competence asks them to review how satisfied they are with how they have performed over the years, including whether they achieved the occupational goals they set for themselves. The Morality subscale also asks that they reflect on whether they feel they have lived their lives morally. The Household Management subscale similarly requires that they engage in a life review, evaluating the extent to which they have been able to provide the necessities for those who have been dependent on them.

The Cognitive Abilities subscale is somewhat different from the items that tapped intelligence on the preceding two instruments (for college students and for adults in the world of work and family). It focuses more on particular cognitive abilities, such as being able to remember what one needs to, being mentally alert, and having the mental skills to solve problems that confront them. Two new subscales, Leisure Activities and Health Status, were designed to assess current satisfaction with activities that contribute to their sense of well-being and an evaluation of whether they have done what they could to maintain good health. Finally, two somewhat more general subscales were included to tap Life Satisfaction (Have life choices given them a sense of purpose, meaning, and inner peace?) and Reminiscence (How much do they enjoy looking back on their life, reviewing past memories, and sharing these past experiences with others?). There are 13 specific domains in all, in addition to a Global Self-Worth subscale. (We are currently in the process of administering this instrument to a variety of samples, after which we will examine its factor structure.)

Although it is always possible to think of additional domains, as well as further differentiate the existing domains, we feel that this life-span battery does reflect important differences in the structure and content of the network of self-evaluations as individuals move into new periods of development. The fact that seemingly analogous constructs are defined somewhat differently at different life stages is inevitable if one is to remain developmentally sensitive to psychological changes in the meaning of these self-evaluations. This issue is not unique to the assessment of self-representations, but to most constructs that developmentalists have sought to measure across portions of the life span. Nevertheless, similar constructs can be compared across age levels as a general indication of possible developmental changes. In making such comparisons, it is critical that mean scores be analyzed and reported according to the 4-point scale that has been utilized at every age period (rather than total scores, since the number of subscale items varies somewhat across instruments, given that we need more items at the younger ages for purposes of reliability). Comparisons across age groups will only have meaning if a common metric is employed. (Unfortunately, certain investigators have reported total scores based on the erroneous assumption that they are more sensitive because the range appears broader. Statistically, there will be no difference, and thus keeping scores on the intended 1- to 4-point scale will make any given set of findings much more interpretable.)

Other investigators have developed multidimensional measures, although typically these have primarily been restricted to older children and adolescents or young adults. For example, another popular multidimensional instrument for use with children has been developed by Marsh. The Self-Description Questionnaire–I (Marsh, 1988) initially included the domains of Physical Abilities, Physical Appearance, Peer Relations, Parent Relations, and General School Performance, and is appropriate for children. The Self-Description Questionnaire–II (Marsh, 1990), developed for adolescents, added the domains of Opposite-Sex Relations, Same-Sex Relations, Honesty, and Emotional Stability. The Self-Description Questionnaire–III, appropriate for older adolescents and young adults (Marsh, 1991), taps 13 dimensions of the self-concept. In addition to the discrete domains tapped by these instruments, each also contains a General Self-Concept Scale, tapping content similar to our Global Self-Worth Scale and Rosenberg's (1979) Self-Esteem Inventory. The Multidimensional Self-Concept Scale, developed by Bracken (1992), is the most recent such measure for use with children. It taps six domains, Social, Competence, Affect, Family, Physical, and Academic, as well as a separate subscale to assess Global Self-Concept. Thus, instruments that combine domain-specific evaluations as well as a global evaluation of one's sense of overall worth have become the measures of choice in the 1990s. For a very comprehensive review of these and other self-concept measures, see Keith and Bracken (1996). The Harter and Marsh scales are also reviewed by Wylie (1989).

THE SHIFT TO HIERARCHICAL MODELS

An appreciation for both global and domain-specific self-evaluations naturally led theorists to speculate on the structure of the relationship between these two types of self-judgments. This, in turn, produced a number of *hierarchical* models in which global self-esteem or general self-concept is placed at the apex and particular domains and subdomains are nested underneath (see Hattie & Marsh, 1996). The original models were more conceptually than empirically derived. For example, Epstein (1973) suggested that the postulates one has about the self are hierarchically arranged, with self-esteem as the superordinate construct. Epstein's second-order postulates include general competence, moral self-approval, power, and love worthiness (see Coopersmith, 1967, who identified four very similar dimensions). Lower-order postulates, for example, those organized under competence, include assessments of general mental and physical ability. The lowest-order postulates under competence include assessments of specific abilities. (There are similar types of subcategories under the other three second-order postulates.) Epstein suggests that as one moves from lower-order to higher-order postulates, they become increasingly important to the maintenance of the individual's self-theory.

A somewhat different hierarchical model can be found in the theorizing of Shavelson, Hubner, and Stanton (1976), who initially identified two broad classes, academic and nonacademic self-concepts, nested under general self-concept at the apex. The nonacademic self-concept is subdivided into social, emotional, and physical domains. Physical self-concept is further differentiated into physical ability and physical appearance. The academic self-concept is subdivided into particular school subjects: English, History, Math, and Science. Self-perceptions at lower levels were hypothesized to have a causal impact on those at the next levels, for example, perceptions of math competence "cause" perceptions of overall academic achievement, which in turn impact general self-concept (Byrne, 1996). Marsh and colleagues have conducted extensive research on this model, employing hierarchical, confirmatory factor-analytic and multitrait, multimethod statistical procedures applied to data from the Self-Description Questionnaires (see reviews in Byrne, 1996; Hattie, 1992; Marsh, 1990, 1993; Marsh, Byrne, & Shavelson, 1992).

Since their initial formulation, Shavelson & Marsh (1986) have proposed an even more differentiated model in which academic self-concept is further subdivided (Marsh, 1993). For example, the initial second-level construct of academic competence has been differentiated into Verbal and Mathematics self-concepts, given their empirical independence. Moreover, other academic domains have been added, for example, Foreign Languages and History under the verbal self-concept, and Science under the math self-concept. There has been some, though not unequivocal, empirical support for the model initially proposed by Shavelson and colleagues, as well as their revised model (see reviews cited earlier).

Song and Hattie (1984) have also modified the original Shavelson et al. model, dividing the academic construct into Perceived Ability, Actual Achievement, and more interpersonal perceptions of self in the classroom (e.g., "I feel left out in class"). The social dimension is divided into Peer and Family self-concepts. A third dimension, presentation of self, is divided into Confidence or Self-Regard and Physical Self-Concept. Factor-analytic procedures provide some support for this hierarchy (see also Hattie, 1992). Yet another, even more complex hierarchical model has been developed by L'Ecuyer (1992). Five overarching central categories are proposed, with each further divided into two intermediate subcategories: the Material Self (Somantic and Possessive), Personal Self (Self-Image and Self-Identity), Adaptive Self (Self-Esteem and Self-Activities), Social Self (Social Attitudes and Sexuality), and Self/Non-Self (References to Others and Opinions of Others). Each of the intermediate categories is further divided into "secondary" subcategories. Unlike the efforts described earlier, in which subjects are presented with structured questionnaires that include items tapping each dimension, L'Ecuyer analyzes the spontaneous self-descriptions of subjects. Although the hierarchical nature cannot be directly tested through factor-analytic procedures, L'Ecuyer presents profiles of the percentage of individuals generating self-descriptions at each of the three levels (Central, Intermediate, and Secondary) for men and women, observing that this procedure can be broadened to account for developmental differences across the life span.

In summary, the hierarchical models that have become popular have considerable appeal in their organized representation of networks of domain-specific judgments that combine to predict global self-esteem. However, these general frameworks may not be applicable to the structure of self-representations for given individuals or particular subgroups of respondents. For example, a cardinal assumption underlying many of these hierarchical models is that people organize or structure the vast amount of information they have about themselves into predictable subcategories, which they then relate to one another as higher-order clusters. These clusters, in turn, are expected to generically impact global self-concept at the apex of the model (Marsh et al., 1992). However, one has to ask whether the *statistical* structure extracted for large samples does, in fact, mirror the psychological structure as it is phenomenologically experienced by individuals. The statistical procedures employed do not directly tap the manner in which individual subjects themselves organize their self-constructs. For example, our efforts (Harter & Whitesell, 1996) reveal numerous pathways to global self-worth that represent different combinations of domain-specific self-evaluations and related perceptions of support. Thus, the hierarchical models reflected in statistical solutions may confirm theories in the minds of psychologists but may not necessarily describe the actual self-theories in the minds of individuals (Harter, 1986a; see also Hattie, 1992, for an excellent discussion and critique of hierarchical models). Procedures that directly tap the manner in which subjects organize their own self-constructs, as well as techniques that allow for different constellations of attributes that may be predictive of global self-worth, are required.

For example, with regard to how individuals themselves may cluster self-attributes, Linville (1987) reports that there are clear individual differences in the complexity of the self-structure when subjects are asked to directly sort self-traits. Complexity refers to both the number of levels in the hierarchy and the number of categories or degree of differentiation. Other sorting procedures also reveal categorization principles that differ from those proposed in the hierarchical models described earlier. For example, in asking adolescent subjects to sort self-attributes in central, intermediate, and peripheral categories, Harter and Monsour (1992) found that the *valence* of the attributes was more salient than the particular content domain (academic self, social self, etc.). The vast majority of central attributes were positive in valence whereas negative attributes were relegated to the periphery of one's self-portrait. Showers' (1995) findings point to other interesting individual differences in how subjects organize self-attributes that are positive and negative in valence. Certain individuals employ what she terms "evaluative compartmentalization," in which positive attributes that cut across roles or domains form one category, whereas negative attributes across those same roles form a separate category. In contrast, others employ "evaluative integration," in which attributes are categorized by role (me with friends vs. me with my boss). Within each separate role, there are both positive and negative attributes.

Indeed, there is a growing literature describing an increasing number of alternative models of the cognitive organization of self (see reviews in Greenwald & Pratkanis, 1984; Higgins & Bargh, 1987; Kihlstrom & Cantor, 1984; Klein & Kihlstrom, 1986; Wyer & Srull, 1989). Certain researchers have developed the notion of self as a hierarchical category structure, building upon the initial formulation of Rosch (1975) and Cantor and Mischel (1979). Others have viewed the self as a dynamic system of schemas, a memory structure in which certain attributes are more closely linked to the self than others (Markus, 1977; Markus & Sentis, 1982; Markus & Wurf, 1987). Others claim that self-knowledge is organized around "prototypes" that also serve to structure one's perceptions of other people (e.g., Kuiper, 1981; Lord, Gilbert, & Stanley, 1983; see also Rosenberg, 1988). Still others focus on the multiplicity of the self, demonstrating that multidimensional scaling techniques reveal individual differences in how self attributes are organized (e.g., Breckler & Greenwald, 1982). Most recently, controversy has surrounded a variety of models that speak to whether general trait knowledge is represented in memory independently of specific, trait-relevant behavioral knowledge (see Srull & Wyer, 1993).

A review of these issues and models is beyond the scope of this chapter. However, it is clear that while hierarchical models of the self-concept have enjoyed some popularity, increasingly there are alternative theories that are based on the direct examination of how subjects process information about self-relevant and irrelevant attributes. Such an examination may well reveal that there are different hierarchies for different individuals, a topic to which I shall return in evaluating James' formulation on the causes of self-esteem. For James, there was not one common hierarchy across individuals. Rather, self-esteem, at the apex, resulted from a comparison of a given individual's hierarchy of perceived successes in relation to the hierarchy of the importance of success in each corresponding domain. The discrepancy or congruence between these two hierarchies, which differs from person to person, is the critical predictive construct.

MULTIDIMENSIONALITY: A PROFILE APPROACH

A major value of multidimensional approaches to self-evaluation lies in the demonstration that a given individual typically evaluates the self differently in different domains, providing a *profile* of his/her sense of adequacy across relevant life arenas. In fact, multidimensional approaches can only be justified to the extent that the majority of individuals do evaluate themselves differently across domains. In any given data set, one can identify individual children, adolescents, or adults who feel uniformly very positive about themselves across domains. Analogously, there are those who give themselves very unfavorable ratings across the board. However, the majority of individuals report meaningful variations in their perceptions of competence or adequacy in different arenas of their life. An examination of individual scores reveals myriad profiles that cannot easily be reduced to a few common prototypes. In our own work, we have been far more impressed by the variety of profiles that emerge, beginning in middle childhood. The adoption of an idiographic frame of reference, in which one attends to individual profiles, has particular utility clinically, where the diagnostician or therapist wishes to pinpoint perceptions of personal strengths as well as weaknesses. Interventions, in turn, may be designed according to an individual's particular profile.

A profile approach may also be useful in understanding subgroups of individuals who share common features. For example, one can ask whether there are different profiles for males and females. Other investigators may be interested in special groups, such as learning disabled children or adolescents, mentally retarded children, gifted children, or children with particular medical conditions (e.g., asthma, diabetes, cancer, etc.), that may compromise individuals with a particular disorder. Others may be interested in cross-cultural comparisons, or an analysis of subgroups within a given culture. Toward these ends, it is important to determine whether the *content* of the instruments administered is meaningful to the subgroups included, as well as whether the normative *structure* is maintained across subgroups. If one is satisfied that these two conditions have been met, then analyses of differences in subscale means may be open to meaningful interpretation. A few examples of each type of comparison illuminate the potential value of a profile approach, as well as pitfalls that one may encounter in comparing different subgroups.

Gender Differences in Domain-Specific and Global Self-Evaluations

There is now an emerging body of literature that has examined gender differences in subscale scores among older children, adolescents, and college students. For the most part, the findings are quite consistent with regard to a number of gender differences as well as similarities. The major pattern to be documented is that females consistently report more unfavorable perceptions of their *appearance* or looks and their *athletic competence,*

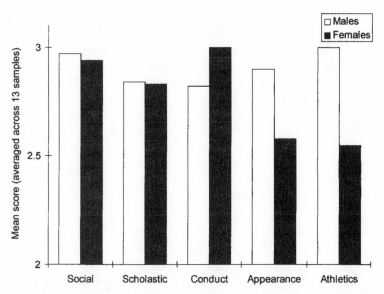

FIGURE 5.2. Domain scores for male and female older children and adolescents.

the two dimensions that define the physical self. Across numerous studies from our own laboratory, the mean scores of females on these two subscales fall within the range of 2.3 to 2.6, whereas scores for males typically fall within the range of 2.8 to 3.3. Moreover, these gender differences are highly significant (p's from .01 to .0001).

Figure 5.2 summarizes the data across 13 samples (four from elementary school, five at the middle school level, and four at the high school level). The pattern is the same across all samples. As the figure reveals, males' scores reveal much less variability across domains, hovering at or just below 3.0 on the 4-point scale. The profile for girls shows greater variability in that although scores for social acceptance, scholastic competence, and conduct are at or slightly below 3.0, the scores for physical appearance and athletic competence are near the midpoint (2.5) for the scale.

Moreover, this pattern has been found to be highly robust across different countries where gender differences for physical appearance and athletic competence are similar in magnitude and highly significant. Thus, in addition to other findings in the United States (see also Hagborg, 1994) the more favorable perceptions of physical appearance and athletic competence by male children and adolescents has been found in other English-speaking countries, namely, *England* (Fox, Page, Armstrong, & Kirby, 1994), *Australia* (Trent, Russell, & Cooney, 1994), and *Ireland* (Granleese & Joseph, 1993). The very same pattern has been documented across a range of non-English-speaking countries, including the French-speaking areas of *Switzerland* (Bolognini, Plancerel, Bettschart, & Halfon, 1996; Pierrehumbert, Plancherel, & Jankech-Caretta, 1987), *Italy* (Pedrabiss & Santinello, 1992; Pedrabissi, Santinello, & Scarpazza, 1988), *Holland* (van Dongen-Melman, Koot, & Verhulst, 1993), *China* (Meredith, Abbott, & Zheng, 1991; Stigler, Smith, & Mao, 1985), *Japan* (Maeda, 1997) and *Korea* (Rhee, 1993).

The very same gender pattern favoring males on both perceived athletic ability and attractiveness persists at the college level. Our own data reveal that female students feel significantly worse about their appearance (M = 2.57) and their athletic competence (M = 2.67) than do males (M's of 2.88 and 3.00, respectively). These same gender differences have been reported in other college samples as well (Crocker & Ellsworth, 1990; Klein, O'Bryant, & Hopkins, 1996; McGregor, Mayleben, Buzzanga, Davis, & Becker, 1992; McGregor, Eveleigh, Syler, & Davis, 1991).

Interpretations of the gender differences in perceived athletic competence have focused on the fact that, historically, sports has been largely a male domain, with far more opportunities for athletic competition that would allow boys to develop their physical skills. Moreover, male sports figures represent powerful role models that male children and adolescents are eager to emulate. Despite the gains that some females have achieved in entering the world of sports, women athletes have not, for the most part, been viewed as role models for those girls and female adolescents in the mainstream culture.

Clearly, in the United States, the current female role models are glamorous women who are extremely thin, an image that is not consistent with the muscular, mesomorphic body types of most female athletes. Moreover, images of female attractiveness are very punishing in that they are unattainable by the vast majority of girls and women in the culture. As a result, most females fall far short of these ideals, resulting in the pattern of findings obtained for perceived physical appearance, namely, that females feel particularly inadequate. Males, on the other hand, can be judged attractive not only on the basis of their physical features but by virtue of the fact that they have money, status, or power. (A magazine poll of women just after the Gulf War had ended revealed that General Norman Schwartzkopf was judged to be the sexiest man in America!).

The overall pattern of gender differences obtained for both athletic competence and physical appearance is qualified by an examination of particular subgroups of females. For example, in the study of college students by Crocker and Ellsworth (1990), the investigators separately examined a subgroup of Physical Education majors. They found that the females in this group reported significantly higher perceptions of their athletic ability than did the normative sample as a whole. Moreover, among Physical Education majors, the female students did not differ from the male students. The advantage conferred by the Physical Education program did *not*, however, transfer to the domain of physical *appearance*, where females continued to feel significantly worse about their looks than did males. Marsh and Jackson (1986) report a similar pattern in that female athletes, beginning at the high school level, reported higher physical ability than did nonathletes, although the groups did not differ significantly in their perceptions of their physical appearance.

We have also found across several adolescent samples that *gender orientation* impacts the perceptions of females in particular. Those females endorsing a feminine orientation (where they identify with feminine sex-role stereotypes but reject the masculine attributes) report more negative perceptions of their athletic ability (M = 2.41) and their physical appearance (M = 2.43) than do androgynous females who endorse both feminine and masculine items (M's = 2.92 and 2.87, respectively). The scores of these androgynous females do not differ significantly from those of either masculine or androgynous males, for whom scores range from 2.92 to 3.18 across the two subscales. Thus, feminine girls are at particular risk for unfavorable evaluations of their physical selves. To the extent that they view athletics as a male domain, they are likely to avoid sports activities that would allow them to develop physical skills. However, their primarily feminine orientation would appear to lead them to emphasize the importance of physical attractiveness. Attentiveness to this domain may well serve to highlight the difficulty of attaining the impossible standards of beauty that are touted by the culture. As a result, they judge their appearance quite unfavorably relative to the judgments of androgynous females and to both androgynous and masculine males.

Femininity, therefore, will represent a liability in each of these physical domains to the extent that it is not combined with masculine attributes. It should be noted that the feminine girls also reported significantly more negative perceptions of their scholastic competence (M = 2.80) compared to their androgynous female peers (M = 3.14). Eschewing such masculine attributes as assertiveness and competitiveness, while identifying primarily with such interpersonal attributes as connectedness and concern for others, may divert their attention from academic pursuits. However, such a feminine orientation leads to perceptions of social acceptance and behavioral conduct that are comparable to those of androgynous females, as might be expected given its interpersonal focus.

With regard to gender differences in other domains, at the college level, significant gender differences favoring males have also been found for perceived *creativity* (Klein et al., 1996; McGregor et al., 1992; McGregor et al., 1991). In our own data, the gender difference in creativity approaches significance. Thus, while females do *not* differ from males in their perceptions of either general intellectual ability or scholastic performance, they do judge their creativity to be inferior relative to the ratings of male college students. The gender socialization literature (see Basow, 1992; Beale, 1994; Block & Block, 1980; Eisenberg, Martin, & Fabes, 1996; Ruble, 1988, 1998) emphasizes that boys receive more encouragement and opportunities for exploration and inventiveness that may, in turn, lead to males' enhanced perceptions of creativity at the college level. (Because the domain of creativity has not been included on the instruments for older children and adolescents, researchers have not yet determined whether there are gender differences at younger ages).

Across some samples in this country and abroad, gender differences in perceived behavioral conduct favor girls. Two studies at the college level report that females score higher on the morality subscale. However, other studies find no gender differences in conduct or morality. Moreover, when differences are obtained, as in our own samples, they are much smaller in magnitude than the highly consistent gender differences found for athletic competence and physical appearance, favoring males. With regard to global self-worth, studies in this country as well as abroad reveal either no gender differences, or a small, but nonsignificant difference, favoring males. Thus, males and females evaluate themselves similarly with regard to their perceptions of overall worth as a person, where scores typically hover around 3.0. In summary, the pattern clearly reveals markedly more favorable self-evaluations for males with regard to perceptions of both athletic prowess and physical attractiveness. At the college level, males also report greater creativity than do females. These differences have been documented across numerous samples and are exacerbated when comparisons are made between feminine girls and males of either androgynous or masculine orientations.

Cross-Cultural Comparisons

It has become increasingly common for investigators in other countries to administer self-concept scales such as our own to children and adolescents in their own culture. As noted earlier, the finding that males feel better about their athletic competence and physical appearance than do females has been exceedingly consistent across countries. However, there are potential pitfalls in administering measures developed for a given culture to those from other countries. At a minimum, any meaningful interpretation requires that these instruments show comparable psychometric properties. However, attention must also be directed to culturally relevant content, because domains and/or items within a given subscale may need to be tailored to each culture.

Across the studies in non-American countries, the factor pattern itself has been shown to be quite robust. It has been replicated in other English-speaking countries, namely, *Canada* (Crocker & Ellsworth, 1990) and *Australia* (Marsh, 1990; Trent et al., 1994). It has also been replicated in non-English-speaking samples from *Quebec* (Boivin, Vitaro, & Gagnon, 1992; Gavin & Herry, 1996), *Switzerland* (Pierrehumbert et al., 1987), *Germany* (Asendorpf & van Aken, 1993), *Italy* (Pedrabissi et al., 1988), *Greece* (Makris-Botsaris & Robinson, 1991), *Holland* (van Dongen-Melman et al., 1993; van Rossum & Vermeer, 1994), *Japan* (Maeda, 1997; Sakurai, 1983), *Korea* (Rhee, 1993), and *China* (Stigler et al., 1985). For the most part, the reliabilities have been good to adequate. In certain countries, particular items have attenuated the reliability of a given subscale and have not loaded on their designated factor (although the overall subscale structure has been demonstrated). Some of these item difficulties may reflect translation issues. However, the existence of such items should serve as a red flag that a given instrument may require revisions at the item level in order to be culturally sensitive to potential differences in how the domains are best defined in a given country.

There are further cautions about the use of our instruments in countries such as China and Japan. For example, Meredith et al. (1991) have reported that only 20 of the 36 items on the Self-Perception Profile for Children factored appropriately. Moreover, in both this Chinese sample as well as the sample studied by Stigler et al. (1985), reliabilities were far from acceptable. The Global Self-Worth subscale was particularly problematic in both studies (alphas of .57 and .54). Lee C. Lee (personal communication, April 5, 1987) found similar problems with a Chinese American sample and thoughtfully concluded that the concept of global self-worth as defined in the American mainstream culture may not be an appropriate construct to include on an instrument examining meaningful self-perceptions among the Chinese. The Meredith et al. (1991) study reported relatively low reliabilities across all subscales (ranging from .44 to .61) suggesting that there exist items that are inappropriate for each of the domains.

Meredith, Wang, and Zheng (1993) have also argued that there are additional domains of relevance to Chinese children that are not included on our American instruments. As a first step, they added several other possible dimensions and asked Chinese children to rate their *importance*. Among these additions were items tapping group orientation (e.g., willingness to help others), social conduct (e.g., respect for parental and teacher authority), and social acceptance (e.g., engaging in behaviors such as getting good grades that would meet with peer as well as adult approval). Such an approach is commendable in that it addresses culturally sensitive issues involving the inclusion of domains that are most relevant for a given culture.

Of further concern is that in Chinese (Stigler et al., 1985), Japanese (Maeda, 1997; Sakurai, 1983), and Korean (Rhee, 1993) samples, the means are considerably lower than are scores in U.S., Canadian, Australian, and European samples. (The domain of social acceptance is perhaps the only exception.) Stigler et al. (1985) offer two possible interpretations for the low scores of his Chinese sample. The first is that the Chinese appear to display a *self-effacing* style that leads them to be more modest in their report of personal qualities. The second is that our structured alternative format, in which we contrast statements about "Some kids" versus "Other kids," implicitly demands a form of social comparison with others. Stigler and colleagues observe that such social comparison is frowned upon in China, where individual differences in competence are downplayed. Thus, Chinese children's unwillingness to report that they may be superior to others leads to a pattern of low scores that may not truly reveal their private perceptions of personal adequacy. These same interpretations may well apply to other Asian countries such as Japan and Korea.

In summary, the use of our instruments would appear to be particularly problematic in Asian cultures where (1) the content of certain items may not be relevant or meaningful, (2) other culturally sensitive content is needed, and (3) response tendencies (e.g., a self-effacing style coupled with an avoidance of social comparison) may require different item content, a different response format, as well as an instructional set to maximize the report of a true evaluation of one's perceived competencies.

It should be noted that we have never recommended the use of our instruments in other countries, particularly in cultures in which the self may be construed differently, or in which perceptions of self may not be that central to individuals' functioning. Rather, we urge that investigators adopt a more culture-specific perspective, focusing on the very meaning of self-constructs and their potential correlates for a given culture. An emphasis on correlates and consequences of self-perceptions is particularly essential, since it is important to address the issue of whether self-judgments do, in fact, have any predictable impact on other systems (e.g., behavioral, emotional) of interest; that is, investigators in any country, our own included, need to be clear about the purpose of examining self-perceptions and should attend to their functional role.

The need for such an approach in China is particularly pressing. The intellectual vacuum created by the Cultural Revolution extended to the field of psychology, where for two to three decades, progress and productivity was effectively halted. This vacuum has exacerbated the current search for methods, measures, and paradigms from Western countries that may be applicable. As I observed at a recent conference in Beijing, many Western psychologists are eager to share their theoretical and methodological wares with their Chinese colleagues. However, in our zeal to be benevolent (or our less than benevolent quest for fame!), we need to guard against imposing frameworks and related instruments that may be inappropriate for a given culture either because they do not adequately tap the construct in question, because the construct may not be that critical to the functioning of individuals within that culture, or both.

Special Groups of Children

There has been increasing interest in examining the self-concepts of special groups of children that have a variety of physical, medical, or intellectual impairments. Elsewhere (Harter, 1986a; Harter & Silon, 1985; Harter, Whitesell, & Junkin, in press), we have presented an analysis of how one needs to consider both similarities and differences among mentally retarded and learning-disabled youth. For example, when we administered the original version of our instrument for older children, the Perceived Competence Scale for Children (Harter, 1982a), we found that the two competence domains (Scholastic and Athletic) combined to form one factor, distinct from Social Acceptance, and that the Global Self-Worth subscale was very unreliable (Harter & Silon, 1985). These items simply did not make sense to retarded children. Thus, the picture is very similar to what we have obtained for younger normal children who would be at approximately the same mental age as the retarded children we sampled.

The picture for learning-disabled children is decidedly more complex. In an initial study in which we administered the Perceived Competence Scale for Children to learning disabled students, we found that the Scholastic Competence subscale items split into two factors, one that represented more specific skills, and one that reflected more general intelligence. Our interpretation was that this pattern reflected the messages that teachers and parents give to such children, namely, that although they are smart, they may have deficits in particular areas that will impact their performance in certain school subjects, for example, reading, spelling, or math. Thus, we developed the Self-Perception Profile for Learning Disabled Students (Renick & Harter, 1988) in which we included one subscale to tap General Intellectual Ability, and four separate subscales to tap specific school subjects. Factor-analysis reveals that all five of these scholastically oriented subscales define separate factors.

Children with various medical disorders (e.g., asthma, cancer, diabetes) also present particularly interesting challenges with regard to their self-perceptions. There would appear to be the implicit assumption among many who work with such groups of children that the compromising nature of their condition should result in less favorable perceptions of their competence or adequacy across certain domains tapped by our instruments. However, these assumptions have not been supported in the empirical literature.

We adopted such a framework in examining the self-perceptions of a group of children who were hospitalized as part of an inpatient treatment program for chronic asthmatic children. These children were under heavy medication, including steroids, which have a number of side effects that include the stunting of growth and bodily distortions such as swelling of the face. It was our general expectation that in a number of spheres, for example, athletic competence, social acceptance, and physical appearance, these children would score significantly lower than normative samples. Surprisingly, the findings provided absolutely no support for these predictions, given that there were no significant differences in the mean subscale scores for any of the domains we examined. We were perhaps most astounded by the physical appearance scores of these asthmatic children, which were equivalent to our norms.

A similar pattern of findings is beginning to emerge among studies examining children who are physically disabled (Sherrill, Hinson, Gench, Kennedy, & Low, 1990), who have cancer (Katz, Rubinstein, Hubert, & Blew, 1988; Spirito, Stark, Cobiella, Drigan, Androkites, & Hewett, 1990), who are suffering from diabetes (Hagen et al., 1990; Liakopoulou, Korvessi, & Dacou-Voutetakis, 1992), and who are hearing impaired (Hopper, 1988); that is, the profiles of these children across the domains that our instruments tap do not differ significantly from our means in normative samples, nor from normative control groups if they were included in these studies. Often, investigators are at a loss to interpret such findings, as we were, given the implicit assumption that actual deficiencies associated with a particular disorder should be linked to more negative self-evaluations. Thus, how is one to interpret the equivalent scores of such special groups of children?

There are a number of possible interpretations that, while speculative at this point, require empirical attention, since different pathways to equivalent scores may dictate different reactions to dealing with such children or may require different intervention strategies. Our own thinking about the lack of differences in self-perceptions between severely asthmatic children and our normative samples led us to hypothesize about five possible reasons for equivalent profiles that may also be operative among other groups suffering from various medical conditions.

1. *Similar social reference group.* It may well be that children with medical conditions are comparing themselves to others with that same condition, rather than to children in their school or neighborhood. This may be particularly relevant if they are in an inpatient program or a camp for others with the same disorder. As a result, scores would be higher than if these

children had compared themselves to normal children (i.e., those without the disorder) as their reference group. Relative to children *with* the same disorder, they may feel that they are functioning quite adequately. Moreover, they may be receiving positive feedback and encouragement from peers confronted with similar challenges.

2. *Conscious distortion or socially desirable responding.* Another possibility, which we entertained with our asthmatic sample, was that such children were purposely not presenting an accurate picture of their actual self-perceptions. They simply may not have felt comfortable expressing their true feelings to test administrators whom they did not know, or, perhaps they consciously chose to present themselves in the most favorable light possible. Although our question format has been found to be effective in offsetting social desirability response tendencies among most children without special problems, it may well be that its effectiveness is limited among children with medical conditions, who need to defend against limitations that lead to an underlying negative self-image.

3. *Unconscious denial.* At another level, children with such conditions may have been unconsciously denying their inadequacies; that is, they may unwittingly distort the self-portrait they present given their defensive need to protect or enhance the self, in order to avoid the painful realization that they do have limitations.

4. *Confusion between the real and the ideal self.* A related explanation is that such children blur the boundaries between their actual level of competence or adequacy and their desired or ideal level of competence or adequacy. For example, within the realm of physical appearance, asthmatics may have been presenting a picture of the way they would *like* to look, which was perhaps how they actually did look before they were put on medication. Thus, in this realm, there may be two distinct bodily self-images (real and ideal), and on our self-report measure they opt to present the idealized perception of the self. They may also harbor the belief that were they to be taken off medication, they would return to their former physical self.

5. *Healthy adjustment to self-standards.* The most optimistic interpretation, perhaps, is that these children have come to grips with the limitations that their medical condition has imposed and have adjusted their standards accordingly; that is, the portrait that they present of the self does not represent distortion, denial, or confusion, but an adaptation to reality and the belief that, given the constraints associated with their condition, they are actually doing quite well. Such children would appear to eschew social comparison in favor of a focus on how they are coping relative to their disorder. As a result, they are able to maintain positive self-evaluations that are both healthy and functional as they meet the challenges imposed by their condition.

This discussion highlights the potential complexity of the self-evaluative judgments of children who are coping with medical disorders, as well as the difficulty in interpreting their profile of scores. The hypotheses we have entertained underscore the need to go beyond the standardized administration of self-concept measures when we are dealing with special populations; that is, we cannot be content merely to ask such children to fill out our questionnaires. For children with intellectual deficits, physical handicaps, and medical conditions such as asthma, diabetes, cancer, obesity, and so on, the processes through which self-perceptions are formulated, maintained, and enhanced are undoubtedly very complex. As a result, we need to design assessment procedures that will do justice to this complexity, that will directly address the various dynamics contained in the preceding hypothesized reasons. We need to develop sensitive techniques that will allow us to test these hypotheses, which in turn will allow us better to understand the processes underlying the self-evaluations of children with limitations. Finally, as argued in the previous section on cross-cultural comparisons, we need to be clear about the *purpose* for examining these processes; that is, we need to make explicit a model that identifies both the causes and consequences of such children's self-perceptions in order to design effective interventions that will allow them to better cope with their condition.

CONCLUSION

There has been a major shift away from purely unidimensional models of self-evaluation to multidimensional frameworks that better capture the complexity of self-evaluative judgments. However, these newer frameworks preserve the construct of global self-esteem or self-worth. In fact, the identification of both domain-specific evaluations and global self-esteem has led theorists to develop hierarchical models in which combinations of domains are nested under global self-esteem at the apex of the network. It was suggested that many such hierarchical models represent conceptual schemes that allow *theorists* to organize these constructs. The manner in which given individuals organize their self-perceptions would appear to be far more idiosyncratic.

Multidimensional models have also dictated the construction of a variety of self-report instruments to tap relevant domain-specific self-perceptions across the life span. Our own battery now spans early childhood through late adulthood. The value of these more differentiated instruments is that they allow one to examine the profile of perceived strengths and weaknesses in particular individuals as well as particular subgroups of individuals. Considerable attention has been devoted to an examination of gender differences across domains where the pattern clearly reveals that males view themselves more favorably in the domains of athletic competence and physical appearance. Cross-cultural comparisons further reveal that samples of Western children and adolescents report more positive self-evaluations across most domains than do those from Eastern cultures. However, these differences may reflect cultural styles as well as the use of instruments that may be inappropriate for the Asian countries in which they have been administered.

A different set of challenges faces investigators who seek to examine the self-perceptions of special groups with medical disorders, where their generally positive self-perceptions are open to a range of interpretations. It is urged that we move beyond the standardized administration of instruments designed for normative, Western samples to any and all groups of children. Rather, we need to develop assessment procedures that are sensitive to the underlying processes through which self-perceptions are formulated as well as shared with others. Finally, we must attend to the particular relevance of self-perceptions in the lives of particular subgroups of individuals, as well as develop models that will address the causes of such perceptions and their functional role with regard to correlates and consequences.

Discrepancies between Real and Ideal Self-Concepts

In addition to developing self-representations of their actual attributes, what has been termed the *real* self-concept, individuals construct representations for what they want to be, or feel that they should be, namely, a concept of their *ideal* self. In this chapter, attention shifts to the relationship between self-evaluative judgments of one's actual perceived competence or adequacy across domains and one's personal ideals within each domain. The implications of discrepancies between real and ideal self-concepts are of particular relevance, since failure to achieve one's ideals will result in negative outcomes such as anxiety, low self-esteem, and depression. An analysis of developmental processes underlying the ability to construct such discrepancies is first presented, including the implications of different types of discrepancy constructs. James' (1892) formulation regarding the origins of self-esteem represents a variant on this theme in that the discrepancy between perceived success in a given domain and the *importance* attached to success was identified as a major determinant of one's level of global self-esteem. Findings from our own laboratory clearly support James' formulation.

However, there has been controversy within the literature on the value of a Jamesian approach. There are those who have questioned the usefulness of importance ratings and associated discrepancy scores in predicting global self-worth, whereas we have documented the utility of such an approach, as becomes evident. An analysis of the contribution that domain-specific evaluations make to the prediction of global self-esteem also ushers in the issue of the relative contribution of particular domains. Are some domains more predictive of self-esteem or self-worth than others? This issue is discussed, drawing upon findings both in this country and abroad, with a special emphasis on the role of perceived physical appearance, because it is the domain most highly and consistently associated with global evaluations of self. The implications of the inextricable link between perceptions of one's outer self (physical appearance) and one's inner self (self-worth) are explored, including clinical implications for those young women with eating disorders.

DEVELOPMENTAL PERSPECTIVES

The real/ideal terminology initially found its way into the adult clinical literature through the efforts of Rogers and his colleagues (Rogers & Dymond, 1954). In Rogers' view, the magnitude of the disparity between one's real and ideal self was a primary index of maladjustment. This construct was operationalized in a number of measures for adults, the most popular instrument being a Q-sort task designed by Butler and Haigh (1954). More recently, *developmentalists* have become interested in the real/ideal disparity construct.

One developmental issue concerns the age at which children are able to develop a sense of the ideal self that can then be compared to perceptions of the real self. The emergence of this ability is a reflection of cognitive advances as well as processes of socialization. As observed in Chapter 2, young children appear to confound their judgments of their actual competencies with their desired competencies, leading to overestimations of their virtuosity; that is, they cannot yet distinguish between these two types of evaluations. Thus, their self-descriptions include such claims as "I'm a really fast runner, I can run faster than my father!"; "I can count to a million!"; "Everybody in my school wants to be my friend!"

During early to middle childhood, children begin to develop separate representations for their skills and the importance of such abilities. However, the cognitive limitations of this period render young children incapable of simultaneously comparing two concepts such as self-evaluations and judgments of importance (see Fischer, 1980; Higgins, 1991), namely, real and ideal selves. During middle childhood, cognitive advances in the ability to differentiate constructs about the self come to be applied to the distinction between one's actual and desired characteristics. Moreover, the newfound capacity to compare these representations leads to the potential for children to realize that there may be a discrepancy between their real and ideal self-concepts. If this discrepancy reflects the fact that the real self-concept falls short of one's ideals, then negative affective outcomes may ensue.

In addition to an appreciation for the cognitive structures necessary to create such a discrepancy, developmentalists have been interested in those social experiences that shape the content of the ideal self. With development, children become increasingly cognizant of the standards and ideals that socializing agents hold for their behavior. Not only do they become sensitive to these external standards and ideals, but also they are typically very motivated to match and display these expectations in their behavior. Higgins and colleagues (Higgins, 1991; Moretti & Higgins, 1990) attempt to integrate the cognitive and social contributions, in offering a stage model that relies heavily on Case's (1985) framework, but that also incorporates features of other developmental formulations (Damon & Hart, 1988; Fischer, 1980; Piaget, 1960; Selman, 1980). According to Higgins, the ability to construct ideal self-representations, which he terms "self guides," emerges in middle childhood. Prior to this stage, children develop representations for what *others* wanted them to do.

The advance in middle childhood is that children come to *internalize* the expectations of significant others in the form of self-guides that can now be compared to their perceptions of the real self. As Higgins notes, this ushers in a potential vulnerability if there is a discrepancy between one's ideal self-guides and one's view of self. This liability is enhanced by the fact that the child can now conceptualize the self in terms of dispositional traits that may be viewed as relatively stable over time or situation. Consider the child whose parents have extremely high academic standards for their son or daughter, ideals that the child internalizes but is realistically unable to meet. Such a discrepancy will take its toll on global feelings of self-worth and may also be associated with hopelessness about improving one's scholastic performance, particularly if the child believes that intellectual abilities are fixed or immutable (see Dweck & Leggett, 1988). In other cases, it is societal standards that come to be internalized in the form of self-guides. For example, my own findings reveal that failure to meet punishing cultural standards of attractiveness leads to large discrepancies for many females that erode self-worth and lead to negative affective reactions (Harter, 1993).

In addition to specifying the particular cognitive structures necessary to construct such discrepancies beginning in middle childhood, Higgins also predicts that different types of discrepancies will produce different forms of psychological distress. Discrepancies between actual and ideal selves in the form of how one *wants* to be produce dejection-related emotions (e.g., sadness, discouragement, depression). For example, adolescent females who want to meet the standards of beauty demanded by the culture, but who fail to do so, will become despondent and depressed. In contrast, discrepancies between one's actual self and the self one should or *ought* to become produce agitation-related emotions such as feeling worried, threatened, or anxiously on edge. Thus, children who feel that they should excel academically, but who are unable to meet their achievement goals, will typically experience anxiety.

Developmentalists have also been interested in whether there are age-related changes in the *magnitude* as well as the implications of real/ideal disparities. In a seminal series of studies, Zigler and his colleagues (see review in Glick & Zigler, 1985) challenged Rogers' assumptions that self-image disparity is necessarily indicative of maladjustment, suggesting an alternative developmental framework. Their findings reveal that in children and adolescents, the discrepancy between one's real and ideal self-images increases with development, as indexed by age, as well as by a broad array of measures of cognitive maturity.

One plausible interpretation for increases in the discrepancy between real and ideal self-images with development comes from the work of Leahy and colleagues (see Leahy & Shirk, 1985). For these investigators, developmental increases in *role-taking* ability are critical. From a symbolic interactionist position, taking the role of others toward the self may lead one to construct more realistic (typically less positive) views of the self and/or to internalize increasingly higher standards of behavior. In consort, these two shifts would lead to greater disparity between self-evaluations and one's standards. The findings of Leahy and colleagues reveal that higher self-image disparity and a more positive ideal image were associated with greater role taking (see also Oosterwegel & Oppenheimer, 1993).

What are the implications of the fact that discrepancies increase with development? Higgins predicts that the *magnitude* of these discrepancies is critical in that if it is relatively large, it will represent an index of maladjustment, consistent with Rogers' initial clinical claims. Zigler and colleagues (see Glick & Zigler, 1985; Rosales & Zigler, 1989), in an attempt to reconcile the developmental findings with Rogers' maladjustment position, observe that there may be a point beyond which the discrepancy does become debilitating. They also note that one needs to consider not only the discrepancy per se but also the absolute level of real and ideal ratings, since the same discrepancy associated with a negative sense of one's real self may produce more distress than if it was associated with a more positive evaluation. For example, an adolescent who feels that he/she is relatively competent (e.g., real self-concept of 3 on a 4-point scale) with an ideal to achieve at even higher levels (e.g., an ideal self of 4) may experience fewer negative reactions than a child who feels he/she is performing poorly (e.g., real self-concept of 2) relative to his/her positive, ideal level of performance (e.g., 3). Thus, the absolute magnitude of the discrepancy may take on different meaning depending upon where these values fall upon the scale.

Certain theorists have also emphasized the positive function of discrepancies in motivating behavior. Rosales and Zigler (1989) argue that some degree of real–ideal differentiation is necessary as a source of motivation. Bandura (1990) also describes how people actually produce discrepancies by creating challenging standards that then mobilize them toward a goal. Subsequent goal attainment then reduces the discrepancy, leading the person to set even higher standards. In these more recent efforts, it is apparent that the field has moved away from views that emphasize either implications for maladjustment *or* the developmental underpinnings of self-discrepancies and their function, toward a more thoughtful consideration of both.

Closely related to the concepts of real and ideal selves is another distinction between real and *possible* selves (Markus & Nurius, 1986; Oyserman & Markus, 1993). Here, we can appreciate the legacy of James (1890), given his characterization of "immediate and actual" selves as well as "remote and potential" selves. Possible selves represent both the hoped-for and dreaded selves, and function as incentives that clarify those selves that are to be approached as well as those to be avoided. Markus and her colleagues contend that possible selves have a very important *motivational* function (see also Epstein, 1973, and van der Werff, 1985). From their perspective, it is most desirable to have a balance between positive expected selves and negative feared selves, so that positive possible selves (e.g., obtaining a well-paying job, wanting to be loved by family, hoping to be recognized and admired by others) can give direction to desired future states, whereas negative possible selves (e.g., being unemployed, feeling lonely, being socially ignored) can clarify what is to be avoided (cf. Ogilvie & Clark's [1992] concept of "undesired" selves). Markus and colleagues report findings supporting these motivational functions.

Finally, the manner in which the ideal self is defined may be critical to the outcomes anticipated or obtained. Rosenberg (1979) observes that the distinction between one's idealized self-image and one's "committed" self-image is frequently overlooked. The committed image is what we take seriously; it is not merely a desirable fantasy. Thus, an academic may have a fantasized image of winning a Nobel prize, whereas his/her committed image is to obtain tenure. Rosenberg suggests that in earlier work, where subjects were asked what they would "ideally" like to be, we have no idea whether they responded in terms of a more fantasied ideal or the self that they were earnestly committed to become. For example, a large discrepancy between the evaluation of one's talents as a faculty member and one's fantasy of winning the Nobel prize will have fewer negative psychological consequences than a large discrepancy between one's perceived academic talents and one's perceptions of the likelihood that one will obtain tenure. Oosterwegel and Oppenheimer (1993) suggest that some of the inconsistencies in this literature stem from the fact that certain measures may pull for the more fantasied ideal, whereas other instruments, including their own, may be more likely to induce a consideration of more committed ideals.

THE JAMESIAN DISCREPANCY MODEL

There is clear convergence between the self-image disparity work and James' (1892) model emphasizing the need to consider perceptions of success in relation to pretensions, namely, aspirations or intentions to be successful. For James, the congruence or the discrepancy between these two dimensions was very functional in that it represented the primary antecedent of global self-esteem. According to this formulation, individuals do not scrutinize their every action or attribute; rather, they focus primarily on their perceived adequacy in domains where they have aspirations to succeed. Thus, the individual who perceives the self positively in domains where he/she aspires to excel will have high self-esteem. Those who fall short of their ideals, creating a discrepancy between perceived successes and their pretensions, will experience low self-esteem.

It is critical to appreciate that, from a Jamesian perspective, inadequacy in domains deemed unimportant to the self should not adversely affect self-esteem. For example, an individual may judge the self to be unathletic; however, if athletic prowess is not an aspiration, then self-esteem will not be negatively affected. Thus, the high-self-esteem individual is able to *discount* the importance of domains in which he or she is not competent, whereas the low-self-esteem individual appears unable to devalue success in domains of inadequacy.

There is a growing body of literature revealing that individuals do differentially value some domains more highly than others, beginning in middle childhood. One can observe this emphasis in Kelly (1955), who postulated that in the self-theory there were core constructs more critical to the evaluation and maintenance of one's identity than were peripheral constructs. More recently, Markus and Wurf (1987) have also argued that self-descriptions differ in importance. Their findings reveal that some attributes possess high personal relevance and function as central or core characteristics, whereas other characteristics are less personally relevant and more peripheral. Other findings (Harter & Monsour, 1992) indicate that adolescents can construct a self-portrait in which they differentiate the most central or important self-descriptors from those that are less, and least, important. Moreover, beginning in middle childhood and beyond, our evidence reveals that individuals typically evaluate the importance of the domains included in our self-perception profiles differently.

With regard to testing the Jamesian hypothesis more specifically, Rosenberg (1979) provided some initial documentation that the importance of a domain will determine the degree to which success and failure affect overall self-evaluation. Focusing on the centrality of one characteristic, likability, he found that among those who cared about being likable, the relationship of perceived likability and global self-esteem was much stronger than for those to whom this quality mattered little. With adult subjects, Tesser and his colleagues have demonstrated that if a dimension is highly relevant to one's self-definition, performance judged to be inferior will threaten one's sense of self-esteem (Tesser, 1980; Tesser & Campbell, 1983).

In our work, we have directly examined the Jamesian hypothesis across an age span from 8 to 55 (where self-worth is synonymous with the term "self-esteem"). With regard to operationalization, individuals evaluate their adequacy or competency across age-relevant domains and also rate the *importance* of each domain. We opted to have participants rate importance rather than to make judgments about their ideal self for two reasons. First, the construct of importance would appear to better mirror James' concept of pretensions or aspirations. Second, the construct of importance is closer to Rosenberg's concept of the "committed ideal" and avoids the confound with a fantasied ideal that may not represent the individual's day-to-day aspirations.

Support for James' Formulation

Our findings have revealed precisely what James hypothesized. By way of illustration at the level of individual children, Figure 6.1 presents two older children, one with high self-worth (Child A) and one with low self-worth (Child B). These children were selected for illustrative purposes, because although they differ markedly in the level of global self-worth, the scores that define their profile across the individual self-concept domains are quite similar. How is it, one might question, that they can look so similar in their domain-specific self-evaluations yet report such disparate levels of global self-worth? James' (1892) formulation on the role of importance provides a partial explanation. In Figure 6.1, it can be seen that Child A, with high self-worth, judged scholastic and athletic competence to be relatively unimportant. Thus, such a child can *discount* the importance of areas in which he/she is not competent, while touting the importance of domains in which he/she is doing well. Conversely, Child B is unable to discount the importance of scholastic and athletic competence, leading to a vast discrepancy between very high importance judgments and very low competence/adequacy evaluations in these two domains. From a Jamesian perspective, this discrepancy, therefore, should take its toll on global self-worth.

We have now documented this pattern systematically, with group data from older children, adolescents, college students, and adults in the world of work and family (Harter, 1990a). We have employed several data-analytic strategies, each of which tells the same story. We have constructed actual

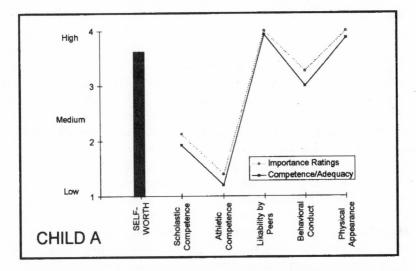

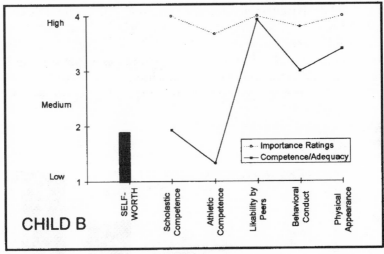

FIGURE 6.1. Profiles of two young adolescents with similar competence/adequacy scores for specific domains but very different levels of global self-worth.

discrepancy scores between importance ratings and competence judgments in each domain. Averaging these across domains, initially, we have determined that the larger the discrepancy, that is, the more one's importance ratings exceed one's perceived adequacy or competence, the lower one's self-worth. Across numerous studies, these correlations typically range from .55 to .72. Employing a second procedure, in which we have examined self-worth as a function of the average absolute competence/adequacy judgments for *only* those domains rated very important or sort of important, a systematic, linear relationship emerges (see Figure 6.2). Thus, relatively low self-worth is reported for those acknowledging that they lack competence or adequacy in domains for which they have aspirations of success, namely, those who are unable to discount the importance of domains in which they feel inadequate. As perceived success in domains deemed important increases across groups, parallel gains in self-worth are reported. Employing this second strategy, we find that the relationship between competence in important domains and self-worth ($r = .70$) far exceeds the correlation between competence in unimportant domains and self-worth ($r = .30$), a difference that would be predicted from a Jamesian perspective.

The value of James' formulation is controversial, however. Certain investigators, notably Marsh and associates (1986, 1993; Marsh & Hattie, 1996), have argued that importance ratings add little if anything to the prediction of global self-esteem or self-worth, on the basis of findings revealing that merely correlating competence/adequacy scores with self-esteem (ignoring importance) yields values that are not significantly different from those based on procedures in which importance is taken into account. Such investigators conclude, therefore, that a model ignoring the role of importance is more parsimonious. We do not contest the findings, which are consistent with our own; rather, we question the conclusions.

Why might merely correlating competence/adequacy scores with glo-

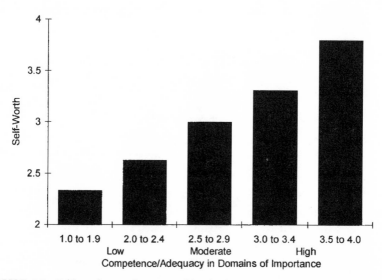

FIGURE 6.2. Self-worth as a function of level of competence/adequacy in important domains.

bal self-worth result in values comparable to those based upon correlating competence/adequacy scores with global self-worth for just those individuals rating domains as important? The answer lies in the fact that since the vast majority (75%–80%) of older children and adolescents rate these domains as important, the two correlations will be based on virtually the same group of participants. Only a small subset (20%–25%) will be lost in the second case, given that relatively few children and adolescents are able to discount the importance of the domains we have selected. It is our contention that the more parsimonious *empirical* model in which importance ratings are ignored may obscure the actual psychological processes through which an individual formulates a sense of his/her worth as a person; that is, such evaluative judgments are not necessarily parsimonious (see also Pelham & Swann, 1989). Therefore, ignoring the role of the value attached to success across domains may ignore the complexity of the processes underlying these judgments.

However, to empirically demonstrate this claim, procedures that are more sensitive to these processes among particular subgroups of individuals need to be employed. Toward this end, we have approached this issue employing four different approaches. First, a more appropriate statistical test of the value of the Jamesian hypothesis lies in a comparison of the correlations with self-worth of domains rated as competent or adequate in importance or central and those rated as *unimportant* (among that subset of individuals). As noted earlier, in our own work, the magnitude of the differences between these two correlations (.70 vs. .30) is quite convincing, suggesting that the importance construct does make a difference. Second, according to the Jamesian formulation, discrepancies between relatively high importance ratings and relatively low competence/adequacy ratings should be greater for low-self-worth individuals compared to high-self-worth individuals for whom there is greater congruence between their aspirations and their perceived successes. This assumption should result in lower correlations between importance ratings and competence judgments for low-self-worth compared to high-self-worth individuals. We have obtained this pattern at both the middle school and high school level, where the correlation for low-self-worth individuals is .19 versus .42 for the high-self-worth individuals.

Third, an even more direct test of the role of importance, including the discounting process, involves a comparison of the importance attached to domains in which individuals feel incompetent or inadequate, among high- and low-self-worth groups. According to James, while high-self-worth individuals may and do have domains in which they feel inadequate, they should be able to discount the importance of these domains. In contrast, low-self-worth individuals should give higher ratings of importance to domains in which they feel inadequate. Thus, we examined importance ratings for only those areas in which both low- and high-self-worth participants reported that they felt incompetent or inadequate. To examine the generality of this principle, we included normally achieving, learning-disabled, and behaviorally disordered groups of adolescents (Harter et al., in press). We first identified high- and low-self-worth individuals within each educational group. We then selected only those domains in which members of both groups indicated that they felt incompetent or inadequate, and examine the importance ratings attached to those domains.

Our findings directly supported the Jamesian hypothesis. As can be seen in Figure 6.3, high-self-worth adolescents were better able to discount the importance of domains in which they felt they had weaknesses; that is, their importance scores were significantly (p < .0001) lower than the importance scores of the low-self-worth adolescents. Moreover, this pattern was observed across all three types of students. Thus, these findings provide further confirmation for James' contention that the inability to discount the importance of areas in which one reports personal limitations is a characteristic of low-self-worth individuals.

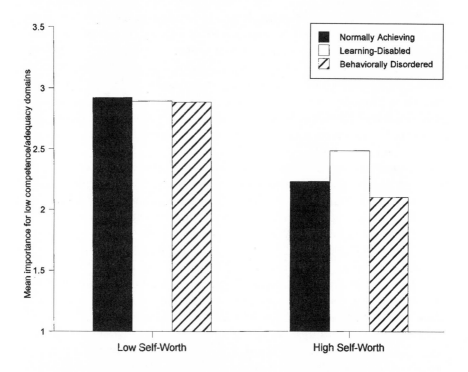

FIGURE 6.3. Mean importance ratings of low competence/adequacy domains for high- and low-self-worth individuals within three different educational groups.

Finally, we have also employed more direct qualitative procedures in which older children are asked to respond to cameo descriptions of hypothetical students, procedures that reveal that the children are consciously aware of how importance and the discounting process contribute to overall feelings of worth (Harter, 1986a). Each child was presented with a vignette, the content of which paralleled the domain in which he/she had previously reported feeling the least adequate, in order to make the vignettes credible and personally meaningful. The story child (same gender as the participant) initially feels that being skillful at activities in this domain is very important; however, the child later comes to learn that he/she lacks competence at these activities. For example, for the domain of sports, the scenario is one of a child who feels that being successful on the soccer team is very important; however, as the season progresses, the child comes to realize that he/she simply is not a good soccer player. The participant is then asked to indicate which of two decisions the story character makes: (1) that the activity is not that important after all (demonstrating that the child can discount the importance of domains in which he/she is not competent), or (2) that the activity is still very important even though he/she is not very good at it (demonstrating that the child is unable to discount a domain of incompetence, continuing to maintain its importance).

For purposes of analysis, participants were divided into high-, medium, and low-self-worth groups. We found that 80% of the high-self-worth children indicated that the story child would decide that the domain was no longer important. Among those with moderate levels of self-worth, 45% supported the discounting decision, whereas 55% indicated that the story character would continue to feel that the activity was important. Among the low-self-worth group, only 30% felt that the story character would discount the importance of the activity, whereas the majority of these participants (70%) reported that the story child would continue to feel that the activity was important, despite the fact that his/her incompetence had been demonstrated.

The actual importance ratings that participants gave for their own least competent domain were consistent with this pattern. The high-self-worth children felt that their least competent domain was only of moderately low importance (M = 2.6 on the 4-point scale). The moderate-self-worth group claimed that their least competent domain was somewhat more important (M = 3.3), and the low-self-worth group reported that their least competent domain was even more important (M = 3.6) compared to the other two groups. Thus, across several indices, our findings support James' contention that it is competence or adequacy, relative to the importance of successes, rather than perceived competence/adequacy alone, that best predicts global self-worth.

From a more applied or clinical perspective, a comparison of the profiles of competence/adequacy scores and importance ratings of individual children and adolescents may be invaluable in planning intervention strategies to bolster or maintain self-worth. Consider the student profiled in Figure 6.4, a 15-year-old male with a history of poor academic performance and conduct problems. He reports relatively low competence/adequacy scores, below the midpoint of 2.5 in four domains (Cognitive Competence, Athletic Competence, Behavioral Conduct, and Romantic Appeal) and relatively high scores (3 or above) in the remaining four domains (Appearance, Likability, Close Friendship, and Job Competence). If one were to consider competence/adequacy judgments only, ignoring importance, an intervention might be targeted at improving competence/adequacy in the four lowest domains. In contrast, a focus on the relationship of these scores to importance ratings would dictate a different strategy. For the cognitive domain, one would attempt to reduce the large discrepancy by the two strategies implicit in James' formulation, namely, increasing cognitive competence, reducing the importance attached to such success if these aspirations were unrealistic, or both. A similar strategy could be employed with regard to the discrepancy in the domain of romantic appeal. Although perceptions of athletic competence are also quite negative, this domain is not important to the individual and thus unlikely to erode self-worth. Thus, this domain would not require specific attention.

In the conduct domain, where both sets of ratings are quite low, a

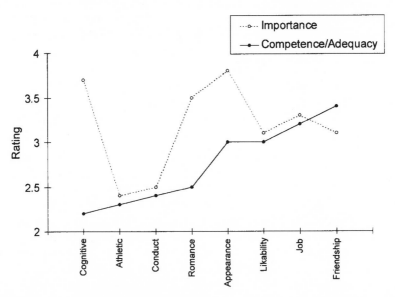

FIGURE 6.4. Profile of competence/adequacy scores and importance ratings for one student to illustrate implications for enhancing self-worth.

different strategy may be dictated to the extent that educators, parents, or mental health workers feel that appropriate conduct is desirable and should be valued. One may first want to *create* a discrepancy by heightening the student's perception of the importance of good conduct, after which strategies to reduce the discrepancy by improving the individual's conduct would be employed. Finally, in the domain of appearance, although the absolute level of this student's perceptions is not low, there is a large discrepancy due to the extreme importance attached to this domain. Thus, rather than ignore this arena given the relatively favorable evaluation, a consideration of the importance rating would suggest interventions to reduce the discrepancy (e.g., by pointing out that the punishing standards for appearance that many adolescents adopt are unrealistic and that qualities other than one's outer self should be critical to one's sense of personal worth).

Such an approach obviously presents greater challenges to those developing intervention strategies to improve self-worth since they require attention to the particular profiles presented by each individual. As recent findings indicate (Harter & Whitesell, 1996), there are multiple pathways to low self-worth and associated correlates such as depression (to be discussed in Chapter 8), and therefore it is essential to identify the specific pathways for given individuals. The point of this chapter is that a focus on the relationship between self-evaluations and the importance of corresponding domains can provide critical insights into precisely where and how one should intervene to enhance the self-worth of individuals lacking a sense of personal esteem.

Why Should Low Self-Worth among Certain Individuals Persist?

If the psychological system is adaptively programmed to reduce discrepancies between importance and perceived incompetence, beginning in middle childhood, why do such discrepancies exist initially as well as persist, leading certain individuals to experience low-self-worth? That is, both the Jamesian and recent self-discrepancy formulations have now identified the relevant processes that could potentially be engaged to enhance self-worth. James clearly asserted that for the low self-esteem individual, there were two potential routes to self-esteem enhancement. One could lower one's aspirations by discounting the importance of success in areas where one was deficient. Alternatively, one could raise one's level of actual competence or personal adequacy (e.g., through skills training or other efforts to overcome one's limitations). Both of these strategies will serve to reduce the discrepancy between competence and importance; decreasing this discrepancy should, in turn, increase one's level of self-worth.

Although such intervention strategies are theoretically compelling, they may not be that plausible or realistic given the actual lives of children and adolescents. Several factors would appear to mitigate against their utilization and therefore their potential effectiveness. There are two psychological roadblocks to discounting the importance of the specific domains we have selected in the face of perceived inadequacy. First and foremost, these domains were initially chosen because most children and adolescents, in interviews, identified these areas as very important; that is, we are living in a society where scholastic competence, athletic competence, physical attractiveness, social acceptance, and appropriate behavioral conduct are highly valued and sought after by the majority of youths in the cultural mainstream. Thus, personal aspirations and standards in these domains are typically quite high, making it difficult for those feeling inadequate to discount their importance.

Second, these domains are valued by significant others, notably parents and peers. Our own findings reveal that children and adolescents judge scholastic competence and behavioral conduct to be most important to parents, and social acceptance, physical appearance, and athletic competence to be most important to peers. Moreover, importance to others is highly correlated with importance to self, and competence in domains important to others is just as highly correlated with self-worth as is competence in domains important to the self (Harter & Marold, 1993). Thus, it would appear to be extremely difficult for children and adolescents to discount the importance of domains that represent standards set by significant others whom they wish to please (see also Baumeister, 1990), despite feelings of inadequacy in these areas. Thus, for both of these related reasons, the discrepancy between high importance and low competence or adequacy will be difficult to reduce by lowering one's aspirations.

Increasing one's competence and corresponding self-evaluations as a strategy for reducing this discrepancy would also appear to be problematic for many youth. First, there are undoubtedly natural limits to the extent that many children and adolescents can increase their actual competence or adequacy. Although a given individual may be highly motivated to improve his/her scholastic performance, athletic ability, or physical appearance, there may be little that an individual can realistically do given certain ceilings on intellectual and physical potential.

Second, there may also be limitations placed on *perceived competence*, given the standards imposed by social comparison. As noted in Chapters 2 and 3, studies have shown that the process of comparing the self to others for the purposes of self-evaluation begins in middle childhood and increases as one matures. Our own research has demonstrated that the use of social comparison is rampant in the five domains that we have selected. Children within regular classroom settings can rank-order with great precision the competence level of every member of their class. Interestingly, we have also documented the use of social comparison among learning-disabled children (Renick & Harter, 1989) as well as intellectually talented children within segregated classes for the gifted. Beginning in middle childhood, therefore, most children adopt the cultural preoccupation with how individuals are different from one another, with competition, with who is the best, with who ascends to the top. Thus, how one measures up to peers and societal standards becomes the filter through which judgments about the self pass.

One may well espouse the value of social comparison, since it presumably provides individuals with the necessary guidelines or standards by which to evaluate themselves and improve performance. Supposedly, comparison with others offers a welcome anchor to help ground people in reality and foster the accuracy of self-evaluations. However, since most of life's activities are graded on a curve, particularly the domains we have selected, relatively few individuals can occupy the prestigious positions at the top of the ladder. Thus, even if an individual, motivated to improve, does demonstrate actual gains, compared to his/her own past performance, he/she will likely fall short relative to the punishing peer standards that provide the metric for self-evaluation. As a result, it becomes difficult to greatly increase one's perceptions of competence relative to others as a potential route to reducing the discrepancy between importance and competence that contributes to low self-worth. I return to these issues in Chapter 12 on intervention strategies.

ARE SOME DOMAINS MORE PREDICTIVE OF SELF-WORTH THAN OTHERS?

In shifting to multidimensional, hierarchical models of the self, many investigators have understandably been interested in whether some domains are more predictive of global self-esteem or self-worth than others. The pattern of findings is quite similar in the United States and in other countries. Table 6.1 presents, by domain, the range of correlations and the average correlation across 13 U.S. samples from our own work (see also Hagborg, 1994) as well as from nine samples from other countries. These other countries include *England* (Fox et al., 1994), *Ireland* (Granlese & Joseph, 1993), *Australia* (Trent et al., 1994), *Canada* (Crocker & Ellsworth, 1990), *Germany* (Asendorpf & van Aken, 1993), *Italy* (Pedrabissi et al., 1988), *Greece* (Makris-Botsaris & Robinson, 1991), *Holland* (Van Dongen-Melman et al., 1993) and *Japan* (Maeda, 1997).

As can be seen in Table 6.1, the range of correlations as well as the average correlations are strikingly similar in our own U.S. samples and in

TABLE 6.1. Correlations of Domain Competence/Adequacy Scores and
Global Self-Worth across Samples in the United States and Abroad

	Range of correlations		Average correlation	
Domain	Harter's U.S. samples	Other countries	Harter's U.S. samples	Other countries
Physical appearance	.52–.80	.54–.65	.65	.62
Scholastic competence	.34–.54	.33–.48	.48	.41
Social acceptance	.34–.58	.32–.51	.46	.40
Behavioral conduct	.32–.50	.41–.47	.45	.45
Athletic competence	.23–.42	.24–.38	.33	.30

those from other countries. Physical appearance correlates most highly with global self-worth; athletic competence consistently bears the lowest relationship to global self-worth, and falling in between are scholastic competence, social acceptance, and behavioral conduct. Not only does physical appearance correlate the most highly, but the correlation is remarkably high. Other investigators examining the link between perceived appearance and self-worth or self-esteem among children and adolescents have obtained similar relationships (Lerner & Brackney, 1978; Lerner & Karabenick, 1974; Lerner, Orlos, & Knapp, 1976; Marsh, 1987; Padin, Lerner, & Spiro, 1981; Pomerantz, 1979; Simmons & Rosenberg, 1975). Most recently, we have turned our attention to the relationship between perceived physical appearance and self-reports of behaviorally manifest self-worth among young children, ages 4 to 7 (Nikkari & Harter, 1993). Even at this young age, physical appearance headed the list in terms of the domain most highly correlated with self-worth.

Moreover, in our own work, we find this relationship to be just as high in special populations such as the intellectually gifted and the learning disabled, where one might anticipate that scholastic performance would bear a stronger relationship to self-worth, given the salience of academic performance in defining such groups. In the same vein, we find the correlation between appearance and self-worth is equally high among adolescents identified as behaviorally disruptive, exceeding that of the correlation between behavioral conduct and self-worth (Harter et al., in press). In a master's thesis (Lee, 1993), we examined the self-perceptions of children in Special Olympics before and after the actual athletic events. Given the focus on the domain of sports, we anticipated that perceived athletic competence would be most predictive of global self-worth. However, in this sample as well, physical appearance was the domain most highly correlated with self-worth, comparable to other samples.

Numerous findings in the adult literature, including our own work with college students and adults in the world of work and family, also reveal that perceived physical appearance and self-esteem or self-worth are inextricably linked (Adams, 1982; Berscheid, Walster, & Bohrnstedt, 1973; Davies & Furnham, 1986; Feingold, 1992; Franzoi & Shields, 1984; Hatfield & Sprecher, 1986; Jackson, 1992; Korabik & Pitt, 1980; Lerner, Karabenick, & Stuart, 1973; Longo & Ashmore, 1995; Mathes & Kahn, 1975; McCaulay, Mintz, & Glenn, 1988; Messer & Harter, 1989; Mintz & Betz, 1988; Neemann & Harter, 1987; Rosen & Ross, 1968; Ryckman, Robbins, Thornton, & Cantrell, 1982; Silberstein, Striegel-Moore, Timko, & Rodin, 1988). Moreover, self-esteem has been found to be more highly related to perceived attractiveness than to actual physical attractiveness (see Feingold, 1992).

Certain investigators (see Boivin et al., 1992; Makris-Botsaris & Robinson, 1991) have suggested that in studies employing our instruments, the high correlation between perceived appearance and global self-worth may be spurious given the manner in which the physical appearance items are worded. They argue that many of the appearance items make reference to *satisfaction* with one's appearance (e.g., "happy with the way I look," "like my physical appearance the way it is," etc.), whereas this is not the case for most of the items on the other domain subscales. Since the global self-worth items also make reference to satisfaction (e.g., with the self as a person, with how one is leading one's life, etc.), these investigators raise the issue of whether the common focus on satisfaction may be inflating the correlation between global self-worth and perceived physical appearance relative to the other domains. We have addressed this issue empirically, and our findings do not support this interpretation. One of the physical appearance items does not make reference to satisfaction, namely, an item that states that one thinks one is good-looking (or does not). Thus, we independently correlated this single item with the global self-worth subscale across numerous samples and compared those correlations to the remaining items that do contain the satisfaction language. The item referring to "good-looking" correlated just as highly with self-worth (average correlation of .54) as did other satisfaction items (average correlation of .52). Thus, using the item that these investigators would deem more appropriate did not produce a different pattern. However, their point deserves attention, and in future revisions of the instrument, care will be taken to alter the wording of items so as to remove this potential confound.

The pattern of findings reveals, therefore, that at every developmental level (through middle-aged adults), the evaluation of one's looks takes precedence over other domains as the number one predictor of self-worth, causing us to question whether self-worth is only skin-deep. Why should one's *outer,* physical self be so tied to one's *inner* psychological self? One possibility is that the domain of physical appearance is qualitatively different from the other arenas we have tapped in that it is an omnipresent feature of the self, it is always on display for others or for the self to observe. In contrast, one's adequacy in such domains as scholastic or athletic competence, peer social acceptance, conduct, or morality is not constantly on display for evaluation, but rather is more context-specific. Moreover, one has more control over whether, when, and how personal adequacy in these other domains will be revealed.

Studies indicate that others begin to react to the ever-present display of the physical self when one is an infant and toddler (Langlois, 1981; Maccoby & Martin, 1983). Those who are attractive, by societal standards, are responded to with more positive attention than those judged to be less physically attractive. Thus, from a very early age, the physical or outer self appears to be a highly salient dimension that provokes evaluative, psychological reactions that may well be incorporated into the emerging sense of one's inner self. Moreover, findings reveal that even young children are well aware of the cultural criteria for attractiveness (Cavior & Lombardi, 1973).

Clearly, a critical contributing factor involves the emphasis that contemporary society places on appearance at every age (see Adams, 1982; Andersen, 1992; Elkind, 1979; Hatfield & Sprecher, 1986; Kilbourne, 1994; Nemeroff, Stein, Daiehl, & Smilack, 1994; Silverstein, Perdue, Peterson, & Kelly, 1986). Movies, television, magazines, rock videos, and advertising all tout the importance of physical attractiveness, glamorizing the popular role models one should emulate, for males and females. Standards regarding desirable bodily characteristics such as thinness have become increasingly unrealistic and demanding for women within the past two decades (see Garner, Garfinkel, Schwartz, & Thompson, 1980; Heatherton & Baumeister, 1991; Jackson, 1992; Wiseman, Gray, Mosimann, & Ahrens, 1992). An examination of contemporary women's magazines (e.g., *Family Circle, Woman's Day, First for Women*) reveals that the standards are paradoxical and punishing for women. All of these magazines relentlessly insist that women simultaneously (1) attend fiercely to their appearance (hair, face, and particularly weight) while they (2) cook a vast array of fattening foods for themselves and their family! Moreover, articles and ads specifically preach that altering one's looks, often in the form of an invasive cosmetic overhaul to approximate rather narrowly defined cultural stereotypes of beauty, will enhance one's self-esteem. These stereotypes have become even more unattainable given the use of computer-generated magazine models in which combinations of physical features are artificially combined.

Although the media are also increasingly emphasizing the importance of appearance for men, it would appear that there is still more latitude in the standards of attractiveness for men. Moreover, for men there is not the singular focus on physical features (e.g., face, hair, body, weight) as the criteria for attractiveness and the pathway to acceptance and esteem that one finds for women. For men, intelligence, job competence, athletic ability, wealth, and power, are all routes to positive evaluations of appearance in the eyes of others as well as the self.

The difficulty for females of meeting the cultural stereotypes of physical beauty appears to be brought home over the course of development, the closer one comes to adopting one's role as a woman in this society. Our own data, averaged across seven different samples (see Figure 6.5), reveal that for females of predominantly Caucasian origins, perceptions of physical attractiveness systematically decline with grade level, whereas there is no such drop for males. Thus, in middle childhood, girls and boys feel equally good about their appearance; however, by the end of high school, females' scores are dramatically lower than those of males. Others also report that dissatisfaction with appearance among females begins in middle childhood (Maloney, McGuire, & Daniels, 1988; Mellin, 1988; Salmons, Lewis, Rogers, Gatherer, & Booth, 1988; Stein, 1996). The adult literature further documents the fact that females are typically more dissatisfied with their appearance than are males (Adams, 1982; Birtchnell, Dolan, & Lacey, 1987; Cohn et al., 1987; Davies & Furnham, 1986; Fallon & Rozin, 1985; McCaulay et al., 1988; Mintz & Betz, 1988; Silberstein et al., 1988; Stager & Burke, 1982). However, this literature also reveals variability across subcultures in this coun-

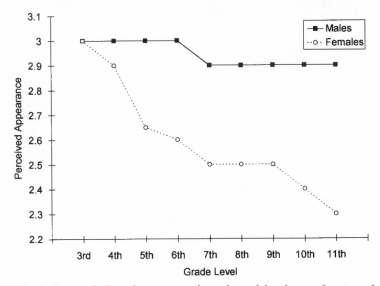

FIGURE 6.5. Perceived physical appearance for males and females as a function of grade level.

try. Noteworthy, in this regard, is the finding that African American women rate their appearance more highly than do women in Caucasian samples.

Gender differences in self-worth also widen with development, paralleling the trajectories for physical appearance. Beginning in junior high school and continuing into high school, self-worth is consistently lower for females compared to males. Decreased perceptions of attractiveness among females would appear to contribute to the lowered self-worth of females, as other investigators have also suggested (Allgood-Merton, Lewinsohn, & Hops, 1990; Nolen-Hoeksema, 1987; Simmons & Blyth, 1987). Our data further reveal that the importance of physical appearance increases over childhood and adolescence for both males and females; however, these differences are greater for females than males. Among female elementary school children, the importance ratings of physical appearance are 2.80 compared to 3.04 during middle school, and 3.34 among female high school students. Thus, decreasing perceptions of one's attractiveness coupled with increasing importance should, according to a Jamesian perspective, lead to bigger discrepancies that would result in declines in self-worth for females. However, in our own data, females' self-worth does not decline as dramatically with age as does perceived physical appearance. Rather, there is another mediating factor, namely, the perceived directionality of the link between appearance and self-worth.

The Directionality of the Link between Appearance and Self-Worth

According to the Jamesian perspective, domain-specific evaluations are the *antecedents* of global self-worth or esteem. Recently, the directionality of these links has been questioned. Brown (1993b), for example, argues that self-esteem is an affectively based, fluid construct that generalizes to specific domains. Thus, if one's self-esteem is high, it imbues the self with many positive qualities. He reports findings that are consistent with such a claim but not conclusive. In our own work, we have also been concerned with the directionality of the link between domain-specific self-evaluations and self-worth, focusing on the domain of perceived physical appearance. This domain was selected since the correlations between appearance and self-worth range from .52 to .80 across samples, clearly demonstrating a strong link. Rather than take a stance on which directionality best captures this relationship, we have examined adolescents' *perceptions* of the directionality of this link (Harter, 1993).

The robust relationship between perceived appearance and perceptions of global worth as a person raised an intriguing question: Which do adolescents feel comes first? That is, does perceived appearance precede one's sense of self-worth; that is, does it *determine* one's sense of worth as a person? Or, conversely, does self-worth influence perceptions of appearance, such that if an individual feels worthy as a person, he/she will favorably evaluate his/ her looks?

We have begun to research this issue by putting the question, this choice, directly to young adolescents (Zumpf & Harter, 1989); that is, we have asked them to indicate which of these two options best describes the nature of the link between their appearance and their self-worth. Our findings reveal that one group of adolescents (approximately 60%) acknowledges that the evaluation of appearance precedes or determines their sense of self-worth, whereas the remaining 40% endorse the opposite orientation, reporting that their sense of self-worth determines how much they like the way they look. Converging evidence indicates that those in the first group, whose appearance determines their self-worth, also report that appearance is more important, that they are more preoccupied with appearance, and that they worry more about how they look compared to the group whose self-worth precedes judgments of appearance (see Harter, 1993).

Moreover, there is a particularly distressing pattern for *girls* in the first directionality subgroup that is basing self-worth on appearance. Adolescent females who report that appearance determines their sense of worth as a person (1) feel worse about their appearance, (2) have lower self-esteem, and (3) also report feeling more affectively depressed compared to females for whom self-esteem precedes judgments of appearance (Harter, 1993; Zumpf & Harter, 1989). Thus, those adolescent females espousing the Jamesian model in which self-evaluations in domains of importance (e.g., appearance) determine their self-worth are more at risk for low self-worth and associated maladaptive outcomes. Sadly, this is the orientation that is underscored by our society, by the media. The irony, therefore, is that endorsement of a Jamesian perspective with regard to the domain of physical appearance represents a psychological liability for females, in particular, undermining their evaluation of both their outer and inner selves.

Another major liability can be observed in the eating-disordered behavior of females, for whom the incidence is much higher than for men (e.g., Greenfeld, Quinlan, Harding, Glass, & Bliss, 1987; Raciti & Norcross, 1987; Rand & Kuldau, 1992; Striegel-Moore, Silberstein, & Rodin, 1986). In addition to considerable body dissatisfaction and body distortion, studies report that eating-disordered females report much lower self-esteem than normal comparison groups (Baumeister, 1991a; Crowther & Chernyk, 1986; Danis & Harter, 1996; Gross & Rosen, 1988; Heatherton & Baumeister, 1991; Mintz & Betz, 1988; Mizes, 1988; Williamson et al., 1995). There are numerous theories of the dynamics of eating-disordered behaviors, ranging from psychoanalytic interpretations, family-systems approaches, brain–behavior links, and so on. A discussion of these processes is beyond the scope of this chapter. However, one framework is particularly relevant to the themes in this chapter. Baumeister and colleagues have developed the thesis that symptoms such as binge eating represent an attempt to escape from unflattering images of oneself. Such an escape narrows one's attention and deconstructs normal cognitive functioning, which in turn disengages normal inhibitions about overeating. There is considerable evidence that eating-disordered women also experience depression in addition to low self-esteem (Crowther & Chernyk, 1986; Gross & Rosen, 1988; Heatherton & Baumeister, 1991; Kaye, Gwirtsman, George, Weiss, & Jimerson, 1986; Mizes, 1988; Vanderheyden, Fekken, & Boland, 1988). Such a finding is not surprising given the inextricable link between low self-esteem and depression, a topic to which I return in Chapter 8.

The application of James' discrepancy model to the perceptions of eating-disordered females can be observed in a study conducted in our own laboratory (Danis & Harter, 1996), where both anorectic and bulimic college students were included. As Table 6.2 reveals, both groups report that their physical appearance is highly important to them (significantly more so than for a normative sample in the same university). Both also evaluate their physical appearance quite negatively, leading to discrepancies between the importance, and their self-evaluations, of their looks. Of interest is the fact that this discrepancy is greater for the bulimic women given their lowered perceptions of attractiveness. One interpretation of this difference between the two eating-disordered groups is that the anorectic women may feel more in control of their physical appearance given that their weight (in this study and in the literature) is lower than that of bulimics; this index of success may translate into more positive perceptions of appearance relative to the bulimic group. However, the general perception among anorectic women that they are still not meeting societal standards of thinness results in much lower evaluations of their appearance relative to our normative college sample. Global self-worth scores are consistent with the magnitude of the discrepancies in that the bulimic women not only reported a greater

TABLE 6.2. Perceptions among Eating-Disordered and Normative Samples of College Women

	Anorectic	Bulimic	Normative
Importance of appearance	3.57	3.62	2.99
Perceived appearance	1.67	1.26	2.57
Discrepancy	1.90	2.36	.42
Self-esteem	2.66	2.06	3.17
Affect/mood	2.79	2.14	3.20

discrepancy but also significantly lower self-worth than did the anorectic women. Finally, the greater self-reported depressive affect of the bulimic women is predictable given their lowered self-esteem, a general relationship that is explored further in Chapter 8.

CONCLUSION

The evidence reviewed in this chapter provides strong support for models that link discrepancies between perceived adequacy and ideal self-images or aspirations for success to outcomes such as self-worth. These processes become operative in middle childhood, when the ability to compare two representations, one's real and ideal self, emerges. There is considerable evidence for James' discrepancy model in that the more ratings of importance exceed perceptions of competence or personal adequacy, the lower one's overall sense of self-worth. Implicit in James' formulation are interventions for enhancing self-worth, either by increasing one's competence or by discounting the importance of areas in which one has perceived weaknesses. However, there are challenges to effecting such changes in the lives of individuals with low global self-worth.

In addressing the specific predictors of self-worth, it becomes instructive to determine the relative contribution of the domains we have identified. The pattern is very robust in both this country and abroad. Physical Appearance consistently emerges as the best predictor, with correlations ranging from .52 to .80; Athletic Competence bears the lowest relationship to global self-worth, with Scholastic Competence, Social Acceptance, and Behavioral Conduct falling in between. Somewhat surprisingly, the correlations between perceived Physical Appearance and global self-worth are comparable in special groups such as learning-disabled students, gifted students, behavior-disordered youth, and children in Special Olympics, where it might be expected that other domains related to their group membership (e.g., Scholastic Competence, Behavioral Conduct, or Athletic Competence, respectively) would be more salient and therefore more highly related to self-worth. The inextricable link between perceptions of appearance and self-worth is particularly problematic for females given unattainable cultural images of physical beauty. Those females who explicitly base their self-worth on their perceptions of their looks are particularly at risk. In the extreme, large discrepancies between the importance of appearance and evaluations of attractiveness among eating-disordered women are associated with extremely low self-worth as well as depressed affect. The relationship between self-worth and affect is explored in Chapter 8, after a consideration of the social sources of self-worth in Chapter 7.

Social Sources of Individual Differences in Self-Evaluation

As observed in Chapter 1, several historical scholars, James Mark Baldwin (1897), Charles Horton Cooley (1902), and George Herbert Mead (1925, 1934) set the conceptual stage upon which the drama of the self in social interaction was enacted. For these *symbolic interactionists*, the self was primarily a social construction crafted through linguistic exchanges (i.e., symbolic interactions) with others. Thus, the personal self develops in the crucible of interpersonal relationships with significant others. Recently, there has been a resurgence of interest in these formulations that emphasized how interactive processes, initially with caregivers, profoundly shape the developing self (see Bretherton, 1991; Case, 1991; Cicchetti, 1990; Harter, 1998a; Sroufe, 1990).

Of particular interest in this chapter is how the messages or approval or disapproval that caregivers communicate to the child are incorporated into the child's sense of worth as a person. Thus, the focus is on those processes through which the child comes to adopt the *opinions* that significant others are perceived to hold toward the self, reflected appraisals that come to define one's sense of self as a person. For each of the symbolic interactionists, there was an implicit internalization process through which the child came to adopt and eventually to own personally the initial values and opinions of significant others. Cooley, in his "looking-glass-self" formulation, was perhaps most explicit in observing that significant others constituted social mirrors into which the child gazes in order to detect his or her opinions toward the self. These perceived opinions, in turn, are incorporated into the evaluation of one's worth as a person. For Mead (1925), the attitudes of different significant others toward the self were psychologically averaged across these individuals, resulting in the "generalized other," which represented their shared perspective on the self.

Although the symbolic interactionists pointed to critical processes in the normative construction of the self, they did not alert us to the fact that self-development, so dependent upon social interactions, could go awry. Caregivers who provide nurturance, approval, and support that is positive will provoke the child to internalize favorable images of self. However, caregivers lacking in nurturance, encouragement, and approval, as well as socializing agents who are rejecting or punitive, will produce children with very negative self-evaluations. Liabilities also emerge for those who remain drawn like a magnet to the social mirror as a source of self-evaluation, seemingly unable to incorporate the standards and opinions of others in a personal sense of self that guides behavior. Each of these liabilities is explored here.

This chapter begins with a discussion of how an appreciation for the impact of the opinions of others on the *content* and *valence* of self-evaluations requires an understanding of developmental changes that permit the internalization of others' attitudes toward the self; that is, at what age do children come to appreciate others' perspectives on the self? After reviewing these developmental prerequisites, attention turns to how particular child-rearing practices shape the specific content of children's self-representations to produce individual differences in the valence of their evaluations of self. Why do some children come to view themselves as capable and lovable, whereas others see themselves as incompetent and unworthy? Those working within an attachment theory framework have contributed heavily to our understanding of these processes, particularly in demonstrating how caregiver styles can influence the child's working model of self.

Given that the child develops in multiple social contexts, it becomes important to consider how different significant others may impact his/her global sense of worth as a person; that is, what is the relative importance of approval from parents and peers, including both classmates and close friends? For those children who fail to receive parental approval, can support from a special adult in one's life, for example, a grandparent or coach, compensate for the absence of parental support? Moreover, how do different *types* of support (e.g., approval, emotional support, instrumental support) differentially influence the internalization process? The manner in which support is communicated to the child and the accuracy of the perceptions of others' opinions toward the self are also complex issues that are discussed.

In the previous chapter, evidence for James' model of the antecedents of global self-worth or esteem was presented. It was demonstrated that perceptions of competence or adequacy in domains deemed important were a powerful predictor of self-worth. However, support from significant others represents another critical source of self-worth for the developing child and adolescent. James' explanation is not incompatible with a looking-glass-self model of self-worth; it is merely incomplete. Thus, evidence for an additive model, in which both Jamesian and looking-glass-self processes combine to produce an individual's level of self-worth, is presented. Just as there were limitations on the extent to which an individual could reduce the discrepancy between the importance of success and perceived competence given James' model, there are limitations on the extent to which one can garner the desired approval of significant others, liabilities that are discussed.

The issue of the *directionality* of effects that was introduced in the earlier discussion of James' formulation (do perceptions of personal adequacy impact self-worth or does self-worth influence these perceptions?) can also be applied to Cooley's looking-glass-self formulation; that is, although Cooley assumed that the opinions and approval of others served as the basis upon which self-worth was established, might the directionality be reversed at some point in development such that one's perceptions of self-worth determine the perceived level of approval from others? As becomes evident, adolescents differ in terms of which directionality they consciously endorse, and these differences in their metatheory have powerful correlates. For example, our own findings reveal that preoccupation with how the approval of others dictates one's self-worth has debilitating consequences.

The fact that these many social processes increasingly occur in multiple social contexts with different significant others as one moves into adolescence adds to the complexity of the construction of a sense of one's worth as a person. Although global self-worth remains a phenomenal reality in the network of self-representations beginning in early adolescence, individuals may develop a more differentiated perception of their worth as a person across different relationships. Thus, how much one likes oneself as a person with one's parents may differ considerably from how much one likes oneself as a person with particular subgroups of peers. We have labeled this construct "relational self-worth," since self-worth typically varies as a function of the particular relational context. Moreover, the level of relational self-worth in a given interpersonal context can be understood from a looking-glass-self perspective; that is, approval from significant others within a given context is directly related to perceptions of worth in the corresponding context. The relationship between relational self-worth and global self-worth, including implications, is explored, as is the very viability of the global self-worth construct itself.

DEVELOPMENTAL PREREQUISITES

The capacities to engage in looking-glass-self processes as well as to construct working models of self do not emerge at one particular point in development but evolve gradually over the course of childhood. Rudimentary skills begin to appear at about 2 years of age. Stipek et al. (1992) report that toward the goal of anticipating positive parental responses and avoiding negative reactions, 2-year-olds begin to develop an appreciation for parental standards. In addition, they show some initial ability to evaluate whether they have met these standards. Thereafter, children gradually begin to internalize the standards of parents, allowing them to engage in self-evaluation, independent of adults' reactions. As observed in the chapter on self-conscious emotions, children will be more likely to internalize parental standards if there is a strong, positive affective bond. Further contributing to looking-glass-self processes is the increasing ability throughout childhood to appreciate the parents' evaluative perspective toward the self. Through increasing perspective-taking skills, children come to recognize that not only do parents have standards that they expect to be met, but also that parents form an evaluative opinion about the child (Higgins, 1991; Leahy & Shirk, 1985; Oosterwegel & Oppenheimer, 1993; Selman, 1980).

Other formulations, such as Selman's (1980), as well as the seminal observations of Gesell and Ilg (1946), reveal how the internalization process will be transformed as children further develop their capacities for self-awareness during early and middle childhood. Despite the fact that the Gesellian approach has been criticized for being atheoretical and lacking in rigor, the acquisition sequence that is identified provides rich descriptive material, although children are reaching the stages identified at earlier ages. The different stages of self-awareness, articulated by Selman and illustrated by Gesell and Ilg, can be translated into I-self and Me-self processes (see also Harter, 1983). During early childhood, the I-self cannot directly or consciously evaluate the Me-self. However, the I-self does seem to be able critically to evaluate others. As Gesell and Ilg pointed out, at this stage, the child seems preoccupied with the conduct and correctness of his/her friends' behavior, frequently pointing out their faults.

At the next level, the I-self observes *others* evaluating the self due to improved perspective-taking skills but cannot yet evaluate the Me-self critically (see also Leahy & Shirk, 1985). This level portrays the beginning of the looking-glass process in that others serve as the reflective surface providing appraisals that will eventually be incorporated into one's self-definition, namely, the Me-self. Gesell and Ilg describe how, at this stage, children worry about what others might think of them and are careful not to expose themselves to criticism. They are concerned about their actions, ashamed of their mistakes, and cringe when they are laughed at or ridiculed.

At the following level, the standards and opinions of others begin to become incorporated, and through the additional advance of social comparison skills, the I-self can determine whether the Me-self is meeting these standards. At this stage, Gesell and Ilg (1946) describe the child as "increasingly aware of himself as a person" and "more conscious of himself in the ways in which he differs from other people" (p. 176). He is "interested in evaluating his own performance . . . and he wishes to live up to his notion of the standard that other people have for him. Since his performance is often only mediocre and his notion of other's standards are extremely high, there is often a discrepancy here which leads to tears and temporary unhappiness" (p. 176).

At the final level during middle childhood, the I-self comes to directly evaluate the Me-self, having internalized both opinions and standards. At this stage, Gesell and Ilg highlight the emerging capacity for self-criticism. The child is described as anxious to please, but also apprehensive, sensitive to correction, and very sensitive to embarrassment. At this stage, "they may underrate themselves as persons, lack confidence, and remark: 'Oh, am I stupid,' or 'I'm the dumbest,' tossing off self-critical remarks" (p. 208).

Higgins' (1991) developmental model points to further refinements in this process. He describes an interesting shift from the child's *identification* of parental standards to their *internalization*. In the stage of identification, the young child identifies the standards and opinions of others whom he/she wants to please and attempts to regulate his/her behavior accordingly. However, in middle childhood, the child comes to internalize the standards of others in the form of self-guides, as well as to internalize the opinions that others hold about the self with regard to the ability to meet these idealized goals and be the right kind of person (Grusec, 1983; Kohlberg, 1976). Higgins notes that from a self-regulatory point of view, the ability to make self-attributions and to respond critically to one's actions independent of others' opinions of them is the essence of what has been termed the child's new capacity for "internal control."

Connell and colleagues (Connell & Wellborn, 1991) suggest a similar sequence using somewhat different terminology. They have applied their analysis to the child's motivation to engage in schoolwork. Initially, the child performs on the basis of *external* motives (e.g., "The teacher or my parents will get mad at me if I don't do my schoolwork"). At the next, intermediate level of *introjection*, the motive is more internal in that if the child doesn't perform, his/her self-esteem will be threatened and/or lead to a sense of shame. At the third level, the desire to perform is even further internalized in that it is actively adopted as a genuine goal of the *self*. Damon and Hart's (1988) analysis also converges in that they describe a normative-development shift from self-attributes defined in terms of external social standards toward self-attributes that reflect personal beliefs and internalized standards, although they place this shift later than other investigators, namely, at adolescence. Although developmentalists agree that there is a general shift from external to internal sources of self-evaluation, the sense of self will continue to rely to some extent on the recognition and validation of others. Moreover, during periods of new skill acquisition, there will be a return to external standards and feedback, in what Mack (1983) describes as a telescoped recapitulation of the shift from external to internal sources.

CHILD-REARING PRACTICES PRODUCING INDIVIDUAL DIFFERENCES IN THE CONTENT OF SELF-EVALUATIONS

There is considerable evidence from different theoretical perspectives that the quality of caregiving, beginning with the role of parents, has a tremendous impact on the content of the self-system (e.g., how favorably one evaluates the self) as well as how features of the self are organized. Thus, parents who are nurturant, responsive, and approving but demanding of standards will produce children with positive self-evaluations. Traditional psychodynamic theorists such as Sullivan (1953) and Winnicott (1958) placed heavy emphasis on how the quality of mother–infant interactions impacted self-development, a theme amplified in more contemporary treatments of the self (see Stern, 1985). For example, Winnicott described a pattern of "good enough" mothering that would promote healthy self-development. The "good enough" mother responds promptly and appropriately to the infant's demands, thereby promoting feelings of "omnipotence" or power, which certain theorists consider to be a critical precursor of positive feelings about the self (Erikson, 1950; Kohut, 1977). She also responds positively to the infant's mastery attempts. During periods when the infant's needs are met, the "good enough" mother retreats, supporting the capacity for the infant to be alone, which Winnicott considered essential to the development of a stable and positive sense of self. Small failures in parental responsiveness eventually lead to the infant's disappointment in the parent and lessen feelings of omnipotence. However, according to both Winnicott and Kohut, these experiences play a vital role in self–other differentiation, allowing the child that to both separate from the parent and to become more reality oriented (see also Mahler, 1967, 1968).

Similarly, from an attachment theory perspective, a working model of *self* can only be considered within the context of the caregiver–infant relationship from which it emerged. Thus, as Bowlby (1969) contended, the child who experiences parents as emotionally available, loving, and supportive of his/her mastery efforts will construct a working model of the self as lovable and competent, the pattern for securely attached children. In contrast, insecurely attached children who experience attachment figures as rejecting or emotionally unavailable and nonsupportive will construct a working model of the self as unlovable, incompetent, and generally unworthy. Thus, the *content* of a child's working model of self will be impacted by parental responsiveness.

Within the attachment literature (see Bretherton, 1991; Crittenden, 1990), there has been a further distinction between less than optimal parenting styles that are associated with two patterns of insecurely attached children, those labeled as ambivalently attached and those described as avoidant. Ambivalently attached infants whose caregivers were inconsistently available should construct a working model of the self as ineffective, weak, and uncertain. Those with a history of avoidant attachment, whose caregivers were not available, should develop working models in which the self is unworthy and lacks competence. Sroufe (1990) describes longitudinal data supporting these hypotheses within the contexts of preschools and summer camps. Those with insecure attachment histories manifested lower levels of behaviorally manifest and teacher- or counselor-rated self-esteem than did those with secure attachment histories. Differences in self-confidence were also observed, particularly between the securely and the anxiously attached groups, on problem-solving tasks. Both groups of insecurely attached individuals report forms of social withdrawal from peers (see also Rubin, Stewart, & Chen, 1995).

It should be noted that the *self-presentation* by avoidants on verbal self-report measures is often quite positive; that is, they report high self-esteem. In fact, Cassidy (1988, 1990) reports that as young children, many describe themselves as "perfect" in contrast to ambivalently attached children, whose descriptions were typically negative. Securely attached children generally described themselves in positive terms but also admitted to being less than perfect. Similar patterns have been found for ratings and descriptions of adults (Cassidy & Kobak, 1988). Avoidants appear to idealize the self as well as the parent. These findings have been interpreted as revealing defensively high self-esteem in an attempt to consciously or unconsciously mask feelings of unworthiness.

Of further interest are findings revealing that interactions with caregivers also impact the structure and *organization* of the working model (Bretherton, 1991). Insensitive caregivers who ignore the child's signals will produce insecurely attached children whose working models are less coherently organized from the outset and are less likely to become well integrated. Parental underattunement leads to impoverished working models, since it undermines the infant's ability to attend to and subsequently label his/her affective states and thereby incorporate them into his/her self-portrait (Crittenden, 1988, 1990, 1994). The child may also defensively exclude painful experiences at the hands of insensitive caregivers. At the other extreme, Stern

(1985) observes that parental overattunement (or intrusiveness) represents a form of emotional theft in which the parent accentuates how the infant *should* feel rather than how the infant actually *does* feel. Thus, actual feeling states are not shared but become isolated, contributing to fragmentation or lack of coherence.

Crittenden (1990) further distinguishes between securely attached, and both types of insecurely attached, individuals. Her findings reveal that those with a history of *secure* attachment can access and integrate the various memory systems, can view themselves from several perspectives, and can accept both their desirable and undesirable features. They can also reason more openly with parents about the motives for their misbehavior. These features allow them to evaluate the self more realistically and aid in the construction of a self-narrative (see also Cassidy, 1990). Those with an *avoidant* attachment history, whom Crittenden labels "defended," have less access to their various memory systems given that some features of the true self are held out of awareness, whereas others have been defensively "corrected" (Crittenden, 1988). Those with an *ambivalent* attachment history (labeled "coercive"), also have more fragmented and distorted working models. Their tendency to blame others for their misbehavior robs them of the opportunity to integrate behavioral aspects of the self into their working model. Moreover, the inconsistent parenting that they have experienced prevents them from developing an organized or coherent set of internal representations.

Child-rearing practices continue to be critical during later childhood. Parental approval is particularly critical in determining the self-esteem of children, supporting both the attachment and the looking-glass-self perspectives. Coopersmith (1967) has described how the socialization practices of parents impacted children's self-esteem. Parents of children with high self-esteem (1) were more likely to be accepting, affectionate, and involved; (2) enforced rules consistently and encouraged children to uphold high standards of behavior; (3) preferred noncoercive disciplinary practices, discussing the reasons why the child's behavior was inappropriate; and (4) were democratic in considering the child's opinion around certain family decisions.

More recent evidence also reveals that parental support, particularly in the form of approval and acceptance, is associated with high self-esteem and the sense that one is lovable (see review by Feiring & Taska, 1996). Other studies have built upon Baumrind's (1989) typology of parenting styles, linking them to child and adolescent self-evaluations. For example, Lamborn, Mounts, Steinberg, and Dornbush (1991) report that adolescents of authoritative parents report significantly higher self-concepts in the domains of social and academic competence than do those with authoritarian, as well as neglectful, parents.

More comprehensive models linking family factors to child and adolescent self-esteem have recently begun to emerge. For example, Hattie (1992) presents a model in which such structural features, including social status, are included; however, family psychological characteristics such as expectations and encouragement of the child, rewards and punishments, as well as family activities and interests, play a major role. Feiring and Taska (1996) present a heuristic model that identifies family factors impacting the child's self-representations, building upon attachment theory. For example, they suggest that during childhood, positive interactions between caregiver and child (e.g., affectionate contact upon reunion) coupled with a warm and reliable relationship will foster positive self-representations within the family context (e.g., "I am loved, valued, accepted") as well as more global self-evaluations that transcend family relationships (e.g., "I am worthwhile, secure, and autonomous"). They review isolated findings consistent with pieces of the model but observe that there is relatively little research that comprehensively addresses many of the issues in their framework.

In their review, Feiring and Taska observe that within the family systems literature, attention has recently turned to the impact of siblings upon developing self-representations. Age-related status is one influence in that an older sibling may come to view the self as nurturant or dominant, whereas the young sibling will identify more with the role of being nurtured or dominated. Social comparison with siblings represents another avenue through which the self-concept is impacted, depending upon how one measures up to the siblings with whom one is compared. Deidentification is another pathway to self-definition as children attempt to be *different* than siblings, in part to avoid intense competition.

The field is also beginning to examine how *dysfunctional* families influence the developing child's sense of self. For example, research (reviewed by Feiring & Taska, 1996) reveals that children from alcoholic families report lower self-esteem. Considerable evidence also reveals that children from *abusive* families suffer a constellation of assaults to the self-system (see reviews by Harter, 1988b; Putnam, 1993; Westen, 1993). The disruptions in both I-self functions and Me-self manifestations are the specific topic of Chapter 10.

THE INFLUENCE OF DIFFERENT SOURCES AND TYPES OF SUPPORT ON SELF-WORTH

There is general consensus of opinion that support from significant others is a critical determinant of global self-worth or self-esteem. However, a more differentiated picture is beginning to emerge with regard to support from different sources of support, for example, parents versus peers in either more public or private relational contexts. From a looking-glass-self perspective, one can ask the question: Mirror, mirror, on the wall: Whose opinion is the most critical of all? Another issue involves the particular type of support, for example, approval, emotional support, and instrumental support. Is one type of support more critical to self-worth than others?

In our own research documenting the looking-glass-self formulation, we have broadened the examination of the *sources* of approval to whom children turn. For older children, we have identified four sources of potential support: parents, teachers, classmates, and close friends. We then created self-report items (see Social Support Scale for Children and Adolescents, Harter, 1985c) tapping the extent to which one feels that these others approve of or value the self. Through the construction of such items, we have been able to directly examine the link between the perceived regard from others and the perceived regard for the self (i.e., global self-worth).

Across numerous studies with older children and adolescents, as well as college students and adults in the world of work and family, we have found that the correlations between perceived support from significant others and self-worth range from .50 to .65 (Harter, 1990a, 1993). As anticipated from Cooley's model, those with the lowest levels of support report the lowest self-worth, those with moderate support have moderate levels of self-worth, and those receiving the most support hold the self in the highest regard. Among the four sources of support that we have examined, we have repeatedly demonstrated that for older children and adolescents, perceived classmate and parent approval are the best predictors. Thus, Cooley's looking-glass-self model on the origins of self-worth appears to be clearly documented, with regard to the link between one's perceptions of the approval of others and one's sense of worth as a person.

To date, we have not examined whether *others'* reports of the approval they provide predict self-worth. Interestingly, the literature suggests that there is no consistent agreement between people's self-perceptions and how they are actually viewed by others (Juhasz, 1992; Kenny, 1988; Shrauger & Schoeneman, 1979). Moreover, perceptions of support have been found to be more predictive of self-evaluations than have more objective indices of support (Berndt & Burgy, 1996; Felson, 1993; John & Robbins, 1994; Rosenberg, 1979; Shrauger & Schoeneman, 1979). Thus, Rosenberg concludes that "we are more or less unconsciously seeing ourselves as we *think* others who are important to us and whose opinion we trust see us" (1979, p. 97).

Although types of support other than approval may contribute to self-worth, findings from our laboratory indicate that approval or acceptance is most highly predictive, instrumental support is the least predictive, with emotional support falling in between (Robinson, 1995). From a looking-glass-self perspective, others' approval of the self should be most readily incorporated as approval of oneself as a person, namely, self-worth. Although instrumental and emotional support from significant others should be a welcome sign of caring, they could also serve as a sign of weaknesses rather than strengths, undermining the child's sense of efficacy. Building upon Nadler and Fisher's (1986) model, Shell and Eisenberg (1992) provide an interesting developmental analysis of the conditions under which instrumental aid from others should and should not pose a threat to one's self-esteem. For example, among older children, who have developed trait conceptualizations of self-attributes (e.g., smart vs. dumb), help from others could be interpreted as feedback that they are "dumb," leading to negative self-evaluations and a sense of helplessness. Similarly, if one needs emotional support from others to deal with psychological problems, this may be construed as a sign of weakness that can undermine self-worth.

From a developmental perspective, parental approval has been found to be more predictive of self-worth than is approval from *peers* among *younger* children (Nikkari & Harter, 1993; Pekrun, 1990; Rosenberg, 1979). Rosenberg has observed that the younger children's conclusions about what they are like rest heavily on the perceived judgments of external authority, particularly parental authority. Knowledge of the self is regarded as absolute and resides in those with superior wisdom, a conclusion consistent with Piaget's (1932) observations of children's understanding of rules and sources of moral judgment. Thus, during childhood, parents are considered to be more *credible* sources of information on the self (see also Oosterwegel & Oppenheimer, 1993). According to Rosenberg, respect for parental knowledge declines with development, and peer evaluations rise in importance (see also Pekrun, 1990).

Evidence only partially confirms these claims. For example, although the correlation between peer approval and self-worth has been found to increase with development, the correlation between parental approval and self-worth does not decline, at least through adolescence (Harter, 1990a). This pattern is consistent with the recent conclusions of Oosterwegel and Oppenheimer (1993), who emphasize the importance of parents' opinions of the self well into adolescence. Others also report that while peers become more important as one moves into adolescence, parents continue to remain central; their role may be transformed; however, it is not diminished (see Buhrmester & Furman, 1987; Lamborn & Steinberg, 1993; Ryan & Lynch, 1989). Correlations between parental approval and global self-worth have been observed to decline, however, when adolescents make the transition to college (Harter & Johnson, 1993).

With regard to the role of the appraisals of peer groups on self-worth, the particular type of peer approval differentially influences one's sense of personal worth. At every developmental level we have investigated, namely, middle to late childhood, adolescence, the college years, and early to middle-age adulthood (Harter, 1990a), we have consistently found that support from peers in the more "public domain" (e.g., classmates, peers in organizations, work settings, etc.) is far more predictive of self-worth than is support from close friends. We interpret this finding to suggest that support from others in the more public domain may better represent acceptance from the "generalized other," approval that is perceived as more "objective," or from more credible sources, than the support from one's close friends. This is not to negate the importance of close friends' support, which would appear to be critical as a source of empathy, feedback, and clarification of values. Such close friends' support would seem to function as a secure psychological base from which one can reemerge to meet the challenges of the generalized other, whose acceptance appears critical to maintaining a positive sense of one's worth as a person.

For some adolescents, the opinions of selected subgroups, rather than of mainstream classmates, become critical to their self-definition. For example, failure to meet the standards of the dominant group may produce negative self-attitudes that in turn cause such adolescents to seek the company of teenage groups or gangs, where prevalent societal standards are ignored and delinquent behaviors are admired (Kaplan, 1980). Through these identifications, an individual's level of self-esteem can be elevated. For example, evidence reveals that boys who suffered the biggest reduction in self-esteem when they entered high school were able to restore their self-esteem by engaging in delinquent behavior (Bynner, O'Malley, & Bachman, 1981).

A looking-glass-self perspective can also be applied to the relationship between self-esteem and ethnicity. The majority of comparisons have been made between European American and African American youth. Overall, particularly when socioeconomic status is controlled, the pattern of findings reveals little in the way of systematic differences in self-esteem (see Crain, 1996). Interestingly, among African American youth, the relationship between the attitudes of significant others toward the self (especially family members as well as African American friends and teachers) has been found to be somewhat stronger than among European American youth (Rosenberg, 1979). It has been suggested that not only is the African American community a source of positive self-concept in African American children but also that under certain conditions, the African American family can filter out racist, destructive messages from the white community, supplanting such messages with more positive feedback that will enhance self-esteem (Barnes, 1980). More recent treatments of ethnicity suggest the need for much more complex models that take into account a variety of risk factors, stressors, contextual variables, social support, and relatedness to others in predicting self-perceptions, including their impact on positive and negative outcomes (see Connell, Spencer, & Aber, 1994; Cross, 1985; Iheanacho, 1988; Spencer, 1995; Spencer & Markstrom-Adams, 1990). This is clearly the direction in which the field needs to move in order to thoughtfully address the complexity of the issues involving ethnicity and the self.

The Role of Special Adults

Although parents and peers, particularly those in the more public arenas, have been demonstrated to be particularly important sources of social support, impacting self-worth, alternative sources may also have an influence. Children and adolescents, be they ethnic minorities or Caucasian youth, may profit from the support of special adults. A number of studies (Darling, 1991; Galbo & Mayer-Demetrulias, 1996; Hamilton & Darling, 1989; Darling, Hamilton, & Niegro, 1996; Masten, in press; Munsch, Liang, & DeSecottier, 1996) have documented the fact that a significant percentage of children and adolescents have special adults, defined as a nonparents who provides a variety of types of support including approval, emotional support, instrumental aid, as well as shared time and activities. Findings on the particular *impact* of special adults on outcomes such as self-worth and its correlates have been limited, however. Of particular interest in our own work has been the issue of how support from special adults interacts with the level of support from parents (Talmi & Harter, 1998). Toward this goal, we identified young adolescents (middle school students) at three levels of parental support: high, moderate, and low. At each of the levels, we identified those with and those without special adults. Fully 60% of the entire sample reported that they did have a special adult, who was most typically a relative, a friend's parent or their parents' friend, and those with special adults were represented at each level of parental support. Moreover, perceived support from special adults was uniformly high. As outcomes, we were interested in global self-worth and two of its correlates, hope (hopeful to hopeless) and affect (cheerful to depressed). We first demonstrated that there was a predictable impact of level of parental support on these outcomes, consistent with earlier findings. Those with high parental support reported the most positive outcomes; those with low parent support reported the most negative outcomes, with those receiving moderate support falling in between.

We anticipated that for adolescents receiving moderate to high levels of support from parents, the effect of support from a special adult would be *additive* in that those with special adults would report more positive outcomes that those without special adults. For those with low levels of support, we predicted that the presence of a special adult would serve a *compensatory* function, leading those with a special adult to display more positive outcomes than those without such an adult figure; that is, we reasoned that the support from the special adult may help to offset the negative effects of low parental support.

Although this framework implies that the presence of a special adult will have a facilitative effect at all levels of parental support, we did not anticipate that special adult support would necessarily improve the functioning of all adolescents who had such a figure in their lives. Although support from significant others is a powerful predictor of self-worth, other determinants such as perceived competence or adequacy in domains deemed important (derived from James' formulation) contribute heavily to self-worth; that is, the effects of support from a special adult may be undermined to the extent that these other predictors are operative, namely, that perceptions of inadequacies in domains of importance are taking a major toll on self-worth.

As a data-analytic strategy at each level of parental support, we identified two subgroups: those who appeared to profit from special adult support in that their mean outcome levels were markedly higher than those without special adults, and those who appeared to derive no benefit; that is, their outcome scores were comparable to those without special adults. We anticipated that those adolescents who did *not* demonstrate the additive or compensatory effects of special adult support would report lower levels of perceived competence or adequacy, suggesting that the presence of this additional support could not overcome the impact of another very important predictor of self-worth and selected correlates.

Examination of the perceived competence/adequacy scores across the five domains included (Scholastic Competence, Athletic Competence, Physical Appearance, Peer Likability, and Behavioral Conduct) revealed that for every domain, the self-concept scores of those who did not benefit from special adult support were markedly lower than those who did appear to profit from special adult support. Thus, negative perceptions of competence or adequacy within each of the domains we examined would appear to have contributed to the level of self-worth, hope, and affect of group, over and above the level of perceived parental support, making it virtually impossible for special adult support either to add to, or compensate for, parental support.

These findings are important with regard to their implications for intervention, a topic to which I return later in more depth. Mentoring programs for youth are currently very much in the limelight and have been highly touted as a panacea for troubled youth by the government, by mental health workers, and by educators. However, the findings of our special adult study reveal that not all youth will profit from such an intervention strategy. For those who not only experience low parental support but also feel very incompetent or inadequate, the support of special adults will be insufficient. Rather, additional interventions, targeted to overcome personal limitations and to enhance particular skills, will be needed to enhance feelings of self-worth, hope, and happiness.

Communication of Approval

The manner in which approval from significant adults, be they adults or peers, is communicated is also more complex than initially assumed. Symbolic interactionists, particularly Mead, placed heavy emphasis upon the *direct* communication of others' evaluations in the form of language, evaluations that were then incorporated into a sense of self. Certain theorists (e.g., Ashmore & Ogilvie, 1992) suggest that such a model is too passive and mechanical, arguing that in our interactions with others, we not only encode their verbalizations but also affective, verbal, motoric, and behavioral information about the other as well as the self. Felson (1993), as well as Shrauger and Schoeneman (1979), also notes that the opinions of others may be gleaned through channels other than direct communication. Negative evaluations, less likely to be communicated directly, may be inferred from the absence of positive feedback. Third parties may also serve as a source of information about others' appraisals. In addition, observing how people whose opinions matter evaluate *others* provides indirect information as to how such people evaluate the self. Shared standards and social comparison processes represent another route through which the opinions of others can be inferred; that is, shared *standards* may be communicated directly by others. Individuals then engage in social comparison to determine whether their performance measures up to these standards. If they feel it does not, they conclude that those others whose standards they share must think poorly of them. Conversely, if they meet these standards, then they infer that others must be evaluating them positively. The field lacks an analysis and supportive evidence of the salience of these mechanisms at different levels of development. However, it is likely that the more complex and indirect forms of communication would not be operative until middle childhood and beyond given the cognitive limitations of young children.

LIMITATIONS ON THE ABILITY TO OBTAIN SUPPORT FROM SIGNIFICANT OTHERS

In the preceding chapter, it was observed that there are limitations on the extent to which Jamesian discrepancies can be reduced in the service of enhancing global self-worth. The same general point applies to impact of support on self-worth. Given that for many children and adolescents such support is often not available, it becomes understandable why these individuals suffer from low self-esteem or self-worth. Why is it that these individuals have been unable to obtain the needed support? Why is self-enhancing approval not forthcoming? The answers would appear to lie at the interface of the characteristics of the significant others and the attributes of children and adolescents themselves. With regard to parental support, there is a growing literature on factors (e.g., parental depression, stressful conditions within the family) that lead to parents' inability to provide self-enhancing support.

Our own research has identified another critical facet of support that we have labeled *conditionality* (Harter, Marold, et al., 1992). Conditionality is defined as the extent to which one feels that support is only forthcoming if one meets high parental or peer standards, typically, expectations that are unrealistically high. We have contrasted conditionality to unconditional positive regard (see Rogers & Dymond, 1954) in which one is loved or supported for who one is as a person, not for whether one fulfills the expectations of others that do not respect the child's talents but reflect demands that may be difficult or impossible to meet. Thus, approval is only offered if the child displays behaviors and attitudes that parents and peers unilaterally demand. Our findings have revealed that the more conditional the support, the lower one's perceptions of overall worth as a person. By way of interpretation, conditionality would appear to undermine self-worth because it does *not* validate or signify approval of the self as a person but specifies behavioral contingencies, the psychological hoops through which children must jump in order to please parents or peers. As such, it is perceived as controlling rather than enhancing.

Obviously, child-rearing involves the specification of social rewards for behaviors that are desired by socializing agents, as well as consequences for behaviors that are not desirable. What differentiates these types of natural contingencies from conditionality is that in the former case, caregivers focus on the *behavior*; that is, the message is "I am disappointed with what you did or didn't do," where the child has the capacity to demonstrate the behavior (e.g., not hit one's sister or talk back to parents, clean one's room, do one's homework, etc.). Conditionality, in contrast, demeans the child as a *person* in the face of unilateral demands that represent an unrealistic agenda on the part of parents that is not responsive to the needs and skills of the child and is not negotiable.

The extent to which a parent or peer engages in conditionality represents, in part, a style that parent or peer brings to the relationship. Therefore, the child or adolescent may be at the mercy of a style that undermines his/her own self-worth. However, conditionality also has as its target particular domains of behavior that are displayed by the child or adolescent, domains in which the parent or peer has specific standards of performance. Hypothetically, then, the child or adolescent has only to meet these standards in order to obtain the needed support that will promote high self-worth. Why, then, should devaluation of one's worth exist or persist?

Our answer to this question lies partially in an analysis of the particular domains that peers and parents identify as critical performance arenas for children and adolescents. To obtain such information, we have asked our child and adolescent participants to rate the importance that classmates and parents attach to the five domains we have explored. Our raters report that *peers* place the most importance on the physical appearance, likability, and athletic competence of others their age. In contrast, our raters report that their *parents* place more importance on the scholastic competence and behavioral conduct of their children. Thus, in order to obtain the approval of one's peers, one has to be good-looking, likable, and athletically talented. In order to obtain the approval of one's parents, one has to excel at schoolwork and manifest commendable conduct. However, such goals may be unattainable for some children given natural limits on their abilities and personal makeup. The fact that the conditional expectations of others are often unrealistically high further exacerbates the likelihood of not meeting these expectations in the service of garnering support.

THE CONTRIBUTION OF JAMES AND COOLEY: AN ADDITIVE MODEL OF SELF-WORTH

In the previous chapter on discrepancies within the self-system, evidence bolstering James' formulation, namely, that competence in domains of importance was a critical antecedent of perceived overall worth as a person, was presented. This formulation does not conflict with Cooley's looking-glass-self perspective. Rather, support represents an additional source of self-worth. Our findings reveal that both James' and Cooley's formulations, taken together, provide a powerful explanation for the level of self-worth displayed by older children and adolescents (Harter, 1987, 1990a). As can be seen in Figure 7.1, the effects of these two determinants are additive. At each level of social support (representing the average of classmate and parental approval), greater competence in domains of importance leads to higher self-worth. Similarly, at each level of competence in domains of importance, the more support one garners from classmates and parents, the higher one's self-worth. Those individuals with the lowest self-worth, therefore, are those who report both incompetence in domains of importance and the absence of supportive approval from others. Those with the highest

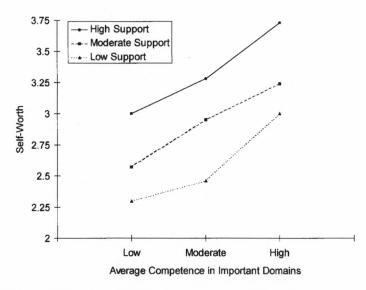

FIGURE 7.1. Additive effects of competence/adequacy in domains of importance and social support on self-worth.

self-worth report the highest levels of competence in domains of importance, as well as the highest level of parental and peer support.

More recently, we have become interested in the *importance* attached to *support* from different sources; that is, just as competence in domains deemed important is critical to James' formulation, by the same logic, might not *support* from sources judged to be *important* be a better predictor of self-worth than support alone? There may be very legitimate reasons why children would discount the importance of support from particular sources, particularly if it were not forthcoming. As discussed earlier, there are a number of reasons why children may not be able to garner the support of significant others. To address this issue, we constructed items tapping the importance of approval or acceptance from each of the primary sources in our model (e.g., parents, teachers, and peers). Analogous to our data-analytic strategy in examining James' hypothesis, we have examined the correlations between support from important versus unimportant sources. The pattern of findings is quite similar. We find that support from important sources correlates much more highly with self-worth (r = .52) than does support from sources deemed unimportant (r = .22). Thus, the same processes appear to be operative for both formulations in that importance of success in particular domains, and the importance of support from each source, contributes to our understanding of the level of self-worth.

THE DIRECTIONALITY OF THE LINK
BETWEEN SUPPORT AND SELF-WORTH

In our treatment of James' formulation on self-esteem, we addressed the issue of the directionality of effects; that is, do domain-specific evaluations (of appearance) serve as antecedents of self-esteem, or alternatively, as some (e.g., Brown, 1993a) have argued, does self-esteem influence domain-specific evaluations? The same issue is relevant to the links between support and self-esteem. A number of investigators have questioned the assumption that the inferred appraisals of others' support necessarily *precede* self-evaluations such as global self-esteem (Felson, 1993; Juhasz, 1992; Leahy & Shirk, 1985). The alternative is also plausible, namely, that self-evaluations may be driving one's perceptions of the opinions of others. Felson (1993) reports a series of studies revealing that children who like themselves assume that their parents' and peers' reactions to them are favorable, leading to an alternative interpretation that he terms the "false consensus effect." It is likely that both effects, the internalization of others' opinions and the assumption that if one likes the self, others in turn will manifest their approval, may be operative. Such reciprocity was acknowledged by Felson and Zielinski (1989), who inferred that "support increases self-esteem, which increases support (or perceived support), which in turn increases self-esteem" (p. 219).

In our model-testing efforts, however, there is reason to be cautious about inferring the directionality of effects postulated. Statistical modeling procedures applied to group data collected at any given point in time do not necessarily simulate the psychological processes underlying the sequence in which perceptions about the self and others unfold. Often, in path analysis, reversing the order of the relevant components (e.g., support and self-worth) will provide just as adequate a fit to the data.

Our own interest in the directionality of these components provoked us to examine what proportion of adolescents *consciously endorse* Cooley's looking-glass-self formulation (Harter, Stocker, & Robinson, 1996); that is, how many adolescents actually acknowledge that they need the approval of others in order to approve of the self? This issue becomes particularly relevant during adolescence, since at this stage, young people begin to form metatheories about the causal nature of the links between constructs that involve the self and others. Therefore, we first asked young adolescents to endorse one of three possible orientations with regard to the direction of peer approval and global self-worth: (1) peer approval precedes self-worth (i.e., perceptions of peer approval are the basis on which judgments about one's worth as a person are formed); (2) self-worth precedes approval (i.e., how much one likes oneself as a person will determine how much approval one will receive from peers); and (3) there is no connection between peer approval and self-worth (i.e., how much one likes oneself as a person has little or nothing to do with approval from peers). After making their choices, participants were asked to provide their own description of a situation that exemplified the directionality orientation they selected.

Participants' spontaneous descriptions clearly validated their orientation choice. Those adopting the looking-glass-self perspective, in which approval precedes self-worth, gave examples such as the following: "When I meet new kids and they approve of me, then I look at myself and say 'I'm not so bad,' and it makes me feel good"; "When other kids make you feel left out, you don't feel good about yourself"; "When people praise everything you do, then you start to really like yourself as a person"; "If other people don't like me as a person, then I wonder if I am a good person because I care about what people say about me."

Those who endorsed the opposite directionality orientation (self-esteem precedes approval), gave the following types of examples: "In seventh grade I didn't like myself as a person, so I didn't have very many friends, but then in eighth grade I felt confident about myself and then I found that I had many more friends"; "You have to appreciate yourself first, as a person; if you wait for other people to make you feel good, you could be waiting a long time!"; "I just like myself and then other people like me too"; "The way I figure it, if you can't like the person you are first, then how do you expect other people to like you?"

Those who saw no link between approval and self-worth gave explanations such as follows: "I really don't care if someone doesn't like me because its their problem"; "Well, somebody said I was stupid. Go ahead, let them think I'm stupid, who cares!"; "The popular people were mean to me, but I kept my head high and ignored it because I like the way I am, its me"; "If someone doesn't like me, they can't make me feel bad if I'm confident enough about myself. What they think doesn't matter."

A major goal of this investigation was to determine whether these three orientations were associated with a predictable pattern of meaningful correlates. More specifically, we sought to examine the general hypothesis that there were certain liabilities associated with the endorsement of a looking-glass-self perspective at this developmental level. We anticipated that those adopting a looking-glass-self orientation would report greater preoccupation with others' opinions, lower support, more fluctuating support, as well as lower and more fluctuating self-worth compared to members of the group who felt that their self-worth would impact the opinions of others. We also anticipated that looking-glass-self subjects would be more likely to be socially distracted from schoolwork. The findings confirmed this pattern of predictions.

Those endorsing the looking-glass-self perspective reported significantly greater preoccupation with peer approval than both the Self-Worth to Approval group as well as the No Connection group, who reported negligible preoccupation. Moreover, teachers rated the looking-glass-self students to be more socially distracted in the classroom. To the extent to which the looking-glass-self adolescents are the most preoccupied and therefore the most cognizant of classmate approval, it was predicted that they should be more likely to detect *fluctuations* (real or imagined) in peer approval than the other two groups, which they did. Since, by definition, the looking-glass-self adolescents are basing their personal sense of worth on approval, the greater self-reported fluctuations in approval were predicted to result in greater fluctuations in self-worth than for the other two groups, which the results corroborated. Looking-glass-self subjects also reported a lower *level* of peer approval. Such individuals, given their preoccupation with approval, may engage in behaviors that do not garner peer support; for example, they may try too hard to elicit peer approval and in so doing will annoy or alienate their classmates. To the extent that the looking-glass-self participants experience lower approval, their self-worth should also be lower than the other two groups, which it was.

Of particular importance are the earlier *developmental* precursors of the three directionality orientations that we identified. Here, we share with many developmentalists, particularly those with an attachment perspective, the view that early relationships with caregivers provide working models that children may carry into relationships with peers (Kobak & Sceery, 1988). With regard to those adolescents who endorse the looking-glass-self orientation, we can only speculate that the developmental history of these individuals may have been characterized by more disapproval, inconsistent or fluctuating approval, or support that was *conditional* upon meeting the demands of others (see Harter, Marold, et al., 1992, for findings on the negative effects of conditional support among adolescents). Such a history could lead to preoccupation and concern over support, perceptions of lower and fluctuating support, which in turn would lead to lower and fluctuating self-worth. A critical assumption is that because such individuals have not received adequate approval of the self from *others*, they have not experienced the kind of validating support that could be internalized as approval of the *self*.

With regard to the development of process through which one's level of self-worth is initially constructed, we are postulating that, during early and middle childhood, approval that validates the self is a critical precursor of high self-worth, as Cooley and others postulated. Thus, the directionality for young children is such that approval initially precedes self-worth, as opinions of others are internalized (which findings from Nikkari & Harter, 1993, support). However, certain caregiver practices, for example, consistency of approval, clear and appropriate links to behavior that the child can perform, in an atmosphere that facilitates the child's adoption of parental values and standards, leads the child to internalize both appropriate and attainable standards and a sense that he/she can achieve them. To the extent that the child comes to personally own these standards and feels that he/she is meeting them, the perception that one's competence or adequacy commands the support of others will be fostered; that is, such a history will lead older children and adolescents to develop a metatheory that their own capacities cause others to approve (and disapprove) of the self.

In constructing a developmental model of the three directionality orientations, it is also necessary to speculate on the caregiving history of those adolescents who reported *no connection* between others' opinions of them and their opinions of themselves. One hypothesis is that such individuals may have experienced relatively low levels of approval and disapproval. They may have received little attention from socializing agents, ranging from benign to more serious forms of neglect. As noted earlier, many of these individuals insisted that they did not *care* about the opinions of others, suggesting a rather defensive reaction to some form of neglect. It is also likely that there may be subgroups within this particular directionality orientation. For example, within the attachment literature, Bartholomew (1990) has identified two patterns in which adults avoid intimate relationships. One such style, labeled "dismissing avoidance," would seem to apply to the subgroup within our No Connection participants, who reported that they didn't care about the opinions of others. This style is one in which there is a defensive denial of the need for social contact, accompanied by a positive view of the self.

However, there may be less defensive stances that lead to the No Connection orientation as well, leading to another subgroup that may represent a more normative pattern. Such individuals may minimize the need for approval because they are relying on alternative paths to self-worth. For example, our own findings on individual differences in the sources of self-worth have revealed three subgroups of young adolescents: (1) those who rely on social support as well as on competence in domains of importance, the hypothesized cause according to James (1892); (2) those who rely on social support only; and (3) those who rely on competence in domains of importance only. It is this third subgroup that may also find membership within the No Connection directionality group. Such adolescents place considerable emphasis on personal competence and sense of self-adequacy, which is consistent with the pattern of results obtained for the No Connection subjects who were less concerned about approval and less socially distractible in the classroom.

It is important to reiterate that *developmentally*, a looking-glass-self model represents a critical mechanism through which opinions of others come to impact the self initially, and that this is an important and inevitable process. However, the healthiest developmental course would appear to be one in which the standards and opinions of others are eventually internalized, such that actual *self*-evaluations become the standards that guide behavior (see Higgins, 1991). Damon and Hart (1988) come to a similar conclusion, observing that adolescents who do not move to the stage of internalized standards, but continue to rely on external social standards and feedback, will be at risk, since they will not have developed an internalized, relatively stable sense of self that will form the basis for subsequent identity development.

A BUDDHIST PERSPECTIVE ON PREOCCUPATION WITH THE SELF

Our findings have revealed the liabilities of a *preoccupation* with the link between approval and one's evaluation of self, particularly if positive attitudes are not internalized. As such, they raise broader issues about whether this is what the I-self should be doing, namely, scrambling to divine the opinions of others, particularly as one moves toward young adulthood. Is this really how the I-self should ultimately be spending its time? Should this be the I-self's primary job description? Aren't there better things for the I-self to be doing? Appreciating art? Enjoying nature? Practicing the game of inner tennis? Planning and planting one's garden? Openly experiencing other people? Honestly expressing feelings? From a very Western view of the self, people appear to be preoccupied with the self. Witness the large number of professional publications on the topic, not to mention the vast array of books and articles in the popular press that are devoted to enhancing one's self-concept. A judicious selection from this menu is viewed as the contemporary meal ticket to psychological health. However, this is by no means a universal window on self-processes. In fact, it departs dramatically from those perspectives that have grown out of certain Eastern, Buddhist traditions.

Consider the following observation from a Buddhist scholar (Tulku, 1978), who would appear to *begin* with a looking-glass-self perspective, although the implications take a decidedly different turn: "Each of us has a self-image that is based on who we think we are and how we think others see us. When we look in a mirror, we know that what we see there is only a reflection. Even though our self-image has the same illusory quality, we often believe it to be real. Our belief in this image draws us away from the true qualities of our nature. Because the self-image is based on how we wish we were, on what we fear we are, or how we would like the world to see us, it prevents us from seeing ourselves clearly" (pp. 102–103).

Another Buddhist scholar, Trungpa (1976), describes how we attempt to create the illusion that self and other are solid, continuous, and consistent. He writes: "We build up an idea, a preconception, that self and other are solid and continuous, and once we have this idea, we manipulate our thoughts to confirm it, and are afraid of any contrary evidence" (p. 13). From this particular Buddhist perspective, the preoccupation with the self, watching oneself as an external object, is a form of ignorance, labeled "self-observing ignorance." Trungpa notes that self-observation can actually be quite dangerous; it can involve watching yourself like a hungry cat watching mice.

According to Trungpa, we create a *watcher*, which is actually a very complicated bureaucracy that we set up seemingly to protect and enhance the self. In our own parlance, the watcher represents the rather frenetic, and at times desperate, I-self preoccupied with strategies for managing the impression that the Me-self is making upon the world. However, from a Buddhist perspective, one must go beyond this form of self-observation; one must remove the watcher and the complicated bureaucracy that it creates to preserve the permanence of the self. As Trungpa observes, once we take away the watcher, there is a tremendous amount of space, since the watcher and the bureaucracy take up so much room. Thus, if one eliminates the role of watcher, the space becomes sharp, precise, and intelligent. In fact, one does not really need the watcher or observer of the self at all.

One can see in this brief comparative analysis rather divergent views of how the I-self should be occupying its time. From the perspective of traditional Western psychology, the I-self should be gainfully employed in observing and protecting the Me-self, packaging it as a valued commodity in the psychological marketplace. However, from a certain Buddhist perspective, many more fringe benefits will accrue if the I-self averts this myopic gaze, since it represents a distorted lens that obscures one's true nature. Rather, the I-self should direct its energies outward, exercising its capabilities and enjoying life experiences, rather than turning inward in its continued preoccupation with the opinions of the others in the construction of a Me-self that it hopes will be acceptable to the society at large.

It would be instructive to examine the links between the typology revealed in our own findings and in this particular Buddhist perspective; that is, our findings reveal that a preoccuption with the impact of the opinions of others upon the self carries with it detrimental consequences. Those who are less preoccupied with this link and who have decoupled the impact of others' opinions upon their self-worth fare far better in terms of the outcomes we have assessed.

RELATIONAL SELF-WORTH: A LOOKING-GLASS-SELF PERSPECTIVE

For Cooley (1902) and even more so for Mead (1925), self-worth involved a *global* evaluation of oneself that required the individual to psychologically average the perceived opinions of significant others, which Mead labeled the "generalized other." Until recently, self-worth, or self-esteem, has been treated as a unitary construct. However, our own findings suggest that this formulation is in need of refinement in that the impact of different opinions of *specific* others toward the self needs to be considered; that is, differences in self-worth across interpersonal contexts could be expected to emerge during adolescence. Just as adolescents provide different self-descriptions of their attributes in different relational contexts (Hart, 1988; Griffin, Chassin, & Young, 1981; Harter, 1998a; Harter, Bresnick, et al., 1997; Harter & Monsour, 1992; Rosenberg, 1986), so might they be expected to evaluate their worth as a person differently across contexts. Others have also argued that the evaluations of one's worth may vary across situation or time (see Demo & Savin-Williams, 1992; Harter, Stocker, et al., 1996; Heatherton & Polivy, 1991; Kernis, 1993; Leary & Downs, 1995; Rosenberg, 1986). In postulating that self-worth would vary as a function of relational context (e.g., with parents, teachers, peers), we have adopted the term "relational self-worth" (Harter, Waters, & Whitesell, 1998).

From a revisionist, symbolic interactionist perspective, self-worth should vary as a function of relational context to the extent that approval for the self as a person varies across contexts; that is, the internalization process could well be context-specific. We thought it plausible that for many adolescents, the multiple selves that they present with different significant others may well provoke different levels of approval or support. In an initial study with high school students (Harter, Waters, & Whitesell, 1998), we examined the hypothesis that adolescents would report differing levels of self-worth in four contexts: with parents, with teachers, with male classmates, and with female classmates. The findings provided clear support for the fact that many adolescents do judge their worth as a person differently across these four contexts.

Factor analysis revealed a clear factor pattern with high loadings on the designated factors and negligible cross-loadings. As a second index of adolescents' differentiated view of their worth across contexts, we examined the discrepancy between their highest and lowest relational self-worth scores. The findings revealed that a minority of adolescents (approximately one-fourth) reported no variation in self-worth across contexts. However, the vast majority, almost three-fourths of the sample, reported that their self-worth did vary as a function of the particular relational context. The average discrepancy was approximately 1.0, where the maximum potential discrepancy was 3.0. A subgroup analysis revealed that for some adolescents, the discrepancy was relatively small. For others, it was moderate, and for still others, it was relatively large. In fact, there were a few participants who actually reported the maximum discrepancy (e.g., one girl who reported a self-worth score of 1.0 with her parents and 4.0 with her female classmates).

In another study with middle school students (grades 6 to 8), we included a somewhat different set of significant others, namely, mother, father, siblings, classmates, and close friends. Once again, we found a very clean factor pattern with extremely high loadings on the designated factor with negligible cross-loadings. Thus, from a developmental perspective, relational self-worth is clearly a meaningful construct that is present in early adolescence. In a subsequent study on the effects of the support of mother and father among high school students (Buddin, 1998), self-worth with mother and self-worth with father also defined very distinct factors.

In order to examine the findings within a looking-glass-self framework, we further hypothesized that approval for the self as a person should be highly related to self-worth within the corresponding context. The pattern of results confirmed the more specific prediction that support within a given type of relationship would be more highly correlated with relational self-worth in that context compared to relational self-worth in the other three contexts. Moreover, approval from individuals in a specific context was more highly predictive of relational self-worth in that context than of global self-worth. Thus, the findings suggest a refinement of the reflected appraisal process in that support in the form of validation or approval from particular significant others will have its strongest impact on how one evaluates one's sense of worth as a person with those particular others.

Given this more differentiated approach, it becomes important to address what the concept of *relational* self-worth implies for the construct of *global* self-worth? Is the latter to be replaced, if not buried, in the contemporary shift to relational and multidimensional frameworks? Such an internment is unlikely given the voluminous literature that has identified numerous correlates and consequences of global self-worth or self-esteem. Moreover, global self-worth is a powerful phenomenological reality in the lives of children, adolescents, and adults (Harter, 1997). In addition, an interesting pattern has been revealed in the studies described earlier, a pattern that indicates there is considerable utility in retaining the long-standing concept of an overall judgment of one's worth as a person.

More specifically, we sought to determine whether there were subgroups of adolescents for whom relational self-worth in one context was more highly related to global self-worth than was relational self-worth in the other contexts. We examined this issue in the study in which relational self-worth was examined across four interpersonal contexts: with parents, teachers, male classmates, and female classmates (Harter, Waters, & Whitesell, 1998). We found that four clear subgroups could be identified. Each subgroup was defined by the fact that relational self-worth in a particular context was markedly and significantly more highly correlated with global self-worth than were the relational self-worth scores in the other three contexts; that is, individuals differ with regard to which relational self-worth score correlates most highly with their global sense of worth as a person. Thus, for some students, relational self-worth with female classmates was more highly correlated with overall self-worth, whereas for other subgroups, it was relational self-worth with male classmates or with parents.

There are different interpretations for such a pattern. It may well be that certain interpersonal contexts are more important or salient to individual adolescents, such that their feelings of worth, bolstered by the approval in that context, generalize to their overall self-worth. Thus, in future work, it will be critical to include measures of the importance of support from those in each context, as we have begun to do in recent studies. Another interpretation involves the "set" that participants bring to our instruments. Although global self-worth questions are assumed to be "context free," we do not know if subjects, when faced with such global items, supply their own context, for example, framing items within a context that is most relevant to their sense of worth as a person. These are important issues to address in future research.

Given that evaluations of overall worth as a person do represent a phenomenological reality for individuals, and that this construct has important correlates and consequences (discussed in Chapter 8), it is important to retain the construct of global self-worth. To the extent that this general evaluation of worth may be highly determined by feelings of worth in a particular context, identifying that context may have important implications for intervention; that is, for those with low global self-worth, the pathway to self-enhancement may well depend upon specific strategies for increasing the support for a given adolescent in the relevant context, which in turn should enhance both relational and global self-worth. Alternatively, intervention efforts may need to be focused on shifting the adolescent's attention to contexts in which support is forthcoming, which should also serve to enhance relational as well as global self-worth. Thus, there would appear to be considerable utility in considering the role of relational self-worth, as well as in retaining the construct of global self-worth.

We have also applied the relational self-worth framework to an understanding of ethnic minority youth (Ahmed & Harter, 1996), specifically to teenagers from India, whose parents came to this country as first-generation immigrants. Such adolescents must move between the multiple worlds of their family of origin, peers of the same ethnicity, and Anglo American peers (see also Cooper et al., 1995). Findings reveal that their self-worth can differ considerably across these three contexts. For the group as a whole, relational self-worth with parents is significantly lower than with either peer group. Given the demands of acculturating to peer culture, while preserving an identification with the familial culture of origin, adolescents are caught in a struggle in which the proximal demands of school and the peer culture may well dominate, leading them to behaviors and attitudes that are disappointing to their parents. These findings bolster our conclusion that we need to view self-worth from the perspective of particular relational contexts.

CONCLUSION

There is clear evidence from research that has emanated from a symbolic interactionist perspective, as well as within an attachment theory framework, that support, particularly in the form of approval, has a clear impact on the self-evaluations, particularly global perceptions of self-worth, of children and adolescents. Evidence from our own research, as well as the findings of other investigators, clearly documents this link. Support in the form of approval and validation for oneself as a person is, understandably, most highly related to self-worth, since self-worth, by definition, includes one's approval of self. Parental support is particularly critical throughout the periods of childhood and adolescence. Although peer support from classmates becomes increasingly important to self-worth as one moves into late childhood and adolescence, the impact of parental support upon perceptions of one's worth as a person does not decline, contrary to earlier renditions of the importance of significant others during adolescence.

Support from special adults may, for some adolescents, either enhance the effects of existing support from parents or compensate for the lack of parental support. These effects will be most positive for those adolescents who feel relatively competent or adequate across such domains as Scholastic Competence, Athletic Competence, Social Acceptance, Physical Appearance, and Behavioral Conduct. Adolescents who do not feel personally adequate in these domains are much less likely to benefit from the support provided by special adults.

To the extent that children and adolescents cannot meet the conditions that adults and peers require in order to grant approval, it will be difficult to maintain high self-worth. Support that is conditional upon meeting the high expectations of parents and peers, expectations that are often unrealistic from the child's or adolescent's perspective, will actually erode feelings of worth as a person.

Support from significant others, particularly from those whose approval is regarded as important, combines with perceptions of competence in domains of importance to impact the level of global self-worth. Thus, rather than pit a Jamesian formulation against a model based upon Cooley's looking-glass-self formulation, in our own research program, we have examined an additive model in which both determinants can potentially contribute to self-worth. Each framework has been found to make relatively equal contributions to the prediction of global self-worth.

Issues of the directionality of influences are relevant to both a Jamesian model and to Cooley's looking-glass-self formulation; that is, these models presume that, in the case of James, perceptions of competence in domains of importance, and for Cooley, perceptions of the opinions of others toward the self are *determinants* of global self-worth. However, an alternative explanation for the correlations between supposed determinants and global self-worth is that perceptions of global self-worth come to influence one's evaluations of personal adequacy in particular domains or of the regard in which one is held by significant others. Our research has revealed that with regard to the directionality of the relationship between perceived approval from significant others and global self-worth, adolescents have different metatheories. Those who endorse a looking-glass-self model, that is, those who contend that the approval of others remains critical to their sense of worth as a person, are more at risk for a constellation of liabilities. Those who appear to have internalized the more positive messages from significant others, such that they believe that how they think about themselves dictates how others will perceive them, fare much better. The dangers of preoccupation with both the opinions of others and their relationship to evaluations of the self have been identified in Eastern, Buddhist writings as well.

Finally, although the concept of global self-worth or self-esteem has been of historical significance and has been the topic of numerous studies that have examined the correlates of overall perceptions of worth (see reviews by Harter, 1983; Hattie, 1992; Wylie, 1979), more contemporary approaches have turned to an examination of how self-worth may differ across situations, including different relational contexts. Our own research has provided evidence for the construct of "relational self-worth," as documented by the fact that the adolescent evaluates his/her worth as a person differently in different relational contexts. From a looking-glass-self perspective, differences in self-worth are predicted by the level of approval that one receives from significant others in that context. The construct of relational self-worth does not replace the concept of global self-worth. Rather, both exist in the network of self-representations. For most adolescents, relational self-worth in one particular context is much more highly related to global self-worth. Although there are different interpretations for such a pattern, identification of that particular context may represent an avenue for intervention among those with low global self-worth.

A Model of the Causes, Correlates, and Consequences of Global Self-Worth

In the preceding chapters, evidence was presented in support of two formulations concerning the determinants of global self-worth. Chapter 6 reviewed findings bolstering James' (1892) contention that overall evaluations of personal worth or esteem are caused by perceptions of competence or adequacy in domains deemed important. Chapter 7 documented Cooley's (1902) looking-glass-self model in demonstrating that the approval of significant others is incorporated into one's overall sense of worth as a person. Moreover, our findings have revealed that both James' and Cooley's formulations, taken together, provide a powerful explanation for the level of self-worth displayed by older children and adolescents. As Figure 7.1 illustrated, the effects of these two determinants are additive. At each level of social support (representing the average of classmate and parent approval), greater competence in domains of importance is associated with higher self-worth. Similarly, at each level of competence in domains of importance, the more support one garners from classmates and parents, the higher one's self-worth. Those individuals with the lowest self-worth, therefore, are those who report both incompetence in domains of importance and the absence of supportive approval from others.

In the present chapter, I move beyond this additive model, offering a more comprehensive framework in which links between particular domains of competence/adequacy and specific sources of approval are forged. Moreover, I will address the potential consequences of one's level of self-worth. If self-evaluations about one's worth as a person do not directly impact an individual's day-to-day functioning, then research into its causes may contribute little to our understanding of human behavior. In our own model

(Harter, Marold, et al., 1992) dimensions of depression have served as the outcomes to be predicted, given the strong correlations between self-worth and depressive reactions. The model also includes suicidal ideation as another potential outcome.

Although theoretically driven models documenting relationships among predictors and outcomes among large groups of youth are useful, the general pathways identified may not speak to the specific precursors for given individuals. Thus, we have focused on the multiple pathways to self-worth and its correlates, particularly among youth at risk for depression. We have identified several different pathways that represent different combinations of predictors. The identification of specific pathways for given individuals at risk is critical in designing intervention strategies that will speak to particular causes of low self-worth and depressive correlates.

Depressive reactions can also be better understood as a combination of emotions that includes anger in addition to sadness. Findings from our laboratory address the affective experience of depression, as well as document the particular causes of depression as reported by adolescents. Finally, adolescents' perceptions of the directionality of the link between low self-worth and depressed affect are examined. The evidence reveals that some adolescents report that low self-worth precedes depressed affect, whereas others describe the opposite sequence in which depressed affect precedes the experience of low self-worth. There are predictable correlates of these two directionality orientations, which in turn suggest that different intervention strategies need to be considered.

THE POWERFUL LINK BETWEEN SELF-WORTH AND DEPRESSIVE REACTIONS

As the preceding chapters have revealed, during the past three decades, considerable attention has been devoted to an analysis of the determinants of self-worth in the lives of children and adolescents. Yet why should we be concerned about self-worth, unless we can demonstrate that it plays a vital role in individuals' lives, unless we can document the fact that it performs some critical function? The efforts of numerous self-worth researchers may well be misguided if self-worth reduces to an epiphenomenon that has little impact on everyday functioning.

Initially, therefore, attention was directed to the potential *mediational* role of self-worth, in an effort to identify constructs critical to the lives of individuals that self-worth might impact. What are some likely candidates? What outcomes of any significance might self-worth influence? A major candidate is one's *mood* or affect, along the dimension of cheerful to depressed. Recent theory and research has placed increasing emphasis on cognitions that give rise to, or accompany, depression. Cognitions involving the *self* have found particular favor. There is clear historical precedent for including negative self-evaluations as one of a constellation of symptoms experienced in depression, beginning with Freud's (1968) observations of the low self-esteem displayed by adults suffering from depressive disorders. Those within the psychoanalytic tradition have continued to afford low self-esteem or low self-worth a central role in depression (Bibring, 1953; Blatt, 1974).

More recently, a number of theorists who have addressed the manifestations of depression in children and adolescents, as well as in adults, have focused heavily on cognitive components involving the self. For example, attention has been drawn to the role of self-deprecatory ideation and hopelessness in depression (Abramson, Metaksky, & Alloy, 1989; Baumeister, 1990; Beck, 1975; Hammen & Goodman-Brown, 1990; King, Naylor, Segal, Evans, & Shain, 1993; Kovacs & Beck, 1977, 1978, 1986), to attributional style (Abramson, Seligman, & Teasdale, 1978; Nolen-Hoeksema, Girgus, & Seligman, 1986; Seligman, 1975; Seligman & Peterson, 1986) and to cognitive and sociocognitive influences as well as self-discrepancies (Baumeister, 1990; Higgins, 1987, 1989; Kaslow, Rehm, & Siegel, 1984; McCauley, Mitchell, Burke, & Moss, 1988; Pyszczynki & Greenberg, 1986, 1987). Higgins' work is particularly relevant, since he finds that discrepancies between what one would *like* to be and what one perceives oneself to be produce dejection-related emotions such as depression.

In our own studies, we consistently find that among older children and adolescents, self-worth is highly related to affect along a continuum of cheerful to depressed (with correlations ranging from .72 to .80). These findings are consistent with those of other investigators (Battle, 1987; Beck, 1975; Kaslow et al., 1984). Of particular relevance to this chapter is our finding that older children and adolescents within our normative samples who report low self-worth consistently report depressed affect (Harter, 1986a, 1990a, 1993; Renouf & Harter, 1990). Among a clinical sample of inpatient adolescents with psychiatric diagnoses of depression, we have also found a powerful link between self-worth and self-reported depressed affect. Among those reporting depressed affect, 80% also report low self-worth (Harter, Marold, et al., 1992).

Thus, in our original model, we concluded that the two causal constructs, competence in domains of importance and social support, served not only to impact one's level of self-worth, but also provoked a powerful emotional reaction that, for the low self-worth child or adolescent, results in a mood state of depression (see Figure 8.1). It should be noted that this model is consistent with a number of sequential models to emerge in the

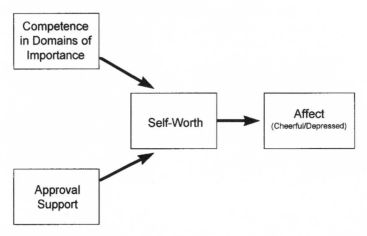

FIGURE 8.1. Original model of the determinants and consequences of self-worth.

1970s, models that have placed considerable emphasis on the mediational role of self-representations. The general character of these models involves the postulation of a chain of events in which self-observation leads to a cognitive self-evaluation, which in turn impacts other motivational, emotional, or behavioral systems. Such models have evolved from learning theory (Bandura, 1977, 1978), from social psychologists (Carver & Scheier, 1991; Dweck & Elliot, 1983; Wicklund, 1975; Wicklund & Frey, 1980), from clinicians with a cognitive-behavioral orientation (Kanfer, 1980; Kanfer & Phillips, 1970), and from personality psychologists who emphasize the primacy of cognitions over emotions (Lazarus, 1982, 1984; Weiner, 1985). (More recently, we have begun to question the unidirectionality of such a sequence, an issue to which I return later.)

MAJOR MODIFICATIONS IN THE ORIGINAL MODEL

In subsequent efforts, we have elaborated upon this basic model with regard to five particular issues, each of which are discussed here (see also Harter, Marold, et al., 1992). First, rather than treating competence in domains of importance as but one construct, we have distinguished between two competence/adequacy clusters of domains: (1) Physical Appearance, Peer Likability, and Athletic Competence, and (2) Scholastic Competence and Behavioral Conduct. Second, we have added direct paths from each of these clusters to the social support variables. Third, we have added *hopelessness* to the model. A fourth modification required that we remove the hypothesized causal path between self-worth and mood. This resulted in the creation of a *depression/adjustment composite* comprised of self-worth, depressed mood, and general hopelessness. Finally, we extended the model to include *suicidal ideation* as one potential outcome of depression, as defined by our composite. This most recent model is presented in Figure 8.2.

Distinction between Two Competence/Adequacy Clusters

Our findings have now revealed the existence of two distinct clusters of domains, given two empirical criteria. First, higher-order factoring of the five competence/adequacy subscale scores reveals two discrete factors. Second, ratings of importance of each domain are applied to self as well as to parents (see Harter, Marold, et al., 1992) for each cluster differ. The first cluster comprises Physical Appearance, Peer Likability, and Athletic Competence, and these domains, particularly Appearance and Likability, were judged to be more important to the self than to parents. The second cluster, Scholastic Competence and Behavior Conduct, formed a separate, higher-order factor, and these two domains were judged to be more important to parents than to the self.

Links between These Two Clusters and Social Support

In our previous models designed to examine James' and Cooley's formulations (e.g., Harter, 1986a, 1987, 1990a), competence in domains of

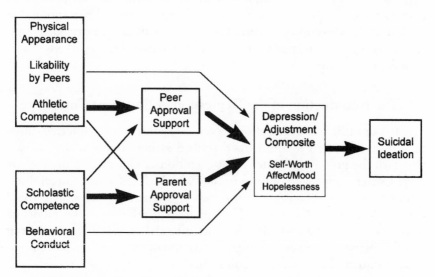

FIGURE 8.2. General model of the predictors of depression/adjustment.

importance and social support were treated as independent contributors to self-worth, and thus paths from the self-concept variables to social support were not included. However, a plausible hypothesis is that one's level of competence or adequacy directly impacts the amount of support that one receives from significant others. More specifically, our findings demonstrate that the first cluster, Physical Appearance, Peer Likability, and Athletic Competence, bears a stronger relationship to peer support than to parent support. As can be seen in the model (Figure 8.2), there is a direct path from this cluster to peer support, reflecting the fact that the more good-looking, likable, and athletically competent one feels one is, the more one reports support, in the form of approval, from peers. Not surprisingly, the cluster comprised of Scholastic Competence and Behavioral Conduct, judged more important to parents than the self, bears a stronger relationship to parental support than to peer support. Thus, if one evaluates the self positively in those arenas valued by parents, one also experiences greater parental approval.

Hopelessness

Following the lead of Beck (1967, 1975, 1987) and his colleagues (Kovacs & Beck, 1977, 1978), we further broadened our nomological network of constructs to include hopelessness, since hopelessness and helplessness have now been clearly implicated in depressive reactions, including suicidal behaviors (see also Baumeister, 1990; Pfeffer, 1988; Rutter, 1986; Schneidman, 1991; Seligman, 1975; Topol & Reznikoff, 1982). Hopelessness is typically defined as the perception that one is unable to control or alter painful life circumstances. Thus, we developed items to tap the general perception that one's future is uncompromisingly bleak. We have discovered that such hopelessness is highly correlated (r's in the .70's) with global self-worth, as well as with depressed affect.

The Introduction of the Depression/Adjustment Composite

In our earlier modeling efforts, a central feature was the inferred causal path from self-worth to affect. As described earlier, we postulated, consistent with the prevailing models, that cognitions about the self directly impacted affect, such that if one was favored with high self-worth, cheerfulness would constitute an affective consequence, whereas low self-worth would provoke feelings of depression. The initial application of causal modeling techniques to our data revealed that such a model provided an excellent fit (Harter, 1986a). However, a thoughtful, comprehensive approach to the use of such statistical procedures requires that one test alternative models, particularly those in which the directionality of effects is reversed.

In our most recent modeling efforts, therefore, we have adopted this approach. In comparing such alternative models, we have discovered that if we reverse the order of self-worth and affect, such that affect is treated as causally *prior* to self-worth, this model fits the data just as well as our original model. This outcome should not be surprising, given that the correlation between self-worth and affect has ranged from .70 to .80 across studies. Moreover, both self-worth and affect correlate equally highly with the postulated antecedents in the model. Therefore, on balance, there were no compelling statistical grounds for asserting that the original directionality, although theoretically derived, truly captured the actual sequence of events.

In light of this discovery, it was incumbent upon us to remove the path from self-worth to affect. As an alternative strategy, we created the Depression/Adjustment Composite, comprised of self-worth, affect, and general hopelessness, given that hopelessness also correlates highly with both self-worth and affect, as described earlier. The creation of the depression composite is not merely a statistical solution, given the multicolinearity of these constructs. Rather, the three constructs that comprise this composite appear to be critical to the identification of individuals at risk for depression. While there may be different antecedents or *pathways* to depression for different individuals (a point to which I return later), a low score on the depression composite for any individual constitutes a psychological red flag that may well be of diagnostic significance.

Suicidal Ideation

Finally, we extended our model to one potential outcome, suicidal ideation. The incidence of suicide among adolescents has tripled in recent decades, leading to efforts to identify the determinants of this major mental health threat to our youth (see Noam & Borst, 1994; Pfeffer, 1986, 1988; Alcohol, Drug Abuse, and Mental Health Administration's report from the Secretary's Task Force on Youth Suicide, 1989). Several broad classes of risk factors implicated in depression and suicidal behaviors have captured the attention of researchers, including biological precursors, epidemiological correlates, and social/psychological stressors. We have been particularly committed to an examination of the third class of risk factors. Evidence to date has revealed a constellation of social/psychological correlates that are predictive of suicidal behavior, including depressed affect, poor self-concept in particular domains, real-ideal discrepancies, low self-worth, hopelessness, and lack of social support (see Baumeister, 1990; Carlson & Cantwell, 1980; Cicchetti & Schneider-Rosen, 1986; Pfeffer, 1986; Rutter, Izard, & Read, 1985).

From a developmental perspective, these particular risk factors become increasingly salient as one moves into adolescence (see Emery, 1983). Self-awareness, self-consciousness, introspectiveness, and preoccupation with one's self-image dramatically increase (see review by Harter, 1990b). Self-worth becomes more vulnerable (Rosenberg, 1986), and adolescents become more aware of the relationship between self-worth, social support, and depressed affect (Harter & Marold, 1993). With regard to the support system, the impact of peer support increases dramatically (Brown, 1990; Savin-Williams & Berndt, 1990). Although young adolescents are beginning to make bids for autonomy from parents, they are nevertheless struggling to remain connected (Cooper et al., 1983; Grotevant & Cooper, 1986; Steinberg, 1990); thus, parent support continues to be critical.

Depressive symptomatology itself increases in adolescence (see Carlson & Cantwell, 1980; Rutter et al., 1985; Shaffer, 1985; Sroufe & Rutter, 1985), and certain associated features such as hopelessness take on increasing importance, since they require a level of cognitive functioning that is not completely developed in younger children (Carlson & Garber, 1986; Kendall, Cantwell, & Kazdin, 1989; Rutter, 1988; Shaffer, 1985). Finally, suicidal behaviors themselves increase dramatically during adolescence (Carlson & Cantwell, 1980; Cantor, 1987; Hawton, 1986; Pfeffer, 1988; Shaffer, 1974, 1985; Shaffer & Fischer, 1981).

While there is a growing body of evidence on the *correlates* of suicidal behaviors, relatively little attention has been directed toward the development of theory-based *models* that identify risk factors representing the antecedents as well as mediators of suicidal behaviors. As Spirato, Brown, Overholser, and Fritz (1989) have observed, we are particularly in need of models that consider antecedent stresses such as family, peer, and school problems, and that include emotional and cognitive states (e.g., depression and hopelessness) that may mediate outcomes such as suicidal behaviors.

Moreover, recently, it has been urged that the field take seriously the study of suicidal behavior and its correlates in *normative* populations of young adolescents (Garrison, 1989). Historically, suicide research has focused on clinical populations. More recently, investigators have demonstrated the fruitfulness of examining the prevalence and antecedents of suicidal behaviors among normative populations including college students (Bonner & Rich, 1987; Rudd, 1989), high school students (Smith & Crawford, 1986) and preadolescents (Pfeffer, Lipkins, Plutchik, & Mizruchi, 1988; Pfeffer, Zuckerman, Plutchik, & Mizruchi, 1984). The period of early adolescence has received relatively little empirical attention. Thus, we sought to extend our efforts, with the goal of determining how the factors we had identified to date, namely, domain-specific self-concepts in areas deemed important, peer and parent social support, and the depression composite (self-worth, depressed affect, and general hopelessness) might function as antecedents and mediators of suicidal ideation in young adolescents.

In extending our model to include suicidal ideation, we have begun to address the links between these constructs, asking what provokes many among our youth to even consider terminating their lives. What cognitive and socioemotional processes conspire to convince an adolescent that life is not worth living? What role do self-representations play in this intrapsychic plot that has such a potentially tragic outcome? What features of adolescents' socialization history cause them to question their worth as a person, and the worth of their life?

The sequential model in Figure 8.2, which provides an excellent fit to the data (see Harter, Marold, et al., 1992), provides a number of clues. Self-evaluations of inadequacy with regard to one's appearance and one's likability, domains judged important to the self as well as to one's peers, appear to attenuate peer support, both of which impact the depression composite (i.e., both of which provoke the personally devastating combination of low self-worth, depressed affect, and general hopelessness). Perceptions of scholastic incompetence as well as negative evaluations of one's behavioral conduct precipitate parental disapproval, and both feelings of inadequacy and lack of parent support, in turn, impact the depression composite. The constellation of low self-worth, depressed affect, and hopelessness, in turn, drives many to consider suicide as a solution, as a form of escape from the painful cognitions and affects concerning the self and the disapproving reactions of others (see also Baumeister, 1990).

The following poignant self-disclosure by one of the adolescents in our studies provides a personal cameo of the model that has evolved in our research:

"I look in the mirror and most days I don't like what I see, I don't like how I look, I don't like myself as a person. So I get depressed, bummed out. Plus, my family has rejected me and that makes me feel pretty lousy about myself. My mother is really on my case because I'm not living up to what she wants me to be. If I get A's in school, she's nice and is proud of me, but if I don't, she doesn't approve of me. You could say how she treats me is conditional on how I do. Mostly she tells me I'm a failure, and I'm beginning to believe it. Doing well in school has always been important to me, but now I feel like I'll never amount to anything. There's no way I'll ever be able to please her; it's pretty hopeless. I don't get much support from other kids either. I probably never will, because I'm an introvert. I don't even try to make friends. So a lot of the time I get depressed, really bummed out. When I'm depressed I feel sad, because other people have hurt me, but I'm also angry at them too, for not caring, for rejecting me. I feel so depressed that I often think about just killing myself. Life is worthless. But so is death. So what's the use?"

Multiple Pathways to Self-Worth and Its Correlates

Although theoretically driven models documenting general relations among predictors and outcomes are very useful, they do not speak to the specific precursors of depressive reactions for a given individual. The inspection of the profile of scores for individuals reveals that not all youth who experience low self-worth, depressed affect, and hopelessness report perceived limitations in both predictive clusters of competence/adequacy, namely, those that are more peer salient and more parent salient. Nor do all adolescents report the lack of both peer and parental support. Thus, we sought empirically to identify subgroups of adolescents that manifest different patterns of predictors, defined by the components in our model, that represented different pathways to depressive reactions (Harter & Whitesell, 1996). From several normative samples of adolescents, we first identified those that reported the constellation of low self-worth, depressed affect, and hopelessness, namely, adolescents who were experiencing self-reported depressive symptomatology. We then looked for subgroups of individuals whose scores represented different combinations of predictors. These efforts have resulted in the identification of six potential pathways to depression. These patterns of pathways differ in the number of predictors of depression. In the first pattern, all four predictors in the general model are relevant. In the second and third patterns, there are three predictors. In the remaining three patterns, there are only two predictors. These patterns, described here and depicted in Figure 8.3, are identified according to the salient predictors. In the figure, variables connected by arrows are the predictors for a given pattern and represent negative evaluations of competence or adequacy and low perceived support. Variables with no connecting arrows are not predictors for that pattern and reflect positive evaluations of competence/adequacy and support.

Four Predictors: Inadequacy in Both Clusters and Low Support from Parents and Peers

For many of our depressed adolescents (41%), all four predictors, the two competence/adequacy clusters and both peer and parent support variables, appear to put these individuals at risk for depressive reactions. These adolescents report that they feel inadequate with regard to their Appearance, Athletic Ability, and their Likability, as well as suffer from limitations in the domains of Scholastic Competence and Behavioral Conduct. Moreover, they report low peer support, particularly from classmates, as well as low parental support. Thus, the general model does capture their experience.

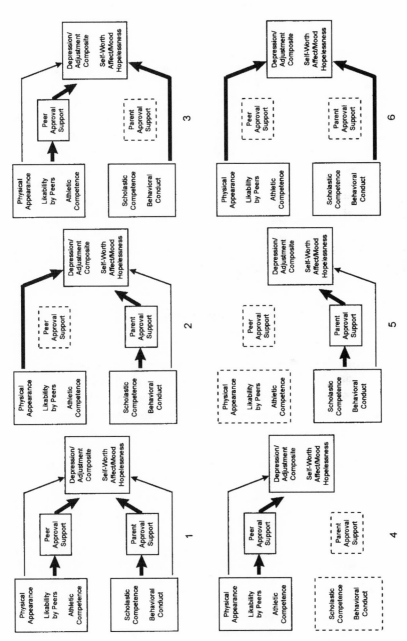

FIGURE 8.3. Six different pathways to adolescent depression.

The adolescent self-description presented here would appear to fit this pattern. He identifies many of the features in our sequential process model predisposing him to thoughts of suicide. This 17-year-old is dissatisfied with his appearance, his outer self, leading him to denigrate himself as a person, to question his essential worth as a human being. As an introvert, he questions his likability, acknowledging that he receives little support from peers. He is dissatisfied with his scholastic performance, a domain that he values, as does his mother, who considers him a failure, a view that he has begun to internalize, leading him to devalue himself further. Interestingly, he labels her reaction as "conditional" (which, as described in Chapter 6, has detrimental effects), and such conditionality further contribute to his feelings of worthlessness. This constellation of precursors ushers in very intense feelings of depression and hopelessness. The toll exacted is tortuous as he wrestles with the question of whether to kill himself and with the uselessness of both his life and death. Such adolescents are clearly at risk not only for the constellation of reactions defining the negative pole of our depression/adjustment composite but also for suicidal behaviors given that their perceptions are so pervasively negative.

Peer-Salient and Parent-Salient Domains as Well as Low Parental Support

A second pattern involves three predictors in our model. These depressed youth report that they have limitations in the peer-related domains of Appearance, Likability, and Athletic Competence as well as in the more parent-salient domains of Scholastic Competence. Moreover, they report low Parental Approval. Their only positive evaluations occur for one predictor, namely, Peer Support. The fact that they report relatively high support from peers requires explanation given that in our general modeling efforts, deficiencies in the more peer-salient domains typically lead to lack of support, particularly from classmates. Perceptions of high peer support in the face of perceived limitations could result from the fact that the assessment of one's adequacy in peer-related domains is unrealistic; that is, the adolescent is evaluating his/her personal qualities too critically, whereas peers are responding to the individual's more objectively manifest positive characteristics. Alternatively, perceived peer support could also be relatively high if the adolescent was overestimating the level of peer approval. For example, it has been demonstrated that aggressive children report unrealistically high levels of support from peers based on their assumption that their aggressive actions are well received, since they are defending themselves against being taken advantage of by others (see Dodge, 1991). Thus, there may be at least two different psychological subpatterns captured by this combination of predictors.

The case example to follow illustrates this second pattern. This adolescent male initially appeared in our normative high school sample and was subsequently hospitalized on the psychiatric unit where we were also conducting research. At the time of his first testing, he reported depressed affect, low self-worth, hopelessness, as well as suicidal thinking. In an interview he told us, "I sure think a lot about killing myself if this life doesn't get much better." His profile revealed that lack of parental support was a particularly salient feature leading to his depressive reactions. He described his parents, both professionals, as busy people who were very demanding and emotionally unavailable. His primary area of interest was dirt-bike riding; however, his parents did not approve of this particular activity and were threatening to take his bike away, in part because of his low grades. They also expressed their disapproval over his appearance, namely, his long hair and his clothing. This young man was also dissatisfied with his appearance, although for different reasons. He was struggling with acne and was also quite short and slight for his age, a factor that also precluded his being selected for school athletic teams. He was aware that these attributes made him less than likable among his peers. His reaction to perceptions of inadequacy was often aggressively to take the offensive. He was disruptive in school and tried to act tough with his male peers. He assumed that classmates respected his toughness, that is, that they approved of him standing up for himself, although there was little objective evidence that his perceptions were realistic. Because his father was in the military, the family moved frequently, thus adding to the difficulty of breaking into school cliques. The school also threatened to suspend him because of an incident in which he was caught drinking alcohol at a school function. This served further to infuriate his parents. He acknowledged that he was a troublemaker, as revealed by his low behavioral conduct score.

Thus, the pattern leading to depression, including suicidal thinking, was precipitated by perceptions of inadequacy in both peer-salient and parent-salient domains, as well as extremely low parental support. At a conscious level, he appeared to be distorting his perceptions of positive peer support in an apparent effort to defend against his feelings of inferiority and lack of parental support. The possibility that he may have been unconsciously aware that peers also frowned upon his behavior could also have contributed to his depressive reactions, including a suicidal gesture. He described how he drove his dirt bike toward the edge of a cliff, but then spun out just before going over. Other incidents clearly indicated that this young man was on a course that may have led to even more serious suicidal attempts had he not been hospitalized.

Three Predictors: Inadequacy in Both Peer-Salient
and Parent-Salient Domains as Well as Low Peer Support

In this third pattern, like the previous profile, the adolescent feels inadequate in both the peer-salient domains of Physical Appearance, Peer Likability, and Athletic Competence and the parent-salient domains of Scholastic Competence and Behavioral Conduct. Consistent with the general model, in which unfavorable evaluations in the peer-salient domains lead to lack of peer support, these adolescents report low levels of peer approval. However, this particular pattern of predictors differs from the general model in that these individuals report unpredictably high levels of parental support. Judgments of parental support could possibly reflect distortions in the adolescent's perception of approval from parents; it could represent socially desirable responding, or it could be quite accurate (e.g., benevolent parents of children with limitations may adjust their expectations and/or be the type of parents who supply considerable unconditional support). The case example involves just such parents.

This 14-year-old girl reports that she does not like herself as a person, displays depressed affect, and is hopeless about her future. Objectively, she has a number of limitations that compromise her ability to function adequately and may understandably lead her to being neglected or rejected by peers. School testing, ordered after several years of poor scholastic performance, revealed an IQ of 87, in addition to mild cognitive deficits in the ability to plan meaningfully as well as anticipate consequences. She is poorly coordinated, making it difficult for her to compete athletically. In fact, she tends to be somewhat klutzy—dropping, spilling, and bumping into things. Moreover, she falls short of the demanding standards of physical attractiveness by which adolescents judge themselves and each other. Although her level of intelligence places limits on her ability to excel, academically, she is nevertheless smart enough to realize that she has limitations relative to other adolescents her age. This realization was apparent in her profile of scores in that she reported unfavorable evaluations in the domains of Physical Appearance, Athletic Competence, Peer Likability, and Scholastic Performance, as well as low peer support. Although she strives to be well behaved, her klutzy behavior leads her at times to accidentally break objects. Moreover, her inability to anticipate consequences often leads her to behave somewhat inappropriately or impulsively in social situations. These factors in turn cause her to rate her behavioral conduct unfavorably.

Her parents, however, are extremely understanding and protective of their daughter. They had tried for years to have a child without success and were thrilled when they learned that the wife was pregnant and that they were going to have a girl. Birth complications ensued; however, the baby was successfully delivered. The parents welcomed the new addition to the family with open arms and were unconditionally accepting of their daughter. They feel that she is doing extremely well, particularly given that complications associated with her delivery may have compromised her ability to function at high levels. They communicate to her the fact that they are pleased with her school performance and forgive the consequences of her occasional clumsiness or impulsivity. They are very thankful that she was not more seriously handicapped and feel that she can live a very normal life in the future. However, they do not understand why, as an adolescent, their daughter has become depressed and evaluates herself so negatively, particularly since her deficiencies are mild. Nor do they understand why she does not seem to profit from their unconditional support, which they feel should compensate for the fact that she is not popular at school; that is, they do not realize the powerful impact of the peer culture and how negative evaluations from the "generalized other" can be psychologically debilitating. There are many such children in our classrooms who are trying to the best of their ability to navigate the rough waters toward scholastic and social success. In fact, those with minor limitations are often more neglected or ostracized than those with severe handicaps, who provoke more sympathy and understanding. The children displaying this pattern are children for whom specific interventions to improve their outlook may not be immediately obvious. Their deficiencies are not so marked as to identify them as candidates for special education programs. Moreover, the fact that they are relatively realistic in their evaluations of themselves and the reactions of others makes their situation all the more poignant.

Two Predictors: Inadequacy in More Peer-Salient Domains Plus Low Peer Support

For these individuals, feelings of inadequacy in the domains of Physical Appearance, Peer Likability, and Athletic Competence are paramount, as is lack of peer support, with which such limitations are typically associated. However, scores are relatively high for the more parent-salient domains, Scholastic Competence and Behavioral Conduct, as are parental support ratings. Thus, personal and social factors most directly related to the peer network would appear to represent the avenue to the depressive features captured in our composite. The more favorable perceptions in the parent salient-domains, typically associated with high parental approval, are not implicated in reactions of depression. Thus, individuals displaying this profile do not seem to be able to draw upon these latter strengths or upon parental support in order to offset their depressive tendencies.

A depressed 15-year-old adolescent female in one of our normative samples displays this type of pattern. Her lowest self-evaluation scores are to be found among the more peer-salient domains, where she devalues her appearance, her peer likability, and her athletic ability. Moreover, she reports low peer support, particularly from classmates. In contrast, she reports high levels of competence/adequacy in the domains of scholastic competence and conduct, along with considerable parental support. In fact, her parents are quite proud of her, since she is a straight-A student and a talented musician. It was reported to us by her school counselor, however, that she does not fit in with her peers at school and has great difficulty forming relationships with others her age. In fact, she is teased by her classmates. In a follow-up interview, she indicated to us that she blames herself for her inadequacies and related lack of peer support, making it even more likely that she would experience low self-worth, depressed affect, and hopelessness about her future.

Two Predictors: Inadequacy in More Parent-Salient Domains Plus Low Parental Support

This pattern represents the mirror-image of the profile just described in that these adolescents report that they feel inadequate in the two domains judged to be particularly important to parents (Scholastic Competence and Behavioral Conduct) and feel that they are receiving minimal parental support. Thus, these would appear to be the salient predictors of their depressive reactions, as tapped by the depression/adjustment composite. In contrast, they report very favorable evaluations in the more peer-salient domains (Physical Appearance, Peer Likability, Athletic Competence) and are experiencing high levels of peer support. However, they do not appear to be able to capitalize on these strengths and related support. Rather, the focus would appear to be on feelings of inadequacy with regard to school performance and conduct and with the associated lack of parental approval.

A 15-year-old male from our normative sample, who was identified as "at risk" given his reports of very low self-worth, depressed affect, and hopelessness, typifies this pattern. His scores for both Scholastic Competence and Behavioral Conduct were extremely low, as were his ratings of parental approval. From the counselor, we learned that this adolescent has been under constant pressure from his family to achieve academically. He has done poorly in school, and several months before our testing, he was placed in a special education class. Perpetually he has gotten into trouble. Thus, his evaluations would appear to be quite realistic. However, his poor school performance and conduct problems have been a great disappointment to his parents given their expectations.

In contrast, his scores in the more peer-salient domains of Physical

Appearance, Peer Likability, and Athletic Competence were quite high, as was his evaluation of peer support. These perceptions would also appear to be realistic in that the counselor reported that he has been observed to do reasonably well with his males peers and has been described as "fun to be with." He has also been relatively successful at sports and was actively involved in wrestling at the time of our testing. However, the causal focus of his depressive reactions appears to be lack of parental support coupled with his perceived inadequacies in domains that are of particular importance to his parents. As described earlier in this chapter, despite adolescent attempts at autonomy from parents, it is also critical that they remain connected and garner support that parents can offer, an outcome that this young man has failed to achieve, thereby leading to his depression.

Two Predictors: Inadequacy in Both Peer-Salient and Parent-Salient Domains

This pattern was of particular interest, since it was unexpected given the empirical links in our general model. These individuals report feeling inadequate in *all* domains, both the peer-salient domains of Physical Appearance, Peer Likability, and Athletic Competence and the parent-salient domains, Scholastic Competence and Behavioral Conduct. However, they also report relatively high levels of support from both peers and parents. Thus, unlike the overall model in which support appears to mediate the effects of domain-specific self-perceptions, in this profile, feelings of inadequacy in the domains we have identified appear to have a direct effect on depressive reactions, bypassing the support, which they report to be quite adequate.

These adolescents appear to eschew the looking-glass-self model of self-worth in which one incorporates the perceived opinions of significant others. Rather, they seem to focus primarily on those Jamesian predictors that involve perceptions of competence, adequacy, or success, particularly to the extent that these are judged important. Of particular interest is why these adolescents seem unable to utilize their perceived high levels of support in the service of elevating their self-worth, mood, and hope. At this point in time, we can only speculate on some possible interpretations. Perhaps these youth do not *believe* the support they report receiving; that is, they may feel that it is not credible given their perceived deficiencies in all domains. Damon (1995) has recently argued that the effusive praise that parents or teachers heap on children to make them feel good is often viewed with suspicion by children and adolescents. Those displaying this pattern may also have developed their own personal standards or have become very self-critical (see Blatt's [1990, 1995] discussion of self-critical depression), placing less emphasis on the standards or feedback of others. Although we do not have data bearing upon these interpretations, the existence of this subgroup indicates that one cannot assume that both the Jamesian and Cooley predictors are relevant to all individuals.

The case of an adolescent male referred to our university clinic, given his expressed suicidal wishes, represents one scenario that can lead to such a profile (see Shirk & Harter, 1996). This 16-year-old had shown signs of self-deprecatory thinking and social withdrawal. Psychological assessment revealed extremely low self-worth (on our adolescent measure) as well as depressive features (particularly, "self-critical depression"). However, his mother reported that he has been a "model son" who was near the top of his class academically, well-integrated socially, and a starter for the high school basketball team. Yet, as the mother observed, he was becoming increasingly hard on himself and felt that he had to be perfect. For example, an A- on an exam would unleash harsh self-criticism and self-punishment. In initial assessment interviews, he indicated that the pressure was not coming from his parents, who were very supportive; they were quite proud of his accomplishments and would be satisfied with a solid B average. Thus, initially, his depressive reactions and associated suicidal thinking were quite puzzling.

During the course of treatment, a much clearer explanation for this pattern, in which he felt he was a failure in most domains despite high peer and parental support, became evident. It was revealed that he had been adopted, although neither he nor his adoptive parents knew the exact circumstances leading the biological parents to relinquish him. However, he was adamant that somehow he had played a role in the process. During a particularly emotional therapy session, he finally acknowledged that "something must have been wrong with me." Thus, beneath his self-critical stance was the belief that he had been flawed; otherwise, his biological parents would have kept him. His belief that he was fundamentally defective generalized to his evaluation of personal inadequacy across numerous domains, limitations with which he had become preoccupied despite strong peer and parental support. Consistent with the previous analysis, approval from others could not be viewed as credible given the belief in his fundamental defectiveness.

From a clinical perspective, initially, adolescents displaying such a pattern represent enigmas to the practitioner until the underlying causes can be illuminated. Another such example involves the case of a 14-year-old diabetic female in one of our clinical samples, who was admitted to a psychiatric inpatient unit due to depression, failure to follow her diet to control her diabetes, and prolonged truancy from school. On our measures, she reported the lowest possible self-worth score, as well as depressed affect and hopelessness. Noteworthy was the fact that she viewed herself as totally inadequate in the domain of Physical Appearance; perceptions of her Scholastic Competence, Athletic Competence, and Behavioral Conduct were also quite low. This young woman came from a very good and caring family, which she verified in her report of high levels of parental support. Peer support was also high. The unit staff was very surprised with her profile of scores, particularly the very unfavorable perception of her appearance, since they described her as "cute, vivacious, and attractive." Yet she did not find these external evaluations credible, nor could she take any comfort in the support provided her. She herself acknowledged that "people tell me I'm cute, but I look in the mirror, and don't believe them."

Subsequent to our testing, the unit staff began to focus more on her seemingly unrealistic concerns about her unattractiveness. In the course of therapy, it was revealed that her perceptions were primarily based upon the abdominal scarring caused by a history of multiple intramuscular injections to control her diabetes. She was preoccupied with this highly undesirable feature of her physical self, which interfered with her attention to other domains and led to more pervasive feelings of inadequacy. Rather than try to convince her that she really was attractive, despite the scarring, the staff initiated a plan whereby she could use an insulin pump, rather than injections, to prevent further scarring. Moreover, she was recommended for surgery to correct the abdominal scarring that had already occurred. This particular clinical example underscores a theme identified in an earlier chapter, where it was observed that females in this culture are particularly vulnerable to negative perceptions of their appearance, especially if they are primarily basing their feelings of self-worth on unfavorable evaluations of their attractiveness. From the standpoint of our identification of particular pathways to depression, this example illustrates the fact that one particular domain can emerge as extremely salient and may be targeted as the point of intervention. Moreover, this case exemplifies the fact that despite high levels of approval, such support cannot overcome the impact of perceived deficiencies that represent the basis for one's perceptions of worth as a person.

In summary, although illustrative cases have been provided for each of the six profiles representing a different combination of pathways leading to depressive reactions defined as low self-worth, depressed affect, and hopelessness about the future, these examples are not necessarily prototypes of these profiles. There can be many scenarios leading to a given profile. Moreover, while it is important to identify the particular predictors leading to an individual's depressive reactions, the instruments allowing one to assess these profiles do not come with a crystal ball. The complexity of the case examples given, coupled with the possibility that, for some individuals, self-reports may represent inaccurate assessments (either consciously or unconsciously), reveals that for purposes of both diagnosis and intervention, the documentation of profiles may not be sufficient; that is, they may not illuminate the underlying causes that lead to a given pattern of predictors. However, they do suggest where one should focus in moving to other standardized assessment techniques, interview procedures, or therapeutic strategies that may further enhance our understanding of these processes.

FURTHER INSIGHTS GLEANED FROM INTERVIEWS WITH ADOLESCENTS

In our interviews with adolescents (from our normative samples) whom we have considered at risk, as defined by low scores on the depression/adjustment composite, a number of other intriguing new themes have emerged. Three such themes are explored in the remainder of this chapter. First, adolescents do not experience depression as profound sadness only, but as an emotion blend of sadness plus *anger*. Second, these interviews have revealed that adolescents identify as the primary causes of their depression actions of *others against the self*. Third, adolescents' portrayals of the link between self-worth and depressed affect reveal that in their phenomenological experience, one component does precede the other sequentially. More specifically, the revelation is that for some adolescents, self-worth is reported to *precede* and provoke depressed affect, whereas for other adolescents, the experience of depressed affect is the springboard to feelings of low self-worth. For example, the first youth we quoted earlier exemplifies the first orientation; when he looks in the mirror, he doesn't like how he looks, he doesn't like himself as a person, which in turn causes him to become depressed. In contrast, other adolescents gave vivid accounts of equally painful events in which significant others reject the self, leading them first to inevitable feelings of depression, followed by disdain for the self as a person. The next step, therefore, in our programmatic effort to better understand the causes and consequences of depression among adolescents was to examine empirically each of these themes more systematically.

DEPRESSED AFFECT AS A COMBINATION OF SADNESS AND ANGER

The first adolescent we quoted at length lamented, "When I am depressed I feel sad, because other people have hurt me, but I'm also angry at them too, for not caring, for rejecting me." Other adolescents voiced similar accounts of their emotional experience when depressed. In a pilot interview study of 12 adolescents from our normative sample, who indicated that they frequently experienced depression, 11 of the 12 spontaneously mentioned that when they were in this emotional state, they felt angry or frustrated, in addition to feeling overwhelmingly sad (Harter & Whitesell, 1989).

According to Freudian (1968) theory, depression is experienced by adults as an affective combination of both sadness and anger. The primary emotion of sadness, typically over the loss of a significant other, is accompanied by anger or rage at being abandoned. However, since it is often impossible or inappropriate to direct such anger toward the lost other, it is defensively directed toward the self. Within the more recent clinical literature, increasing attention has been paid to the co-occurrence of sadness and anger (see Curran, 1987; Gispert, Davis, Marsh, & Wheeler, 1987; Khan, 1987; Rutter, 1989). Moreover, the comorbidity of depressive features and conduct disorder symptoms among certain subgroups of children and adolescents also speaks to the combination of emotions reflecting both sadness and anger (see Puig-Antich, 1982; Shaffer, 1974; Withers & Kaplan, 1987).

Within the developmental literature, recent attention has been devoted to the experience of *mixed emotions* (Donaldson & Westerman, 1986; Harris, 1983a, 1983b; Harter & Buddin, 1987; Harter & Whitesell, 1989). As described in Chapter 2, our own work has demonstrated a five-stage developmental sequence governing the appreciation that one can experience two different emotions simultaneously. These findings indicate that by middle childhood, children acknowledge the simultaneous occurrence of a variety of emotion combinations, including sadness and anger. Thus, it seemed fruitful to extend our inquiry to the phenomenological experience of depression as an emotion blend among young adolescents.

Based on these considerations, we anticipated that among a normative sample, most young adolescents would report that they experience depression as a mix of sadness and anger. With regard to the anger component, a critical question involves the particular target or object of anger. Is anger directed toward the *self*, as psychoanalytic formulations would imply (Asch, 1966; Bibring, 1953; Fenichel, 1945; Freud, 1968; Sandler & Joffe, 1965), or toward *others*? Recent clinical observations of adolescents by Cantor (1987) and Pfeffer (1986; Pfeffer et al., 1984) suggest that at this particular developmental level, depression is often manifest as anger toward others. Based on these observations, as well as on our own pilot studies, we predicted that in describing the emotions they experience when depressed, the majority of young adolescents would report anger toward others, either as the primary target or in combination with anger directed toward the self.

Our first hypothesis, namely, that the majority of adolescents would report anger, in addition to sadness, was supported. Eighty percent of the students sampled selected sadness and anger as the two emotions they most typically experienced when they were depressed. These findings suggest that depression in early adolescence is best characterized as an emotion blend, consistent with several theoretical approaches noted earlier, including the general psychoanalytic formulation (Freud, 1968), developmental theory emphasizing the emergence of the ability to experience two emotions simultaneously (Harter & Whitesell, 1989), and the recent emphasis on comorbidity (i.e., internalizing and externalizing symptoms, or disorders, concurrently) within the clinical literature (Curran, 1987; Gispert et al., 1987; Khan, 1987; Rutter, 1989).

Of further interest was the particular target of anger. We hypothesized, based on the observations of Cantor (1987) and Pfeffer (1986), as well as on our own pilot work, that the majority of adolescents would report anger toward others, either as the primary target of this emotion or in combination with anger directed toward the self. Consistent with these predictions, 39% of the adolescents in our sample reported anger toward others, whereas 40% reported anger toward both others and the self (Renouf & Harter, 1990). These results suggest that there may be at least two patterns of interest. In the first, profound sadness in consort with anger toward others, only, defines the experience of depression. In the second, sadness is accompanied by anger directed toward two targets, other as well as self. These two patterns may have implications for symptomatology and treatment. The first group, primarily experiencing anger toward others when depressed, may be more prone to conduct problems, including aggression toward others. The second group, which experiences anger toward the self in addition to anger against others, may be more prone to self-injurious behaviors, including suicidal thoughts or attempts. These expectations are consistent with the distinction in the clinical literature between "externalizing" and "internalizing" symptoms (see Achenbach, Conners, & Quay, 1985; Achenbach & Edelbrock, 1983). Moreover, these different patterns may bear links to the perceived causes of depression as well as to the sequence in which self-worth and depressed affect are experienced, both of which are discussed here.

THE PERCEIVED CAUSES OF DEPRESSION

From a developmental perspective, it is noteworthy that adolescents within a normative sample do not report the emotional experience more predictable from the psychoanalytic perspective on adult depression, namely, that anger would be primarily directed toward the self. In an attempt to unravel this seeming discrepancy, we next directed our empirical attention to the reported *causes* of depression among young adolescents.

We began with open-ended interviews, asking subjects to "think back to the most depressing thing that has happened to you in the past year" and then to describe that event. The majority of adolescents' responses fell into the following eight categories:

1. Psychological harm to the self by others: For example, "Someone made me feel bad." "They hurt my feelings, teased me, or did something that made me feel bad."
2. Physical harm to the self by others: For example, "Someone physically hurt me or did something to stuff that I own." "They beat me up, hit me, broke or stole something that was mine."
3. Death of someone close: For example, "Someone important to me died, for example, a family member, a friend, or a pet."
4. Separation from someone close: For example, "Someone important to me went away." "My parents got divorced, a friend moved away, or a friend and I broke up with each other [this could also be a boy or girl friend]."
5. Conflict with someone close: For example, "I was not getting along with someone important to me." "I was fighting with my parents, brothers or sisters, friends, boy or girl friend."
6. Rejection by someone close: For example, "I felt rejected by someone important to me, parents, brother or sister, a friend, a boy or girl friend." "Kids at school didn't want to be with me."
7. Loneliness: For example, "I felt lonely and wished I had a friend or a boy or girl friend, or more friends than I had."
8. Incompetence of the self: For example, "I did badly in something or messed up, or there was something I didn't like about myself." "I got bad grades, did something dumb, messed up in sports, or didn't like something about the way I was."

Of interest is that the vast majority of causes generated by adolescents involve negative actions of *others toward the self* (i.e., various forms of psychological and physical harm or insult). (Only the last category explicitly makes reference to negative actions *by* the self.) Intuitively, therefore, it is plausible that adolescents would experience depression as anger toward others. To examine this issue empirically, we next asked a sample of young adolescents to report the level of anger toward others and anger toward the self that they would experience for each of the eight causes (Renouf & Harter, 1990). Table 8.1 presents anger scores, where a 4 represents the highest, and a 1 the lowest level of anger.

As would be expected, the first six causes, clearly representing actions of others against the self, provoked significantly more anger toward others

TABLE 8.1. Anger at Others and at Self as a Function of the Particular Cause of Depression

Cause	Anger at others	Anger at self
Psychological harm to self by others	3.04	1.81
Physical harm to self by others	3.54	2.45
Death of close significant other	3.03	2.45
Separation from significant other	3.19	2.29
Conflict with significant other	3.29	2.50
Rejection by significant other	3.00	2.47
Loneliness	3.12	2.75
Incompetence of self	2.89	2.78

than toward the self. (Loneliness produced only somewhat more anger toward others, and, as anticipated, incompetence by the self produced no differences in anger toward others and the self.) With regard to the first six categories, therefore, the majority of adolescents presumably view others as more responsible than the self for the outcomes of these events, provoking anger directed toward others. It is of interest, in this regard, that recent studies of clinical samples of depressed adolescents have revealed that at this particular developmental level, anger toward others is quite common (Cantor, 1987; Pfeffer, 1986). One could speculate that adolescents may not yet have developed the inhibitions or defenses that would prevent them from expressing their feelings toward the significant others whom they consider to be the cause of their depression-related anger.

In future research, it would be of interest to determine the primary causes of depression for an adult population, including the level of anger directed toward the self and others, in order to determine whether there is a developmental shift between adolescence and adulthood. Adults may well assume more responsibility for their role in negative social interactions and direct greater anger toward the self, consistent with the psychoanalytic position. Alternatively, adults may *experience* anger toward others but are less likely to *express* it; that is, adults may have developed stronger defenses or inhibitions against the display of angry or aggressive impulses toward others. For example, several researchers have reported suppressed anger and hostility in depressed adults (Biaggio & Goodwin, 1987; Frank, Carpenter, & Kupfer, 1988; Riley, Treiber, & Woods, 1989). These issues deserve further study, however, since they suggest that the experience and/or the expression of the components of depression, particularly with regard to the target of anger, may well undergo developmental change between adolescence and adulthood.

PERCEIVED DIRECTIONALITY OF SELF-WORTH AND DEPRESSED AFFECT

As described in an earlier section, in the initial model that provided the impetus for our work, we made the assumption, consistent with a variety of sequential models in the field, that the self-evaluative (cognitive) components *preceded* one's affective reactions. Thus, we postulated that self-worth would be experienced prior to, and would therefore impact, one's emotional reaction of cheerfulness or depression. However, two sources of evidence have cautioned us against making the assumption that such a sequence describes the experiences of all individuals. As noted earlier, a comparison of alternative models through the application of structural equation techniques has demonstrated that a model in which there is a direct path from depressed affect to self-worth fits the data just as well as the original model in which the path was defined as self-worth to depressed affect. Moreover, interview data have revealed that many adolescents experience the depressive affective component prior to low self-worth.

Our interest in this issue is paralleled, broadly, by trends within the field of emotion, where a thrust in the 1980s concerned links between cognition and affect (Frijda, 1986; Izard, 1984; Lazarus, 1982, 1984; Leventhal & Scherer, 1987; Weiner, 1985; Zajonc, 1984). A major debate has surrounded the primacy of these two systems. The most representative proponents of the two camps are Zajonc (1984), who has argued for the primacy of *affect*, and Lazarus (1982, 1984), whose position emphasizes the primacy of *cognition*. Weiner (1985) also represents the latter tradition given his position that self-attributions give rise to distinct emotional states, depending on the specific nature of the attribution. We, too, fell victim to the mentality that one direction took precedence, initially espousing the view that the cognitive judgments inherent in self-worth preceded the affect of depression.

However, proponents of both positions have come to realize that the *directionality* of these links will vary depending on the particular emotions and cognitions in question (e.g., primary vs. secondary or socialized emotions, conscious vs. unconscious cognitive processes, etc.), as well as on particular developmental and individual difference factors (see Leventhal & Scherer, 1987). We concur with the revisionist stance. Our interview data, followed by a more systematic empirical inquiry described next, have required that we alter our position, acknowledging that the directionality of the link between self-worth and depressed affect will differ across individuals. For some, low self-worth will first be experienced, whereas for others, the depressive affect will occur prior to low self-worth.

We have developed a methodology that holds promise for assessing this distinction (Harter & Jackson, 1993; Harter & Marold, 1993). Adolescents are given the task of deciding *which comes first*. They are initially provided with a description in which they are told that students their age often feel that "not liking yourself" and "feeling depressed" go together. However, some students feel that not liking yourself comes first, whereas other students first feel depressed. The subjects are asked to reflect upon whether they first feel that they do not like themselves or, alternatively, whether they first feel that they are depressed. Specifically, they are asked to pick one of the following two options: (1) "I *first* feel *depressed* and *then* that makes me feel like I don't like myself" or (2) "I *first* feel like I *don't like myself* and *then* that makes me feel depressed." After they pick the option that best characterizes their own experience, they are asked to provide a brief written description of an event that represents an example of the sequence they selected.

The findings have been intriguing. First, with regard to the percentages of students endorsing each option across several studies, we have discovered that approximately half of a given sample indicates that the depression component is experienced first, whereas the remaining half indicate that the self-worth component precedes their experience of depression. Moreover, in both normative and clinical samples of adolescents who report that they are depressed, approximately two-thirds of those in the low-self-worth to depressed-affect-directionality group are females, whereas the percentages reverse themselves in the depressed-affect to low-self-worth group, where two-thirds are males.

Content analyses have been illuminating in that the experiences these adolescents describe directly match their choices, providing converging evidence for the meaningfulness of the directionality concept (Harter & Jackson, 1993). There is little overlap in the content of causes or antecedents for each sequence, further suggesting that the distinction between each directionality orientation is very real. What particular causes are cited by members of each group?

Low Self-Worth Precedes Depressed Affect

Students identifying themselves as experiencing this directionality cited examples in which they were dissatisfied with particular *self*-attributes. Three categories consistently emerge across samples: (1) *Physical appearance* heads the list, in that between two-thirds to three-fourths of subjects (typically more females than males) report that they are dissatisfied with some aspect of their looks (e.g., "When I try to do something with my face and hair and it doesn't work out and I think I'm ugly, then I get depressed"); (2) Lack of *competence* is the next most prevalent category (e.g., "I watch the people in sports do what seems to be an easy sport and then when I try it, it doesn't even *look like* the sport so I get depressed"); (3) Dissatisfaction with one's behavior or conduct in *social interactions* is the third most common category (e.g., "First I think I'm not a good friend, and then that makes me feel depressed"). A more complete list of examples is provided in Table 8.1. Thus, the *causes* of depression for adolescents in this directionality group reside in an attribution that finds the self inadequate, incompetent, or wanting.

Interestingly, we find gender differences in the particular themes or concerns that adolescents describe (see Figure 8.4). Girls are significantly more likely to find fault with their *appearance* and their *social behavior* (how they treat significant others with whom they have a relationship) than are boys, whereas the boys cite examples of *incompetence* (typically sports or scholastic performance) and *conduct* (not behaving in ways that are not morally sanctioned, for example, hitting, lying, stealing, acting out, etc.). These findings are consistent with the gender socialization literature revealing that females are particularly attuned to issues involving appearance (Allgood-Merten et al., 1990; Harter, 1998a; Nolen-Hoeksema, 1987; Simmons & Blyth, 1987), as well as relationships and the ethics of caring (Chodorow, 1989; Gilligan, 1982; Huston, 1983; Miller, 1986). Males, on the other hand, are more concerned with achievement and related competencies (Huston,

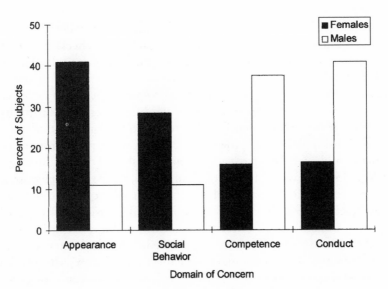

FIGURE 8.4. Gender differences in the particular concerns described by adolescents.

1983; Miezdian, 1991) as well as more rule-bound principles of ethical conduct (Gilligan, 1982; Gilligan, Rogers, & Tolman, 1991).

Depressed Affect Precedes Low Self-Worth

In contrast to the preceding group, adolescents for whom the experience of depressed affect comes first invariably described actions performed by *others against the self.* The vast majority of responses could be captured by three categories (that do not overlap with the categories described by the first group):

1. The most common was *rejection* by others; for example, "I was feeling depressed because all of my friends went to the amusement park, and they acted like they didn't want me to go with them. Then I felt like I was a boring person and I didn't like myself."
2. *Conflict* with others, typically parents, represented another major category; for example, "Every time I get into it with my mom, she always yells at me and then I get depressed and think of things that make me hate myself."
3. Experiences of *loss* of a person or pet, either through death or the termination of a relationship, represents the third most common category; for example, "I usually get depressed because I can't accept my father's dying and then I usually feel that its my fault that he died and I don't like myself."

A more complete list, representing the range of examples, is provided in Table 8.2. In our most recent study, we employed a checklist procedure allowing us to examine the pattern of causes more systematically (Harter & Jackson, 1993). *Peer* rejection and conflict were by far the most common causes of depressed affect (58%), followed by *parental* conflict or rejection (13%) and *loss* (13%). There were no gender differences in this pattern.

While it is certainly plausible that rejection by significant others, loss of a relationship, lack of approval, and conditional support from peers or parents should provoke *depression,* why, in turn, should depression necessarily trigger low self-worth? In our original model, where the direction of effects underlying the robust correlation between self-worth and depression was assumed to flow from lack of self-worth to depression, it was plausible that harsh indictments of oneself as a person, tantamount to loss of self, should cause individuals to become depressed. With regard to the contrasting directionality orientation (depressed affect precedes low self-worth), it is also plausible that loss of another, through rejection, death, or conflict, should provoke *depression.* It is less obvious, however, why depression caused

Table 8.2. Examples of Descriptions for Each Directionality Orientation

Group A. Low self-worth precedes depressed affect

Appearance

"When I try to do something with my face and hair and it doesn't work out and I think I'm ugly, then I get depressed."

"I didn't like it that I was short, so I became depressed."

"I don't like the way I look and then I get depressed because I think I can't change."

"When I look in the mirror, I think I am ugly and then I feel depressed."

"When I can't do my hair the way I want it, and it isn't cute, then it makes me depressed."

"I look in the mirror and don't like something about me, my hair, my body, and I get depressed."

"My nose and my feet are too big, and then I look at other peoples' and its depressing."

Competence

"I watch the people in sports do what seems to be an easy sport and then when I try it, it doesn't even look like the sport, so I get depressed."

"Once I was trying to draw something and I couldn't do it, so I hated myself and then I got depressed."

"I mess up at my school work and then I hate myself and get depressed about it. I'm capable, but I just don't work hard enough."

"I was pitching, and the first two batters I walked, and then I hit the third one with the ball, and then the coach took me out. I was really down on myself and felt depressed the rest of the game."

"I played really bad at soccer and felt like the loss was my fault, so it made me depressed."

Social behavior

"First, I think I'm not a good friend, and then that makes me feel depressed."

"I disobeyed my mom and didn't do my chores, and felt bad about it, and depressed."

"I blew up at my best friend. I got mad at myself for losing my temper and then I felt depressed."

"I first feel like I don't like myself because I yelled at my mom and then I feel depressed."

Group B. Depressed affect precedes low self-worth

Rejection

"I was feeling depressed because all of my friends went to the amusement park, and they acted like they didn't want me to go with them. Then I felt like I was a boring person and I didn't like myself."

"I got depressed because I felt left out of something and then I feel like I don't have any friends and that nobody likes me, and then I didn't like myself."

"I got depressed because people called me a nerd. Half of the people I *know* say I'm a nerd, so I don't like myself and how I act."

"My mom got on my case because of my grades and said she was really disappointed in me, which made me depressed, and then I got disappointed in myself."

Conflict

"Every time I get into it with my mom, she always yells at me and then I get depressed and think of things that make me hate myself."

"I got depressed because I got into a fight with my friend and thought I wasn't a good person."

"My mom got really mad at me for not doing my chores; at first I got mad, and then I became depressed about it, and wondered if I was a good person or not."

(continued)

TABLE 8.2. *Continued*

Loss

"I usually get depressed because I can't accept my father's dying and then I usually feel that its my fault that he died and I don't like myself."

"My grandfather died, and I thought it was my fault cause I didn't visit him often enough."

"My boyfriend broke up with me, and I got really depressed; I wasn't sure what happened, what I had done, and I felt terrible about myself."

---

by actions of others against the self should so predictably produce low self-worth.

Psyszczynski and Greenberg's (1986, 1987) self-awareness theory of reactive depression, against a backdrop of Cooley's looking-glass-self formulation, provides some compelling clues. Self-awareness theory posits that the loss of a significant other may typically signify the loss of central source of self-worth, a contention that finds empirical support. Thus, in addition to a depressive reaction to loss or rejection, one should also experience a loss of self-worth to the extent that the significant other represented an important source of self-worth.

CORRELATES OF DIRECTIONALITY GROUP MEMBERSHIP

The findings presented here document the fact that adolescents in each directionality group systematically cite a different cluster of causes. These differences further suggested that the two groups may predictably be distinguished on a number of potential *correlates* that we had also assessed in the same battery. We examined those correlates that were below the midpoint on the depression/adjustment.

Given that the vast majority of individuals in the low-self-worth to depressed-affect directionality group cite concerns over their physical appearance as the primary cause of their low self-worth, we predicted that on our standardized questionnaires tapping appearance-related issues, this group would report higher levels of concern compared to those in the depressed affect to self-worth-directionality group. The results supported our prediction in that the low-self-worth to depressed-affect group reported greater hopelessness about appearance, more concern over their appearance, and a greater link between appearance and popularity, namely, that how one looks is a major determinant of one's popularity.

Given that the depressed-affect to low-self-worth-directionality group cited examples of actions of the others against the self, we predicted that this group would report lower scores on variables tapping support or approval from significant others than would those in the low-self-worth to depressed-affect group. Findings revealed that the depressed to low-self-worth group reported more conditional peer support, more hopelessness about peer support, greater *worry* over peer support, as well as greater worry about whether they were likable by peers. A similar pattern was obtained for maternal support.

Finally, we anticipated group differences in the *affects* experienced as part of the depressive experience. Both groups were expected to report high levels of *sadness*, that is, sadness should *not* differentiate the two groups. However, the two directionality groups should differ on anger toward the self and anger toward others. We predicted that the low-self-worth to depressed-affect group, given their focus on dissatisfaction with attributes of the self, would report greater anger at the *self*, as well as greater shame, than would the depressed to low-self-worth group. Given that the depressed to low-self-worth group reports actions of others against the self as the cause of their depression, in addition to concerns about support, we predicted that the depressed to low-self-worth group should report greater anger toward *others* than the low-self-worth to depressed-affect group. The findings clearly supported these predictions. Thus, across three types of variables—(1) perceived causes, (2) correlates, and (3) affects associated with depression—we find a predictable pattern of differences, further suggesting that there may be different models or pathways of influence for each directionality group.

TREATMENT IMPLICATIONS

It is highly likely that a knowledge of an individual's directionality orientation may, in conjunction with information concerning a client's presenting problem and diagnosis, have implications for intervention. For those in the low-self-worth to depressed-affect group, a focus on the basis for negative self-evaluations may well be the most fruitful avenue to pursue. Questions such as (1) What are the individual's most salient attributions? (2) How *realistic* are their self-perceptions? and so on, may profitably be posed. In certain cases, the individual may require therapeutic interventions that provoke the alteration of unrealistic self-representations. In other cases, the goal may entail the lowering of unrealistically high expectations of the self. In still other cases, the profile of self-evaluations may highlight areas where skills training may be profitable. Finally, clients may need to shift their investment from a domain in which they are, in reality, not that competent, and may have little potential to improve, to a domain where they can achieve greater success. Each of these strategies should produce, as outcomes, a heightening of self-worth, a reduction in anger toward the self, and the alleviation of depressed affect.

For those endorsing the depressed-affect to low-self-worth directionality orientation, the initial focus of treatment will undoubtedly be conflictual or nongratifying relationships with significant others. Thus, one would want to explore the basis for feelings of rejection, conflict, or loss. Critical questions will include the following:

1. How realistic are these perceptions?
2. Whom does the client see as responsible?
3. What role does the client's own behavior play in this pattern?
4. Can the client realistically expect to obtain support from these others?
5. How critical is the support of these others as a source of the client's self-worth?
6. Are there alternative people to whom one might turn for support that can be more validating or enhancing and less conditional?

In working through these issues, preferably with inclusion of the family in treatment, it is anticipated that there will be an alleviation of the client's depression, his/her anger at others, and an enhancement of self-worth.

CONCLUSION

A major goal of the research presented in this chapter was the construction of a model of the causes, correlates, and consequences of self-worth. With regard to the causes, we built upon the models of James (1892) and Cooley (1902), identifying competence or adequacy in domains of importance and the approval of significant others, respectively. However, rather than treat these determinants as independent influences on self-worth, we have identified and empirically documented the fact that three domains of competence/adequacy (Physical Appearance, Peer Likability, and Athletic Competence) are more directly linked to peer approval, whereas the remaining two (Scholastic Competence and Behavioral Conduct) are more highly predictive of parental approval. In developing a model of the correlates and consequences of self-worth, it was urged that one identify variables that have a direct impact on individual's day-to-day functioning. Depressive reactions, including depressed affect and hopelessness, are among the correlates most systematically related to low self-worth. We have also determined that these depressive reactions are highly predictive of suicidal ideation (although there may be other outcomes as well).

Although our initial sequential model identified self-worth as a determinant of depressed affect, the correlation between these two constructs is so high that it is impossible through causal modeling techniques to determine the directionality of effects, namely, which precedes which. Thus, we have created a depression/adjustment composite in which we have combined self-worth, affect, and hopelessness. Although we cannot statistically determine the directionality of these constructs, findings reveal that the phenomenological experience of adolescents differs with regard to which is experienced as causally prior to the other. For some, low self-worth precedes, that is, provokes, depressed affect. Adolescents endorsing this orientation focus primarily on limitations of the self, for example, perceived unattractiveness or inability to make friends. Adolescents who experience depressive affect prior to low self-worth are more likely to target actions of others against the self at the head of the causal chain; for example, they report being rejected or abandoned by others.

We have also sought to determine how depression is phenomenologically experienced by adolescents as a blend of emotions. For all adolescents, one component is profound sadness. However, the vast majority of adolescents also report that depression combines such sadness with anger. The target of the anger varies, however. For some, the anger is directed toward the self (internalizing symptoms), whereas for others, it is directed toward others (externalizing symptoms). Interestingly, those who report that they experience self-worth as causally prior to depression are more likely to indicate that their anger is directed toward the self. In contrast, those that report that depression precedes self-worth are more likely to report that their anger is directed toward others.

The need to identify multiple pathways to depressive reactions, defined by the constellation of low self-worth, depressed affect, and hopelessness about the future, was underscored. We have empirically isolated six different profiles among our normative samples that point to different patterns of predictors. Case examples provided illustrations of how, for different adolescents, there are different causes for their depressive reactions. These examples by no means exhaust the complex dynamics that contribute to the range of potentially different causes of each pattern. Although the identification of these pathways represents an important first step in pinpointing potential determinants of depressive outcomes among adolescents, typically, further evaluation will be necessary to illuminate the underlying processes that are responsible for negative evaluations of self and/or perceptions of lack of approval from others. Nevertheless, the determination of a particular pathway provides a framework for further diagnostic efforts and possible points of intervention.

The Authenticity of the Self

Building upon the observations of historical scholars who endorsed a symbolic interactionist perspective (Baldwin, 1897; Cooley, 1902; Mead, 1925), contemporary theorists and investigators who have examined self-processes across the life span have continued to highlight the fact that others profoundly impact the formation of one's self-portrait. Although the symbolic interactionists pointed to critical processes in the normative construction of the self, they did not alert us to the fact that self-development could go *awry*; that is, there are liabilities associated with the construction of a personal self that is so highly dependent upon social interaction. As described in Chapters 7 and 8, the most obvious liability involves the internalization of *unfavorable* evaluations of the self by others. Findings clearly reveal that the incorporation of the disapproving opinions of significant others will lead, in turn, to perceptions of personal inadequacy and to low self-worth. This chapter focuses on another liability, namely, the potential for constructing a *false* self that does not mirror one's authentic experiences. Thus, one may incorporate opinions of others toward the self that do not correspond to events as experienced. Alternatively, the demands of significant others, coupled with the need to garner their approval, may lead to the suppression of authentic opinions or behaviors, which may be manifestly supplanted by displays of what others need to observe or want to hear. As will become evident, the creation of a self designed to conform to the wishes and dictates of significant others whom one feels obligated to please may not only compromise the true self, but may also lead to associated negative outcomes such as low self-worth and depression.

Historical roots to an interest in false-self behaviors are briefly summarized at the outset of this chapter. More recently, there has been a resurgence of interest in the causes and manifestations of lack of authenticity, across the life span, as well as sociocultural treatments of how societal and economic changes pose challenges to authenticity for entire generations of individuals. A common form of false self behavior involves the suppression of one's opinions, thoughts, and feelings. Although the seeds of false-self behavior can be sown in early childhood, adolescence is the period during which an awareness of one's false-self behavior becomes particularly acute. In addition, Gilligan and colleagues (Brown & Gilligan, 1992; Gilligan, 1982, 1993; Gilligan et al., 1989, 1991) contend that adolescence is a critical juncture given their observations that many females, in particular, come to suppress their thoughts and feelings, a process they label as "loss of voice." In this chapter, I review Gilligan's analysis for why the voices of adolescent females should go underground. As will become apparent, the school setting is a particularly interesting context within which to examine levels of adolescent voice among both males and females given that it represents a microcosm of the larger society. Moreover, schools have come under increasing scrutiny and criticism for shortchanging girls in ways that may well undermine their desire or ability to voice their opinions.

Despite trenchant analyses by Gilligan and by those who have been critical of the school system in the United States (e.g., Sadker & Sadker, 1994; American Association of University Women, 1992), there has been little empirical work on the causes and consequences of lack or loss of voice as a form of false-self behavior. Thus, our own research group has embarked upon a research program that addresses level of voice in both males and females. It is important to emphasize that in the past literature, there has been no systematic documentation that females actually have lower levels of voice than do males. Gilligan, for example, has chosen to focus primarily on females. However, it is critical to examine the processes that promote or stifle adolescent voices among members of both genders. Moreover, although there has been documentation of gender differences on average for a number of variables that may impact voice, there has been far too little emphasis on the tremendous overlap in the distributions of males and females. Even when differences that may be implicated in level of voice are statistically significant, typically, the effect sizes are quite small.

Nor have theorists, educational observers, and investigators been sufficiently concerned with the potential causes and consequences of the notable individual differences *within* each gender. Our own findings on level of voice reveal that such individual differences represent the major phenomena to be explained; that is, there are no overall gender differences, nor does voice decline with age for girls. Rather, while some adolescent girls lack voice, there are many who report that they are quite capable of expressing their opinions. The same is true for adolescent males in that some stifle the expression of their opinions, whereas others can readily voice their thoughts. In our own research, we have documented two variables that impact level of voice: gender orientation (particularly for females), and the degree to which support for voice influences adolescents' expression of their opinions. Both of these variables contribute heavily to adolescents' ability to voice their opinions.

The chapter concludes with cautions against making sweeping generalizations about gender differences in voice and entertains certain educational implications for enhancing the levels of voice for both genders. For example, although teachers have borne the brunt of the criticism for undermining female students' confidence in the classroom, it will be argued that adolescents come to the school setting with a long history of interactions within the family, as well as with peers outside of the classroom. Moreover, within the context of school, how male and female students treat each other will also impact level of voice. Finally, the focus of the existing educational literature has been primarily restricted to an analysis of how girls are shortchanged in the classroom. We need to redress this imbalance in understanding why certain male adolescents are also at risk for suppressing their thoughts, toward the goal of developing prevention and intervention strategies for both genders.

THE HISTORICAL EMERGENCE OF INTEREST IN FALSE-SELF BEHAVIOR

Avid interest in the distinction between true- and false-self behaviors appears to date from the 16th century (Baumeister, 1987; Trilling, 1971). Trilling describes the obsession with deception and pretense that found its way into politics, philosophy, and literature (e.g., Shakespeare) in England. Baumeister observes that people were particularly worried that others (not they themselves) may be hiding their true selves. With the advent of Puritanism, people became concerned about whether they were deceiving *themselves* with regard to those attributes (piety, faith, and virtue) that were essential if they were to enter into the kingdom of heaven. Emphasis on the hidden parts of the self was exacerbated by Victorian repressiveness; self-scrutiny, coupled with impossibly high moral standards, forced individuals to become self-deceptive. Moreover, Freud's revelations concerning the unconscious led to the conclusion that certain parts of the true self may be inaccessible even to oneself.

The theme of true- versus false-self behavior emerged more explicitly in the clinical literature among those psychoanalytically oriented theorists who built upon Freudian formulations. Horney (1950) described the person's alienation from the real self. Other theorists noted that impostor tendencies represent the need for narcissistic enhancement as a defense against core feelings of worthlessness (Deutsch, 1955; Kohut, 1977). Bleiberg (1984) and Winnicott (1965) focused more on the developmental precursors of false-self behavior. For Bleiberg, false-self behavior resulted from caregivers who did not validate the child's true self, thus leading the infant to become alienated from his/her core self. For Winnicott, parents who are intrusively overinvolved with their infant cause the child to develop a false self based upon compliance (see also Sullivan, 1953). These clinical formulations emphasize the more pathological avenues to the development of a false self.

Within the sociological and social psychological literatures, lack of authenticity among adults is considered to be motivated by attempts to present the self in a manner that will impress or win the acceptance of others. Goffman (1959), in his treatment of the presentation of self in everyday life, described the manipulative motives that compete with our desire to be sincere. Various forms of "facework" communicate to others that we are competent, likable, moral, or worthy of respect, motives designed not only to protect and promote the self but also to curry favor, obtain social currency or power, and preserve critical relationships. Earlier in the same decade, Riesman (1950) distinguished between "inner-directed" individuals who were self-determining and, by definition, more true to themselves, and "outer-directed" individuals whose malleability in the face of social demands marked them as less authentic. A similar distinction has been echoed by Snyder (1987) in identifying high versus low self-monitors. High self-monitors are presumed to suppress features of their true self in order to gain the approval of others. Concern with the social appropriateness of their self-presentations necessarily leads to inconsistency in their self-presentations from one social situation to another. While some condemn the high self-monitor for superficiality if not deceit, Snyder suggests that high self-monitoring reflects the individual's flexibility in coping with the diversity of social roles one is expected to assume. Finally, within the developmental literature, false-self behavior has been considered by some theorists to be a dimension of normative role experimentation during adolescence (Broughton, 1981; Selman, 1980). Thus, a contemporary female adolescent may well don the mantle of Madonna in one situation, but then shift to Kate Moss in another. Elkind (1967) cites an additional motive, observing that the adolescent becomes more self-conscious as it becomes more apparent that he/she is the object of others' evaluations. Thus, adolescents may attempt to obscure their true selves if they feel that they do not measure up to the standards and values set by others whose opinions are critical.

CONTEMPORARY INTEREST IN THE FALSE SELF

Themes that involve lack of authenticity are now being explored across every period of the life span. Lerner (1993) points to the vast vocabulary we have developed to describe deception. Verb forms make reference to fabricating, withholding, concealing, distorting, falsifying, pulling the wool over someone's eyes, posturing, charading, faking, and hiding behind a facade. Adjectives include elusive, evasive, wily, phony, artificial, two-faced, manipulative, calculating, pretentious, crafty, conniving, duplicitous, deceitful, dishonest. Noun forms include hypocrite, charlatan, chameleon, impostor, fake, and fraud. Interestingly, there are common threads in the analyses of lack of authenticity across the life span.

Infancy

As was observed in Chapter 2, from a normative, developmental perspective, the emergence of *language* is a double-edged sword. On the positive side, the attainment of language is potent in the service of union and connectedness, since it provides a common symbol system, allowing for new levels of shared meaning. In addition, verbal representation provides a powerful vehicle through which the child can begin to construct a *narrative* of his/her life, one's "life story" (Stern, 1985), preserved in *autobiographical memory* (see Crittenden, 1994; Eisenberg, 1985; Fivush & Hudson, 1990; Hudson, 1990a, 1990b; Nelson, 1986, 1993; Snow, 1990). However, these theorists also alert us to the liabilities of language. Stern argues that language can drive a wedge between two simultaneous forms of interpersonal experience, as it is lived and as it is verbally represented. The very capacity for objectifying the self through language allows one to transcend, and therefore potentially distort, one's immediate experience.

Moreover, as described in Chapter 2, the narrative that is initially constructed is highly scaffolded by parents who dictate which aspects of the child's experience they feel are important to codify in the construction of the child's autobiographical memory, leading to potential misrepresentations of the child's actual experience (Bowlby, 1980; Bretherton, 1991; Crittenden, 1994). Children may receive subtle signals that certain episodes should not be retold or are best "forgotten" (Dunn et al., 1991). Such distortions may well contribute to the formation of a false self if one accepts the falsified version of experience. Thus, the display of behaviors selected primarily because it meets the needs and wishes of someone else incurs the risk of alienating oneself from those inner experiences that represent one's true self (Crittenden, 1994; Stern, 1985; Winnicott, 1965).

Childhood

Issues involving displays of true- and false-self behavior during childhood have also been related to differences in the socialization experiences of children. For example, Deci and Ryan (1995) contend that a child's true self is fostered by caregivers who love the child for who he/she is, rather than for matching a socially imposed, external standard. In contrast, a false self will emerge to the extent that caregivers make their approval contingent upon the child's living up to their particular standards, since the child must adopt a socially implanted self. Such children display what Deci and Ryan label "contingent self-esteem." Consistent with their analysis are our own findings, revealing that those experiencing support that is *conditional* upon meeting the externally imposed standards of parents and peers display more false-self behavior (see Harter, Marold, Whitesell, & Cobbs, 1996).

Abusive treatment by caregivers also places the child at serious risk for suppressing his/her true self and displaying various forms of false-self behavior (Harter, 1998b). Parenting practices that constitute lack of attunement to the child's needs, empathic failure, lack of validation, threats of harm, coercion, and enforced compliance all cause the true self to go underground (Bleiberg, 1984; Stern, 1985; Winnicott, 1965) and lead to what Sullivan (1953) labeled "not me" experiences. Secrecy pacts around sexually abusive interactions further lead the abused child defensively to exclude such episodic memories from awareness. Thus, sexual and physical abuse at the hands of family members cause the child to split off experiences, relegating them to either a private or inaccessible part of the self. The very disavowal, repression, or dissociation of one's experiences, coupled with psychogenic amnesia and numbing as defensive reactions to abuse, therefore set the stage for the loss of one's true self. Herman (1992) describes a more conscious pathway in that the abused child comes to see the true self as corroded with inner badness and therefore to be concealed at all costs. Persistent attempts to be good, in order to please the parents, lead the child to develop a socially acceptable self that is experienced as false or unauthentic. These themes are developed in more detail in Chapter 10.

Adolescence

The processes just described can and do continue into adolescence. However, other developmental features emerge, making the issue of false-self behavior even more problematic. As described in Chapter 3, the adolescent is confronted with the demand to create *multiple selves* associated with different social roles or contexts. Thus, one may display different selves with father, mother, close friends, romantic partners, peers, as well as don a different persona in the role of student, worker on the job, and athlete (see Erikson, 1950; Griffin et al., 1981; Hart, 1988; Harter & Monsour, 1992; Kolligian, 1990; Smollar & Youniss, 1985). Our own work has revealed that this proliferation of selves naturally introduces concern over which is "the real me." While the creation of multiple selves serves many adaptive functions, certain attributes in different roles are identified by adolescents as contradictory (e.g., cheerful with friends but depressed with parents). During our multiple-selves procedure, a number of teenagers spontaneously agonized over which of these opposing attributes represented the "true self," highlighting the salience of this issue at this point in development.

Although our initial interest focused on the normative, developmental concern that many adolescents express over their false-self behavior, subsequent studies revealed considerable variability in adolescents' reports of the *level* of their own true- and false-self behavior with parents and peers. Thus, we sought to examine certain antecedents of the level of false-self behavior in order to understand these marked individual differences. We looked to features of adolescents' parent and peer *support* systems, given our own previous research on the impact of approval on self-processes and the literature described earlier that implicated certain patterns of support in the display of false-self behavior. More specifically, we predicted that both *level* of support and *conditionality* of support would be important determinants of false-self behavior. Moreover, since a number of pilot subjects spontaneously commented that they felt somewhat hopeless about ever being able to please parents or peers, we also hypothesized that hopelessness may well be implicated in false-self behavior. Employing path-analytic techniques, the best-fitting model revealed that the effect of level and conditionality of support on false self behavior is mediated by hopelessness about obtaining support (Harter, Marold, et al., 1996). Thus, the highest levels of false-self behaviors are reported by those adolescents who feel they are receiving relatively low levels of support that they perceive as conditional, leading them to feel hopeless about pleasing others, which in turn causes them to suppress their true self. It was our interpretation that they did so as a means of garnering the desired support through displays of false-self behavior that they felt others would prefer.

Self-presentation through the use of language stands out as a major vehicle through which false-self behaviors, those perceived to be lacking in authenticity, are displayed. For example, in our own research, we have asked adolescents to describe the meaning of the terms "true"- and "false"-self behavior (Harter, Marold, et al., 1996; Ng, 1993). Subjects provide general descriptions; for example, the true self is the "real me inside," "my true feelings," "what I really think and feel" whereas the false self is described as "being phony," "putting on an act." However, at a more specific level, adolescents typically describe the *verbal* behavior through which their true and false selves are manifest. They define true-self behavior as "saying what you really think," "expressing your true opinion." In contrast, false-self behaviors include "not saying what you think," "expressing things you don't really believe or feel," "not stating your true opinion," "saying what you think other people want to hear." False-self behavior, therefore, is experienced as phony or artificial. Merely verbalizing what others appear to want you to say does not necessarily constitute false-self behavior. It must be accompanied by the phenomenological experience that one's words lack authenticity.

These observations converge with what Gilligan and colleagues (Brown & Gilligan, 1992; Gilligan, 1982, 1993; Gilligan et al., 1989, 1991) have referred to as "loss of voice," namely, the suppression of one's thoughts and opinions. From a developmental perspective, Gilligan finds loss of voice to be particularly problematic for *females*. She contends that prior to adolescence, girls seem to be clear about what they know and most are able to express their opinions forcefully. They are not confused about what they know, about the meaning of what transpires in relationships, and as a result, they can act decisively. However, with the onset of adolescence, many cover over what they knew as children, suppressing their voice, diminishing themselves, and hiding their feelings in a cartography of lies. "The astute, outspoken and clear-eyed resister often gets lost in a sudden disjunction or chasm as she approaches adolescence, as if the world that she knows from experience in childhood suddenly comes to an end, and divides from the world she is to enter as a young woman, a world that is governed by different rules" (Gilligan et al., 1989, p. 3). Many years earlier, Simone de Beauvoir (1952) made a similar point in observing that "young girls slowly bury their childhood, put away their independent and imperious selves, and submissively enter adult existence" (p. 358). Gilligan's analysis of the reasons why girls may lose their voices at adolescence are examined shortly, followed by a discussion of our own findings, which challenge the generality of her claims.

Adulthood

The issue of authenticity during adulthood, particularly for women, has been highlighted by a number of scholars who have spoken to the potential for false-self behavior within close relationships (see Chodorow, 1989; Gilligan, 1982; Jordan, 1991; Miller, 1986). As a starting point, these theorists argue that *connectedness* to others is a commodity that is as essential as the development of autonomy. They argue that relatedness with others brings clarity, reality, and authenticity to the self. However, an overememphasis on connectedness and caregiving may jeopardize authenticity and the development of one's true self. For example, women who adopt a position of subordination in relationships typically "transform" their own needs, seeing others' needs as their own. As Miller (1986) cogently argues, subordination and authenticity are totally incompatible. There is increasing convergence in the literature (Gilligan, 1982; Gilligan et al., 1989; Jordan, Kaplan, Miller, Stiver, & Surrey, 1991; Lerner, 1993; Miller, 1986; Stiver & Miller, 1988) that such women are fearful that if they were to act on their own needs and desires, such an expression of their true self would cause conflict and threaten the relationship. Lerner (1993), in her recent book entitled *The Dance of Deception*, contends that pretending is closely linked with femininity in our culture, providing challenges for women to live authentically. Yet truth telling, she argues, is central to intimacy, self-regard, and joy. Thus, cultural factors conspire to force many women to compromise their true selves, an adaptation that takes its toll in other arenas of their lives.

Sociocultural Analyses

A broader, more sociocultural perspective on how false-self behavior has become a contemporary societal problem has been offered by Gergen (1991). He argues that in the previous period of "modernism," authenticity was a major commodity, as well as an expectation. However, marked advances in technology have vaulted us into an era of *postmodernism*. As noted in Chapter 1, Gergen develops a portrait of the "saturated" or "populated" self, observing that easy access to air travel, electronic and express mail, fax machines, cellular phones, beepers, and answering machines, have all dramatically accelerated our social connectedness and thrust us into a dizzying swirl of relationships.

For Gergen, the demands of multiple relationships split the individual into a multiplicity of self-investments, leading to a "cacophony of potential selves" across different relational contexts. Such multiple selves become increasingly crafted to conform to the particular relationship at hand. As such, they are likely to possess many voices that do not necessarily harmonize, compromising one's sense of an obdurate core self, and casting doubt on one's true identity. Gergen argues that strategically adopting multiple roles for social gain, consciously managing the impressions one wishes to create, depends for its palpability on a contrasting sense of one's *real* self. Such a "pastiche personality" must, in turn, lead the individual to conclude that he/she is not true to oneself. For some, the guise of strategically manipulating others will lead to distress. For others (see Lifton, 1993), such superficiality gives way to an optimistic sense of enormous possibility, particularly if it is successful in enhancing one's social currency.

Gilligan's Analysis of the Motives for Loss of Voice in Female Adolescents

Given that the primary manifestions of false-self behavior are observed in the failure to verbally express one's thoughts and feelings, the remainder of this chapter focuses primarily on such lack of voice. As noted earlier,

Gilligan contends that suppression of voice is most typically observed in females, beginning in adolescence. However, why, according to Gilligan, should adolescent females be particularly vulnerable to loss of voice? For Gilligan, during the developmental transition to adolescence, girls begin to identify with the role of "woman" in the culture, since the onset of puberty makes this impending role more salient. Gilligan argues that teenage girls quickly perceive that the desirable stereotype of the "good woman" is being nice, polite, pleasing to others, unassertive, and quiet. For Gilligan, this juncture creates a conflict for female adolescents. For girls to remain faithful to *themselves*, they must resist the conventions of feminine goodness. However, for girls to remain responsive to *others*, they must resist the values placed on self-sufficiency and self-authenticity. Pipher (1994) concurs, observing that adolescent girls "experience a conflict between their autonomous selves and their need to be feminine, between their status as human beings and their vocation as females" (pp. 21–22). She contends that girls become "female impersonators," who "fit their whole selves into small, crowded spaces. Vibrant, confident girls become shy, doubting young women. Girls stop thinking, 'Who am I? What do I want?' and start thinking, 'What must I do to please others?' " (p. 22). As de Beauvoir (1952) put it, girls who were the *subjects* of their *own* lives become the *objects* of *others'* lives. Alice Miller (1981) described a similar pattern of conflict for girls between being authentic and honest or being loved. If they choose authenticity, they are often abandoned by parents. If they choose to be loved, they abandon their true selves. Pipher describes a similar conflict within the peer arena, where she notes that "girls can be true to themselves and risk abandonment by their peers, or they can reject their true selves and be socially acceptable" (p. 38). I return later to the issue of how *common* such reactions may be among contemporary adolescent females.

Thus, adherence to the "good woman stereotype," putting others' needs and desires ahead of one's own, has been argued to be a powerful motive for suppressing one's voice. Gilligan also contends that in what is still largely a patriarchal society, girls observe that women's opinions are typically not sought after, not valued, and not supported; they notice that the "civilized world" is not equally responsive to the views of men and women. The message to women, Gilligan notes, is to keep quiet, notice the absence of women, and say nothing. Moreover, adolescent girls are subjected to what Gilligan (1993) identifies as societal "voice and ear training," in which it becomes clear what voices people want to hear, and what can and cannot be said in order to avoid being labeled as inappropriate, rude, or wrong. If girls adhere to such training and attempt to emulate the stereotype, their own voices necessarily go underground. Gilligan also claims that many girls observe these stereotypical behaviors in their own mothers, who serve as role models for how women in this culture should act. To the extent that their mothers have endorsed the stereotype and therefore are suppressing their own thoughts and feelings, adolescent girls emulate their mothers and learn not to speak their minds.

In addition, Gilligan describes a constellation of more proximal motives that derive from what she describes as the *relational impasse* in which many adolescent girls find themselves. Given the importance for females of connectedness to others (see Belenky, Clinchy, Goldberger, & Tarule, 1986; Chodorow, 1989; Gilligan, 1982; Miller, 1986; Rubin, 1985), behaviors that threaten relationships are to be avoided at all costs. Thus, beginning in adolescence, many females compromise their authenticity; they take themselves out of "true" relationship in order to preserve connectedness in some lesser form. If they were to speak their minds, express their true voice, it might well cause tension or conflict in the relationship, it might anger the other person; it could hurt the other's feelings, and, at worst, it might lead the other to reject or abandon them altogether. For Gilligan, girls experience this relational impasse as a dilemma involving each of these concerns, which in turn provoke conflict and distress.

There is an even more pernicious outcome of the systematic suppression of one's voice for some females, according to Gilligan. In the early stages, adolescent girls may mask their true opinions but still know what they think. However, after an extended period of such suppression, eventually they come not to know their own minds, reporting that they no longer even have an opinion; that is, they *dissociate*, in Gilligan's terms, from what they know; they come to lose touch with the reality of their own experiences such that they no longer even know or recognize their true selves. Thus, there is not only dissociation from others in taking oneself out of a genuine relationship, but dissociation from one's authentic self.

Gilligan's analysis is quite provocative and represents a very plausible account of the dilemma confronting many adolescent girls at this particular developmental juncture. Her observations, including extensive interviews, dialogues, sentence-completion data, and intense focus group interactions, reveal that for many female adolescents, suppression of voice becomes the only path through which they can preserve relationships. She and her colleagues have also identified a subgroup of "resisters," girls who attempt to reject the stereotype of the good woman and hold on to their voices. Her observations suggest, however, that for resisters, such a stance represents a double-edged sword; that is, although they continue to express their opinions forthrightly, they do so at the risk of being neglected or actively rejected by peers. Such resisters typically experience acute conflicts between their efforts to maintain their authenticity and the social repercussions of adopting such a stance.

Despite this intriguing analysis, Gilligan's efforts have not, to date, resulted in any systematic empirical demonstration of the *prevalence* of loss of voice among adolescent females. Undoubtedly, there are female adolescents who fit these patterns; however, of critical interest is how extensive the patterns identified by Gilligan actually are. Moreover, Gilligan has not yet addressed these issues in adolescent males. Rather, she and her colleagues have committed themselves to understanding female development, particularly the transition from childhood through adolescence to adulthood. In our own work, we have felt it essential to address the question of whether the processes that characterize female development in our culture are relevant to the development of males. I return to this issue in a subsequent section, presenting data revealing that individual differences in level of voice within each gender are very powerful, and that many of the processes that predict lack of voice in females operate similarly among adolescent males.

LACK OF VOICE WITHIN THE SCHOOL SETTING

The school setting would appear to be a particularly interesting context within which to examine levels of adolescent voice among both males and females given that it represents a microcosm of the larger society. Moreover, schools have come under increasing scrutiny and criticism for "shortchanging" girls in ways that may well undermine their desire or ability to voice their opinions. Recent claims of gender bias by the Sadkers (Sadker & Sadker, 1994), as well as a provocative report from the American Association of University Women (1992), point to classroom practices that are especially detrimental to girls (see also Hansen, Walker, & Flom, 1995). Many of these differential practices begin long before adolescence, however, suggesting that processes potentially affecting levels of voice need to be addressed across the entire spectrum of childhood and adolescence, and beyond.

The Sadkers interpret the evidence as indicating that there are gender differences in both the quantity and quality of the attention that boys and girls receive. They indicate that boys receive more positive attention as well as negative attention. With regard to positive attention, boys are reported to receive more praise and reinforcement for their efforts (see also the American Association of University Women, 1992; Baker, 1986; Brophy, 1981; Hansen et al., 1995). However, in more carefully conducted studies, researchers have *not* found that teachers provide more positive attention for boys (Eccles & Blumenfeld, 1985). The classroom observations of these latter investigators reveal that boys are more likely to receive teacher communications concerning what are the proper procedures and behaviors, directives that are often negative. Brophy (1985) concurs, reporting that boys are more likely to be the object of discipline and behavioral monitoring.

The Sadkers and other investigators also report that boys are more likely to be called upon and listened to (see Meece, 1987; Orenstein, 1994; Sadker & Sadker, 1994). The Sadkers further contend that boys receive more individualized attention, more encouragement to develop or embellish ideas expressed in class, and more constructive feedback if they are incorrect (see also Monaco & Gaier, 1992). Others (Barbar & Cardinale, 1991; Brophy, 1985; Jones & Wheatley, 1990; Meece, 1987) have observed that such treatment is particularly likely in math and science classes, leading girls to question their ability at these subjects. In contrast to boys, the Sadkers report that girls receive more reinforcement for being compliant and quiet, for their physical appearance (hairstyles, clothing), and for the neatness of their written work, rather than for the ideas or opinions they may express.

It should be noted, however, that the Sadkers do not present systematic evidence for their claims, nor does their work directly document how school practices impact such outcomes. The American Association of University Women's (1992) report also suggests that the lowered self-esteem and confidence among girls in their own study may be due to just such differential treatment, a cornerstone of their claim that schools are shortchanging girls. However, their report also acknowledges that "there is no social science research to document cause and effect in this matter" (p. 67).

Others (see Delpit, 1993; Maher & Tetreault, 1994; Orenstein, 1994; Sadker & Sadker, 1994) have observed that historically, our educational model has been based upon features more favorable to male stereotypes and socialization. For example, academic *competition,* particularly in large classrooms, favors those males who have been socialized to value and display competitive behaviors (see Eccles & Blumenfeld, 1985; Lockheed, 1986; Wilkinson, Lindow, & Chiang, 1985). The fact that the physical configuration of many classrooms involves rows of desks facing the teacher fosters male stereotypes of autonomy, independence, and individual effort. However, it should be noted that not all males are socialized to display such stereotypical behavior. Moreover, there have been relevant cultural changes in recent years such that many parents and teachers actively foster these characteristics in their daughters and their female students.

Educators have also turned their attention to factors that have been found to be more conducive to learning for females. For example, the newer "cooperative learning" models, which emphasize smaller classroom configurations, in which students can make eye contact, exchange opinions comfortably, and work together toward an educational goal, have been found to produce more favorable outcomes for female students (see review by Kahle & Meece, 1994), although outcomes are partially determined by the specific gender composition of the group (see Webb & Palincsar, 1996; Wilkinson et al., 1995). Moreover, girls are more active and report more positive perceptions of their academic abilities in classrooms that provide them with individualized attention (see American Association of University Women, 1992; Eccles & Blumenfeld, 1985; Eccles, Wigfield, & Schiefele, 1998; Hansen et al., 1995; Meece, 1987; Pintrich & Blumenfeld, 1982). Thus, the newer educational trends would appear to be more conducive to females' expression of opinions.

Stereotypical patterns of dominance and submission can also contribute to level of voice. As Maher and Tetreault (1994) observe, the construction of voice is a function of position in that students fashion themselves in terms of their relationship to the prevailing classroom culture. Thus, those girls who adopt the stereotype that includes subordination to male standards will be most likely to stifle their level of voice. Delpit (1993) concurs, observing that there are codes of power within the school setting, namely, rules that specify how males and females should participate and play out their roles. These rules dictate gender-appropriate linguistic and communicative strategies, as well as forms of self-presentation, including whether and how one expresses oneself verbally. For example, if boys are expected and are allowed to dominate, and if girls are encouraged to be silent, such a pattern will favor males' expression of voice. However, to the extent that many girls no longer buy into these stereotypes, and given that many teachers, sensitized by the gender bias issue, engage in practices to encourage female students to express their opinions, previous codes of power relationships are undoubtedly undergoing change that favors female expression of voice.

However, there will be individual differences in the extent to which teachers reinforce old patterns and gender stereotypes. As Meece (1987) observes, teachers are often characterized as "hidden carriers" of society's gender-role stereotyping; thus, some may encourage traditional roles in the classroom (see also Eccles & Blumenfeld, 1985). Maher and Tetreault (1994), as well as Gilligan (1993), concur, noting that certain women teachers may embody the very attributes that define the good woman stereotype. Some women teachers, they argue, attempt to be the perfect role models for girls, which in part involves teaching them the structure and traditions of the worlds they are entering. Such teachers, according to Gilligan, instruct girls about the necessity of renouncing the self and, in the name of being good women, take themselves out of genuine relationship with their female students. Fine's (1991) observations support these claims in that she finds that many girls learn to shut down what teachers consider to be "dangerous conversation," namely, girls learn to mute their own voices. However, many teachers do not conform to these stereotypes, and there are also assertive girls who fail to adhere to such stereotypical expectations.

Although there are those who would argue that teachers are negatively impacting the voice of girls within the classroom, there are several caveats to be underscored. Many of the claims in the educational literature appear in books (e.g., Sadker & Sadker, 1994) in which compelling empirical research findings and statistical documentation are not provided. While the Sadkers do cite some studies conducted by other researchers, most of the conclusions, including their observations, involve more informal interviews, observations, and anecdotal reports that, while compelling, need to be more systematically demonstrated. (The numerical data from their own investigations have not, to date, appeared in peer-reviewed research journals.) Furthermore, as the carefully conducted classroom observational studies of Eccles and Blumenfeld (1985) have revealed, differences in the educational experiences of males and females are surprisingly small. Based on his own research in the classroom, Brophy (1985) comes to a similar conclusion, observing that teachers react more to students' *behavior* than to their gender. Despite these latter findings, most of this literature focuses on claims about overall gender differences, ignoring the vast individual differences within both males and females.

Moreover, lacking in this literature is evidence on how proposed classroom interactions between teachers and students actually *impact* the outcomes of interest; that is, there are no findings directly *linking* potential practices to consequences such as lack of confidence, voice, or low self-esteem in students. The emphasis has primarily been on how teachers' treatment of male students (as a group), may differ from treatment of female students (as a group) without thoughtful attention to individual differences within each gender; that is, particular female and male adolescents may be treated differentially by teachers, in part because of characteristics that individual students bring to the classroom (see Eccles & Blumenfeld, 1985). For example, teachers respond more negatively to those boys whose classroom behavior is disruptive (Brophy, 1985). Thus, we need to guard against generalizations about how the genders are differentially treated in the classroom. Furthermore, as Eccles and Blumenfeld (1985) cogently observe, there may be arenas in which teachers treat boys and girls quite similarly; however, such common treatment of the genders may affect boys and girls differently. For example, teachers may encourage classroom competition in both genders; however, the effects may be less favorable for some girls, namely, those who buy into traditional female stereotypes.

In addition, we need to attend to student interactions themselves, examining how the genders treat each other. To what extent might voice be undermined if it is not supported by one's classmates? For example, will girls' voices be undermined to the extent that they do not receive support from male classmates? Interestingly, findings reveal that boys either ignore girls or are not responsive to girls' feedback or bids for interaction, a pattern that begins in preschool (Maccoby, 1990, 1994) and continues into elementary school years and beyond (Lockheed, 1986; Webb & Kenderski, 1985;

Wilkinson et al., 1985). These findings also reveal that if boys do attend to girls' behavior, it is often in the form of taunting or teasing. Moreover, many girls experience sexual harassment at the hands of boys, which is often viewed by school officials as harmless instances of "boys will be boys" (see American Association of University Women, 1992; Sadker & Sadker, 1994; Strauss, 1988). Thus, to the extent that some girls' voices are ignored or devalued by boys, girls' expression of their opinions may be stifled. As our own research documents, however, there are individual differences in that certain adolescent males who adhere to masculine stereotypes provide less support for the opinions of those girls who endorse the feminine stereotype.

Finally, in the educational literature, the primary focus has been on causal factors that involve teaching practices in the classroom. There is too little emphasis on the fact that children and adolescents bring very powerful socialization histories from *outside* the classroom to their own school experience (see also Eccles & Blumenfeld, 1985). Family influences, peer interactions, and exposure to the media all impact the attitudes that children display in the school setting. Thus, it behooves us to examine these factors as well, since they undoubtedly color, and interact with, the dynamics within the school context; that is, the student's individual socialization history will influence voice-related behaviors in the classroom, such that gender differences may or may not be observed. As has been argued, gender differences are more likely to be documented in domains where there are stereotypes about each gender that are actively endorsed by girls and boys (see Eccles et al., 1998). For example, Eccles and colleagues find that those girls whose parents endorse the stereotype that boys are more competent at particular school subjects, for example, math, and who come to believe it, will be more likely to lack confidence and to avoid challenge in that domain. Spencer and Steele (1995) have recently documented such vulnerability to stereotypes in their demonstration that females who were told that males do better on a challenging math test did worse than those who were told that males and females perform comparably. Eccles et al. (1998) provide additional evidence that social scripts regarding what is proper behavior for each gender in particular situations, combined with ideal images about what one should be like, represent powerful influences governing the behavior of both genders if these stereotypical scripts are endorsed (see also Archer, 1989).

For girls who buy into such stereotypes, conflict between the scripts defining gender roles and incompatible achievement goals may be created. For example, Orenstein (1994) observes that some girls may fear looking too intelligent, since smart girls are often stigmatized. They fear that to display their intelligence will lead to their social rejection by those boys who either do not value intellectual ability as a female attribute, or may feel threatened lest they feel less competent by comparison. Smart girls may fear alienation from their girlfriends as well, who may view them as showoffs or too academically competitive. Rather than risk social censure, such girls may choose not to express their knowledge or opinions, particularly within the public classroom domain. Bell (1989) has documented these conflicts among one subset of girls who were identified as gifted. These females expressed concern over appearing to be braggarts if they expressed pride in their accomplishments. Even more specific to the issue of voice were these girls' concerns over seeming too aggressive if they attempted to attract the teacher's attention. Moreover, they worried about hurting others' feelings if they were too competitive in achievement situations.

Other girls, for example, those who buy into certain cultural stereotypes about desirable attributes that women should possess, may also stifle their opinions. Certain girls will be at risk for loss of voice if they internalize the message of the larger culture, namely, that women's voices are not valued as much as men's and that a woman's *looks* are potentially her greatest commodity. Much of popular culture and the media perpetuate the stereotype of the desirable woman who should be seen and not heard. Many movies, television programs, magazines, rock videos, and advertisement tout the importance of physical attractiveness, glamorizing the popular role models to be emulated. These media messages assault adolescent and adult females with exhortations that they become thinner and more attractive; in such advertising, there is the implicit assumption that looks are more critical than intelligence and the expression of one's opinion. For example, observe in ads for clothing, perfume, and other women's products the number of *headless* women. If women are depicted with heads, they are often deprived of a cortex. Images of these headless and decorticate females unconsciously communicate the message that women are mindless, brainless, and therefore perhaps should be voiceless. A recent ad depicting a woman applying perfume put it quite explicitly. The caption read: "Make a statement without saying a word." To the extent that females buy into these images and fashion their behaviors accordingly, their voices will necessarily go underground. Males, on the other hand, are typically portrayed as cerebral and forceful, providing role models for the expression of opinions.

By way of summary, in addition to their school experiences, both boys and girls already come to the classroom with individual socialization histories. These backgrounds could potentially lead to a pattern in which girls are more reluctant, and boys more likely, to express their voice *if* they have been socialized to accept and adopt the societal stereotypes for their gender (Eccles & Blumenfeld, 1985; Huston, 1983). However, generalizations based on these assumptions, namely, that the vast majority of girls and boys have been differentially treated by socializing agents, may not be warranted. For example, Brophy (1985) reviews literature demonstrating that individuals of both genders vary considerably in their adoption of the attitudes and behaviors associated with societal gender stereotypes. Moreover, it is often assumed or inferred that the effects of differential treatment, the potential differences between the genders, are not only significant but also large. However, as scholars have noted (see Crawford, 1989; Eagly, 1987, 1995; Eccles & Blumenfeld, 1985; Eisenberg et al., 1996; Ruble, 1988), most gender differences documented in the literature are not large, and for those that may be statistically significant, effect sizes may be relatively small given the tremendous overlap in the distributions for males and females. Furthermore, as Eagly (1995) points out, even when effect sizes are relatively large, the overlap is still considerable, suggesting that the majority of males and females are more similar than different. Thus, what is most striking about a careful analysis of such distributions is the tremendous range of scores within each gender, namely, the *individual differences* among both males and females that should command our attention. In the next section, I review findings from our own laboratory, where we have adopted just such an individual difference perspective with regard to level of voice both inside and outside of the classroom.

OUR STUDIES OF LEVEL OF VOICE: PREDICTORS OF INDIVIDUAL DIFFERENCES WITHIN EACH GENDER

Although it has been claimed by Gilligan and others that many adolescent girls lose their voices, there has been little systematic empirical evidence on whether voice declines developmentally for adolescent females or whether there are gender differences in level of voice. Thus, we embarked upon a program of research to examine predictors and correlates of level of voice among adolescent males and females. Between the ages of 12 and 18, what is the developmental trajectory of voice for girls as well as boys? As an initial framework, we felt it important not to assume that voice was a general construct that transcended particular relational contexts. Rather, we anticipated that one's level of voice may well differ as a function of relational context. Three contexts were school related, namely, voice with male classmates, female classmates, and teachers. Two contexts outside of school were included for purposes of comparison, where we examined level of voice with parents and with close friends. We were also interested in certain variables that might predict *individual differences* in voice. In addition, we addressed the issue of whether lack of voice was considered by teenagers to reflect false-self behavior. Finally, we were interested in whether there were liabilities associated with lack of voice.

As an initial measurement strategy, we were interested in assessing level of voice through self-report procedures. In previous work (Harter, Marold, et al., 1996) we determined that questionnaire methods were quite effective in documenting individual differences in perceived level of true- versus false-self behavior among adolescents. Thus, we built upon this methodology. We first developed questionnaire items that tapped adolescents' ability to "share what they are thinking," "say what's on their mind," and "express their opinions" in different relationships. A sample item is: "Some teenagers usually don't say what's on their mind to (particular persons) BUT Other teenagers do say what's on their mind to (particular persons)." Subjects first select the kind of teenagers they are most like and then indicate whether that choice is *Really true for me* or *Sort of true for me*. Items are scored on a 4-point scale, where 1 equals the lowest level of voice and 4 the highest. The particular *persons* have varied across studies and have included parents, teachers, classmates (male and female classmates separately in one study), close friends, and boys in social situations. Subscales, defined by relationship, have included either four or five items, where we have found internal consistency reliabilities to be consistently high, ranging from .82 to .91 across subscales in three studies (Harter, Waters, Whitesell, & Kastelic, 1998; Johnson, 1995; Waters & Gonzales, 1995).

Before examining the potential predictors of voice, it was important to determine whether lack of voice is actually perceived by adolescents to be false-self behavior (Harter, Waters, & Whitesell, 1997). In our initial studies of voice, we simply *assumed* that lack of voice represents false-self behavior, in large part since adolescents cite the inability to express their opinions as one manifestation of the false self. However, one can imagine other motives for lack of voice that do not imply lack of authenticity. For example, (1) one may be shy temperamentally; (2) one may feel that it is not socially appropriate to express one's opinions in certain contexts; or (3) one may choose not to share certain opinions that are considered private. In our coed sample, therefore, we created items to determine whether adolescents perceive lack of voice as false- or true-self behavior (e.g., "When I don't say what I am thinking around [particular persons] I feel like I am *not* being the 'real me' " vs. "When I don't say what I am thinking around [particular persons], it feels like I *am* being the 'real me' "). A second set of items addressed the extent to which adolescents were bothered or upset by not expressing their opinions in each relationship. Approximately 75% of adolescents of both genders indicated that failure to express their opinions did constitute false-self behavior. By way of converging evidence, 75% also reported that they were bothered by not saying what they really think. The percentages were quite similar across the different relational contexts, bolstering our assumption that, for the large majority of adolescents, lack of voice is perceived as suppression of the true self.

Relational Context

Initially, we were interested in whether there were meaningful differences across five relational contexts—with parents, teachers, male classmates, female classmates, and close friends. We anticipated that an adolescent might be more comfortable sharing his/her thoughts in some interpersonal arenas than in others. For adolescents as a group, we predicted that level of voice would be highest with close friends given that an important function of close friendships is the sharing of intimate thoughts and feelings, particularly during adolescence (see Brown, 1990; Gilligan et al., 1989; Savin-Williams & Berndt, 1990). Level of voice should be somewhat lower with peers in the classroom given concerns such as appearing stupid or alienating others, and with teachers and parents, to the extent that adolescents often feel that adults do not understand or validate their opinions, thoughts, and feelings (see Elkind, 1967, 1984). Our findings (Harter, Waters, & Whitesell, 1997; Johnson, 1995) supported these predictions. For both genders, voice is highest with close friends, followed by classmates of the same gender. However, voice is consistently lower with classmates of the opposite gender, as well as with parents and teachers. For those in the all-girls' high school, voice was lowest with males in social situations (Johnson, 1995). Further evidence (Harter, Waters, & Whitesell, 1997) comes from our factor analysis of voice scores across relationships where we obtain a clear 5-factor solution (voice with close friends, female classmates, male classmates, parents, and teachers) with extremely high loadings (range = .62 to .90, average = .80) and negligible cross-loadings (all 0 to .20). Thus, clearly the nature of the relationship is important in that adolescents are more comfortable expressing their opinions in some relational contexts than in others. Of particular relevance to the school context is the finding that voice is lower with classmates of the opposite gender, as well as with teachers, compared to classmates of the same gender and close friends (who are also predominantly of the same gender).

Thus, the overall pattern reveals that voice is considerably higher among peers of the same gender than among adults (teachers and parents), as well as peers of the opposite gender. These findings are consistent with the peer literature (see reviews by Brown, 1990; Savin-Williams & Berndt, 1990), which reveals that same-gender peers serve critical functions, allowing adolescents to express, as well as clarify, their thoughts and feelings within an atmosphere of support and trust. This pattern also cautions against making generalizations about level of voice given that the degree to which one ex-presses what one thinks is highly dependent upon the relational context.

Does Voice Differ by Grade Level or Gender?

Of particular relevance to Gilligan's thesis is whether voice declines for females across sixth through 12th grades. Gilligan's argument is that girls in our society are particularly vulnerable to loss of voice for the reasons dis-cussed earlier. Our cross-sectional data reveal no significant mean differences associated with grade level for either gender, nor are there even any trends in either the coeducational or all-girls' schools (Harter, Waters, & Whitesell, 1997; Johnson, 1995; Waters & Gonzales, 1995). Voice does not decline within the school contexts (with classmates and teachers), nor does it decline in those relationships outside the school setting (with parents or close friends). Thus, there is no evidence in our data for loss of voice among adolescent females as a group given how we have assessed it. One possibility is that by sixth grade (ages 12–13), the processes cited by Gilligan may already have taken place. However, the mean levels we obtain (average scores of around 3.0 on a 4-point scale) reveal that levels of voice are relatively high among young female adolescents (Waters & Gonzales, 1995), arguing against such an interpretation.

We have also found no evidence for gender differences favoring males. In the middle school, scores were quite comparable for males and females (Waters & Gonzales, 1995). In a second study at the middle school level (sixth, seventh, eighth grades), the findings reveal no gender differences. At the high school level, girls actually reported somewhat higher levels of voice with close friends, females classmates, parents, and teachers than did boys (and comparable scores in the context of male classmates). Thus, the age and gender findings caution against making generalizations about the devel-opmental trajectory of voice for most or all adolescent females, particularly where comparisons with males are implicit. Rather, the most impressive discoveries in our data have been the marked individual differences in level of voice among both male and female adolescents, differences that became the focus of our inquiry as we sought to examine what factors might be responsible. Two such factors seemed to be plausible starting points, namely, gender *orientation* and the level of *support* for voice.

Gender Orientation

One of Gilligan's arguments is that adolescent girls observe and then attempt to adopt the "good woman stereotype" in the culture, part of which encourages an ethic of caring in which females are encouraged to be more sensitive to others' needs and desires than to their own. Moreover, the "good woman" listens empathically to others, often at the expense of speaking her own mind. Yet what percentage of adolescent girls in the 1990s are buying into that stereotype, accepting it as their ideal? To address this issue, we have included a measure of gender *orientation* in which many of the feminine items reflected features of the "good woman" stereotype. We drew items from several instruments in the literature including the Personality Attributes Questionnaire (Spence, Helmreich, & Stapp, 1975), the Sex Role Inventory, developed by Bem (1985), and Boldizar's (1991) adaptation for children and adolescents. Feminine items tap themes that include sensitivity, warmth, empathy, expressions of affection, enjoyment of babies and children, gentleness, and concern for others who are in distress. Masculine items tap dimensions such as competitiveness, ability to make decisions, independence, risk taking, confidence, athleticism, mechanical aptitude, individualism, leadership, and enjoyment of math and science. (Across these instruments, there are a few items that tap voice-like constructs; e.g., assertive vs. shy). However, we did not include these items in our analyses, since they represent potential confounds between the independent variable, gender orientation, and the dependent variable, level of voice.)

We were particularly interested in the hypothesis that among adolescent girls, those displaying a predominantly feminine orientation, endorsing feminine but not masculine items, would report lower levels of voice compared to those displaying an androgynous orientation, endorsing both feminine and masculine items (Waters & Gonzales, 1995). Within our samples, there is clearly a subsample of females who do appear to identify with the good woman stereotype, endorsing only the feminine items, eschewing masculine characteristics (approximately 25% to 35% of our samples of female adolescents). Androgynous females typically represent approximately 60% to 70% of these samples. (There has been an insufficient number of masculine girls, approximately 5%, to make meaningful statistical comparisons.) Hill and Lynch (1983) have argued that at adolescence, there is increased pressure to conform to the prevailing societal gender stereotypes, what they refer to as "gender intensification." Although we do not know at what point in development our participants may have adopted their particular gender orientation, our data suggest that those who endorse feminine but not masculine attributes represent only a *subgroup* of female adolescents; this pattern does *not* characterize the gender orientations of adolescent girls as a group. As others have also observed (e.g., Brophy, 1985), individuals differ considerably in their adoption of societal gender stereotypes.

With regard to level of voice, the findings revealed that femininity does represent a liability for girls in *certain*, but not all, relational contexts (Harter,

Waters, & Whitesell, 1997). Interestingly, feminine girls report significantly lower levels of voice than do androgynous girls in the more *public* context of *school,* namely, with teachers and classmates. Further examination of the data reveals that feminine girls report particularly low levels of voice with *male* classmates compared to female classmates. Among girls in the all-girls' school, the voice of the feminine girls is lowest with boys in social situations (Johnson, 1995). However, in more *private* interpersonal relationships, namely, with close friends and parents, these differences were not obtained, suggesting that femininity is not a liability in these contexts. Dimensions of femininity such as empathy and concern for others may well facilitate expression of voice in such close relationships.

In Figure 9.1, prototypical scores of two individual girls, one feminine and one androgynous, provide examples of how level of voice may vary across each of the five relational contexts. Scores were the same for level of voice with parents and close friends. However, among those in the more public domain of school, namely, with teachers, male classmates, and female class-

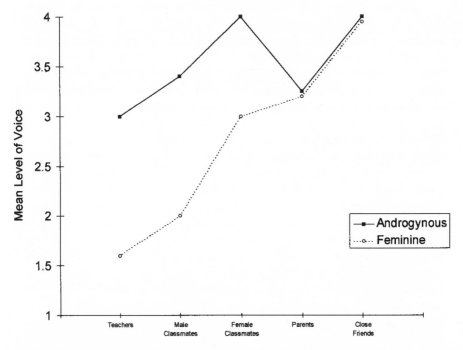

FIGURE 9.1. Voice scores for two prototypical female adolescents, one feminine, one androgynous, across each of the five relational contexts.

mates, voice *levels* are considerably lower for the feminine, compared to the androgynous, subject, although the relative pattern is similar. These findings are consistent with other literature in which there is a distinction between public and private selves. For example, Buss (1980) reports that factors such as social expectations, self-consciousness, and/or anxiety in social situations may cause certain individuals to display public selves that are quite different from the private selves that they reveal to close friends and family. These differences may be very pronounced in certain Asian cultures that prescribe very different displays of self in public and private contexts (Kennedy, 1994).

Our pattern of findings suggests a refinement of Gilligan's position. First, it cautions against making generalizations based on gender alone, since our evidence reveals that it is not gender per se, but *gender orientation* that best predicts level of voice among females. Second, our evidence suggests that a feminine orientation primarily represents a liability for the expression of voice in *public* contexts, namely, in the school setting with teachers and classmates, as well as in social situations with boys. As Meece (1987) observes, public situations in which others can observe and evaluate one's attributes provoke concerns about self-presentation and the appropriateness of one's behaviors and attributes. It is in these more public social contexts that one might expect those highly feminine adolescent females to display behaviors consistent with the "good woman" societal stereotype (Gilligan et al., 1989), leading to their suppression of voice. Thus, the arguments put forth by Gilligan and colleagues, as well as by Pipher (1994) and Orenstein (1994), would appear to be restricted to a particular *subset* of girls, those endorsing a feminine gender orientation, who primarily suppress their voices in those more public arenas where they feel that certain stereotypical feminine behaviors (e.g., being nice and unassertive) are appropriate or demanded.

Pipher observes that "most girls choose to be socially accepted and split into two selves, one that is authentic and one that is culturally scripted. In public they become who they are supposed to be" (p. 38). However, our own findings reveal that such statements need to be qualified, since they do not necessarily represent the reality of "most" girls. Rather, they apply to a subsample of girls who have publicly embraced the good woman stereotype. Whether these girls experience the conflict that Gilligan and others describe is an interesting question for further study, as is the related issue of whether members of this group consider their feminine attitudes to be true- or false-self characteristics. On balance, while the school setting may represent a microcosm of the larger society, females bring different socialization histories to this context, including individual differences in gender orientation which, in turn, impact their level of voice.

As Eccles et al. (1998) observe in their review of achievement motivation in children, it is those girls who buy into gender stereotypes about what is desirable behavior for females, for example, the script that females are less academically competent, who are likely to suffer. Girls who have less stereotypical role models in their own mothers will be more likely to resist these scripts and to demonstrate more confidence in achievement situations. Moreover, they report other studies revealing that parents who endorse such gender-role stereotypes distort their evaluations of their children's abilities in the gender-stereotypical direction (see also Jacobs, 1992; Jacobs & Eccles, 1992).

In our own data, gender orientation functioned somewhat differently for males, among whom we were able to identify both masculine (50%) and androgynous (49%) subgroups. No differences in level of voice were observed with teachers, parents, and female classmates. However, masculine boys reported higher levels of voice with male classmates than did their androgynous counterparts, suggesting that androgyny is a liability for males in this context. In contrast, with close friends, androgynous boys reported higher levels of voice than did masculine boys, suggesting that the possession of certain feminine characteristics allows one to express oneself more comfortably within a more intimate relationship. In our current research, we are examining the hypothesis that voice levels in males will not only be related to gender orientation but also to the particular content of one's thoughts and feelings. For example, masculine males may be better able to voice their opinions about current events, school policies, and emotions such as anger, whereas they may have difficulty expressing fear or sadness ("Big boys don't cry") as well as tender feelings such as love and affection. Gilligan (personal communication, November, 21, 1996) feels that the socialization of males in this cultures causes them to shut down their voices about such affects at a relatively early age. Thus, in these areas we are predicting that girls will actually display higher levels of voice.

The Impact of Support for Voice on the Expression of Opinions

In examining the role of the socializing environment on the self-system, we have adopted a symbolic interactionist perspective, emphasizing the role of the opinions of significant others toward the self. These processes are very salient during adolescence given that it is a period of heightened self-consciousness for both genders (see Harter, 1990a), particularly since it becomes increasingly apparent that one is the object of others' evaluations. Thus, as Elkind (1967, 1984) has observed, adolescents may attempt to obscure their true selves if they feel that their behavior does not measure up to the standards set by others whose opinions are critical and therefore may not meet with others's approval (see also Broughton, 1981; Selman, 1980). Since the level of such support may well vary across relational contexts, we predicted corresponding within-gender individual differences in the level of voice displayed within each context.

The literature reviewed earlier in this chapter, including our own efforts, reveals that lack of parental and peer support in the form of approval serves as a major factor leading adolescents of both genders to suppress their true thoughts and feelings. Thus, if significant others do not validate the child's authentic experiences, the true self goes into hiding as the child increasingly feels compelled to suppress its expression (see Bleiberg, 1984; Deci & Ryan, 1995; Harter, Marold, et al., 1996; Horney, 1945, 1950; Sullivan, 1953; Winnicott, 1965). In our own study, we did not find gender differences in these effects. Building upon that body of work, we reasoned that level of support for *voice*, specifically, should be associated with the level of voice expressed. We created support for voice items that tapped the adolescent's perceptions of others' interest in what one had to say, respect for one's ideas even if there is disagreement, ability to listen to one's opinions and take them seriously, and attempts to understand one's point of view.

We have obtained marked effects that are highly comparable for both genders and can be demonstrated across all relationships. Figure 9.2 presents these effects for our coeducational high school sample, where the scores of females and males have been combined, since there were no gender differences (Harter, Waters, & Whitesell, 1997). As this figure clearly reveals, within every relationship, adolescents reporting low support also reported the lowest levels of voice, and those reporting high support reported high levels of voice, with those reporting moderate support falling in between. As Figure 9.2 reveals, the individual differences in level of voice that are directly related to the amount of support one receives for voice are quite dramatic. Those reporting that others do not encourage or listen to their views have scores around the midpoint of the scale, whereas those reporting high levels of support for verbalizing their opinions have scores near the top of the 4-point scale. Thus, both males *and* females who receive encouragement and support for expressing their views are the adolescents who acknowledge the highest levels of voice; that is, the process is the same for both genders.

There are two possible interpretations of these findings relating support for voice to self-reported level of voice, conclusions about the directionality of effects that are not mutually exclusive. From a symbolic interactionist perspective, support, in the form of encouragement and validation, may promote high levels of voice in adolescents. Thus, such support enhances the adolescent's ability to express his/her opinions. It is also plausible that those adolescents who have relatively high levels of voice are more likely to

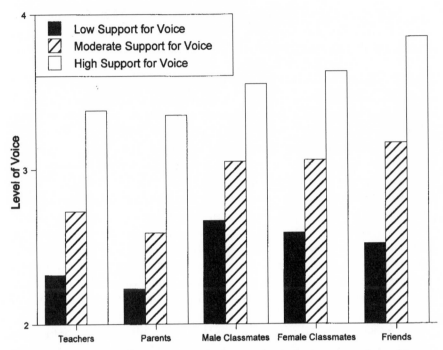

FIGURE 9.2. The effects of support for voice on level of voice across relationships.

be heard and supported. Those remaining more muted create far fewer opportunities to garner support for their opinions, since they are less likely to express them in the first place. It is likely that both of these processes are operative given that they are bidirectional.

Support and Gender Orientation

The pattern of findings also reveals the *additive* effects of support and gender orientation, particularly in more public relational contexts. In the all-girls' high school, we had enough subjects to cross support with gender orientation (Johnson, 1995). Figure 9.3 presents the findings for one such context, namely, voice with teachers. The same pattern was observed for voice with parents, with female classmates, and with males in social situations. The differences associated with the combination of support for voice and gender orientation are dramatic. Those most at risk for lack of voice are feminine girls who also report low levels of support. Those most able to express their voices are the androgynous girls who also report high levels of support.

Although we have crossed gender orientation with support for the purposes of these analyses, forcing them to be orthogonal, one can ask whether certain gender orientations among both females and males are more likely to be supported by teachers and classmates within the school context; that is, whose voices are more likely to be validated? Wigfield, Eccles, and Pintrich (1996) make the general observation that teachers respond differently to students in the same classroom, based upon characteristics that they bring to the educational setting. This issue is particularly germane given claims in the American Association of University Women's report and by the Sadkers (1994) that girls are being shortchanged in our school system. Thus, might some girls as well as boys be shortchanged with regard to support for voice because of their gender orientation?

Our findings (Harter, Waters, & Whitesell, 1997) have revealed that in both coeducational and all-girls' high school settings, the androgynous girls perceived greater teacher support (M = 3.2) than did the feminine girls (M = 2.9). Thus, it is the subset of those endorsing the feminine stereotypes that may be shortchanged with regard to support for voice. In the coeducational setting, androgynous boys reported more teacher support (M = 3.1) than did the masculine boys (M = 2.6). Among the latter group may be those boys who are more likely to be disruptive. Thus, from the perspective of adolescents, teachers provide more approval for androgynous students of both genders relative to those displaying the feminine and masculine stereotypes.

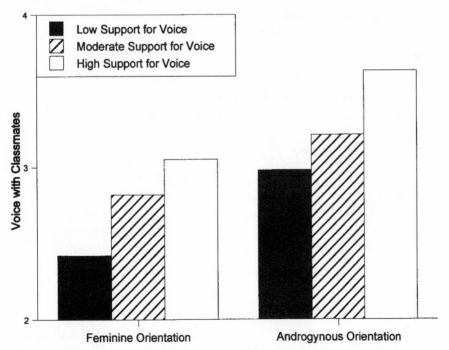

FIGURE 9.3. Level of voice with classmates as a function of gender orientation and support for voice.

However, as Wigfield et al. (1996) urge, we need more detailed classroom observational evidence to determine the precise nature of the link between teachers' behaviors and students' perceptions.

Although teachers have borne the brunt of criticism with regard to differential treatment of the genders, it is also instructive to examine the support provided by *classmates* within the school setting. In the coed setting, feminine girls not only reported less support for voice from teachers but also from both male (M = 2.5) and female (M = 2.9) classmates compared to androgynous girls, who reported more support from both males (M = 3.2) and females (M = 3.3). Among the boys, masculine and androgynous subgroups reported equal levels of support from both male and female classmates. Thus, for female students, it would appear that it is primarily the feminine girls who may be getting shortchanged and who are more likely to be populating the "silent ghetto" in the classroom. While feminine girls may receive support for other attributes, for example, their physical appearance, it is noteworthy that they are receiving less support from males than do androgynous girls for the expression of their opinions in particular. Findings reviewed in an earlier section revealed that boys typically ignore the comments of female students. Our results suggest that the feminine girls are the particular targets of such treatment. From the standpoint of improving the classroom environment for such females, it would be important to consider teacher interventions or educational practices that allow voiceless female students to express their opinions and encourage male students to develop a greater appreciation for what female students have to contribute.

THE LIABILITIES OF LACK OF VOICE AS A FORM OF FALSE-SELF BEHAVIOR

A basic claim of theorists concerned with lack of voice and with false-self behavior is that lack of authenticity has negative outcomes or correlates. Gilligan and colleagues (Gilligan, 1993; Gilligan et al., 1989), as well as others (see Jordan, 1991; Jordan et al., 1991; Lerner, 1993; Miller, 1986; Stiver & Miller, 1988), observe that suppression of the self leads to lack of zest, which, in the extreme form, will be manifest as depressive symptoms and associated liabilities such as low self-worth. In our earlier work with adolescents (Harter, Marold, et al., 1996) we found that those highest in false-self behavior reported the lowest level of global self-worth and the most depressed affect. In a recent study of adult relationship styles (Harter, Waters, Pettitt, et al., 1997), we found evidence for a process model in which lack of validation by one's partner predicted a low level of authenticity within the relationship, which in turn predicted both depressed affect and self-worth. Those who felt lack of validation were considerably more likely to report false-self behavior in the relationship, which in turn was associated with depressed affect and low global self-worth.

In our voice studies, therefore, we anticipated that those low in voice within a given relationship would also report relationship-specific low self-worth within that same interpersonal context (see Chapter 7 for a discussion of the concept of relational self-worth). We examined the relational self-worth scores for those with low and with high levels of voice for each relationship separately. The findings were strikingly comparable for males and females (and are therefore combined) across each context. In relationships with parents, low-voice adolescents had significantly lower self-worth than did high-voice adolescents (M = 2.5 vs. M = 3.4); we found the same pattern in relationships with teachers (M = 2.8 vs. M = 3.3), male classmates (M = 2.6 vs. M = 3.2), and female classmates (M = 2.7 vs. M = 3.2). The link between voice and relational self-worth may well be bidirectional; that is, failure to express one's opinions, one's true self, may erode one's overall sense of worth as a person. Alternatively, if one's self-worth is low, one may feel that one has nothing to say.

In addition to the findings for relational self-worth, similar patterns were obtained for global self-worth as well as affect (cheerful to depressed). Thus, lack of voice, as a form of false-self behavior, is clearly associated with liabilities that in turn may well interfere with adaptive functioning among adolescents. Converging evidence comes from Kolligian (1990), who reports that perceived fraudulence in adults is accompanied by self-criticism and depressive tendencies.

Double Jeopardy for Females Who Are to Be Seen and Not Heard

Feminist scholars have viewed the suppression of voice as distressing for females, particularly given societal messages to the effect that, in comparison to men, women's voices as not as valued and their opinions are not taken as seriously. However, when such messages are coupled with communications about how a woman's *looks* are potentially her greatest commodity, females who buy into these stereotypes may be doubly at risk for negative outcomes. As discussed in Chapter 5, adolescent girls and adult women are particularly vulnerable given the punishing standards of attractiveness that are put forth in the media. Standards regarding desirable bodily characteristics such as thinness have become increasingly unrealistic and demanding for women within the past two decades (see Garner et al., 1980; Heatherton & Baumeister, 1991).

The difficulty for females of meeting the cultural stereotypes for appearance appears to be brought home over the course of development the closer one comes to adopting one's role as a women in this society. Our own data (see Chapter 5) reveal that for females, perceptions of physical attractiveness systematically decline with grade level, whereas there is no such drop for males. In middle childhood, girls and boys feel equally good about their appearance; however, by the end of high school, females' scores are dramatically lower than males' scores. We find similar gender differences in perceived appearance among college populations as well as among adults in the world of work and family, particularly for women who are full-time homemakers.

It is important to realize that not all adolescent girls and women fall victim to this mentality, buying into these media messages. As Pipher (1994) observes, many parents communicate to their daughters their disdain for media values and their resistance to cultural definitions of their daughters as preoccupied with makeup, clothing, diets, and dating. Such parents do not want their daughters to compromise their authenticity in order to become popular. However, what are the consequences for those who *do* adopt the cultural expectations that females should be seen and not heard? We have addressed this issue by dividing female high school students into four groups, based on their levels of voice (high vs. low) crossed with their ratings of the importance of appearance (high vs. low). We examined four correlates, perceptions of appearance, global self-esteem, relational self-esteem, and affect (Harter, Waters, & Whitesell, 1997).

Across every relationship, those most likely to endorse the view that females should be seen and not heard, namely, those low in voice, who rated appearance as highly important, reported the worst outcomes. In contrast, those high in voice, who reported appearance as relatively unimportant, reported the best outcomes, with the other two groups falling in between (manifest in two significant main effects with no interaction). To give one example, those who reported low voice with male classmates and who also touted the importance of appearance, compared to those with high voice who viewed appearance as unimportant, reported lower scores for appearance (M = 2.3 vs. M = 2.9), global self-esteem (M = 2.9 vs. M = 3.4), relational self-esteem (M = 2.65 vs. M = 3.25), and depression (M = 2.9 vs. M = 3.45). The differences were equally dramatic and significant in other relationships (with parents, teachers, and female classmates). Thus, not only does lack of voice bring with it liabilities, but also when coupled with an emphasis on the importance of appearance, it places females in double jeopardy, leading to negative evaluations of both their outer and inner selves.

CONCLUSION

Beginning in adolescence, a concern with false-self behavior emerges. A major manifestation of false-self behavior involves the suppression of one's voice, namely, the failure to express what one really thinks or believes. I began with a summary of Gilligan's contention that females' voices are particularly likely to go underground during adolescence, since to speak one's mind violates society's "good woman" stereotype and may threaten relationships. However, recent literature within the field of education (Sadker & Sadker, 1994; Orenstein, 1994; American Association of University Women, 1992) points to factors within our educational system that occur developmentally much earlier and could potentially contribute to lack of voice among even younger females given claims that schools shortchange girls. Moreover, there are influences outside of the school system—societal expectations, socialization histories, and differential experiences—that boys and girls bring to the classroom that could also impact level of voice within the school setting. Thus, we need to approach generalizations with conceptual caution.

For example, nowhere in this literature has it been empirically documented that there are gender differences in levels of voice showing that females systematically display less voice than do males, nor has it been demonstrated that most girls *lose* their voice at adolescence. Thus, arguments that assume or imply gender differences and their developmental course require systematic empirical study. Moreover, claims suggesting that lack of voice is primarily a problem for females in our society, whether due to general cultural discrimination or potentially linked to gender bias in the classroom, need to be qualified. We can no longer be content with generalizations implying that most or all girls are at risk for lack of voice. Furthermore, we need to attend very seriously to individual differences in level of voice and to identify what causal factors account for lack of voice in *some*, but not most or all, girls. Moreover, there has been virtually no attention to individual differences among males and whether similar or different factors may account for lack of voice in some boys. For both genders, we need to address how potential causes are systematically related to outcomes such as loss of voice, confidence, or self-esteem; that is, we need to document these links directly. To date, we have no documentation of how teachers' interactive styles directly impact these potential consequences. Nor have individual differences in how teachers treat students of both genders, as well as individual students within each gender, been systematically studied.

Our own empirical work has represented an initial attempt to fill in some of these gaps. For example, our results reveal no evidence that girls, in general, lose their voices at adolescence. Rather, they suggest that Gilligan's analysis speaks primarily to a particular subset of adolescent females, namely, feminine girls who report lower levels of voice in *public* contexts (e.g., at school, with teachers and classmates) but not in more private interpersonal relationships with close friends and parents. In contrast, androgynous girls report relatively high levels of voice in all contexts. It will be of interest in future research to determine whether the distinction between femininity and androgyny predicts levels of voice in girls *prior* to adolescence; that is, do feminine girls primarily develop loss of voice at adolescence or might femininity also be a liability even before adolescence? Although, in describing the pattern of findings, we have indicted femininity as the liability, in point of fact, it is actually *femininity coupled with the absence of masculine attributes* that would appear to be detrimental. The combination of both feminine and masculine attributes is most conducive to high levels of voice and acceptance by others among girls.

Our primary focus has been the illumination of individual differences within both female and male adolescents. Support for voice among both genders was found to be a powerful predictor. Thus, consistent with our earlier studies, adolescents who feel that they are not validated, in that others show little interest in or support for what they have to say, report the lowest levels of voice. Interestingly, within the classroom context, androgynous girls and boys report more support for voice from teachers than do feminine girls and masculine boys. Feminine girls also report lower levels of support than all other groups from classmates, particularly male classmates. These findings alert us to the fact that dynamics within the classroom that involve how students treat each other may be just as potent as how teachers are treating their students. Moreover, our results reveal that teachers do not necessarily treat *all* girls, or *all* boys, similarly.

Why should we be concerned about lack of voice? For those individuals of either gender who find it necessary to stifle their opinions, theory and evidence reveals that there are clearly liabilities, particularly when lack of voice is perceived to be false-self behavior. Compromising the self in this fashion is associated with a constellation of negative outcomes, including low self-worth (both global and relational), hopelessness, and depressed affect. Findings from our studies of true- and false-elf behavior (Harter, Marold, et al., 1996) also reveal that those engaging in high levels of false-self behavior report that they no longer know who or what their true self is. Thus, as Gilligan argues, lack of voice not only involves disconnection from others but also disconnection from *oneself*. Such consequences, in turn, interfere with students' ability to attend to the academic tasks at hand, to navigate the challenging journey toward the development of mutually satisfying peer relationships, and to develop an identity that will provide a firm psychological foundation for their transition to adulthood.

Moreover, the negative depressive consequences of lack of voice put the adolescent at risk for self-destructive behaviors, including suicide (see review by Nolen-Hoeksema & Girgus, 1994). Among adolescents in our samples, the liabilities are greatest for those females who not only lack voice but who also emphasize the importance of appearance; in focusing on their outer selves, they face formidable hurdles in trying to meet the punishing cultural standards of attractiveness. Thus, those buying into societal messages that females should be seen but not heard are most at risk. The adolescent literature reveals that many such girls are not only at risk for depression but for eating disorders that can be extremely life threatening (see Gross & Rosen, 1988; Heatherton & Baumeister, 1991; Rand & Kuldau, 1992).

EDUCATIONAL IMPLICATIONS

What are the educational implications of this package of findings? Perhaps the clearest implication is that students need encouragement, validation, and support for expressing their opinions, both from teachers and classmates. Their voices need to be heard. However, in order for students to be supported in expressing themselves, they need the educational opportunities to do so. Models in which teachers merely "instruct," handing down the knowledge to be mastered, will do little to support student voices. Rather, as educators within the cooperative learning movement have suggested, students need opportunities, often in smaller groups, to present their ideas in a context where they will be listened to, heard, and understood (Delpit, 1993; Maher & Tetreault, 1994; Weis & Fine, 1993). Thus, expression of voice must take place within the context of human connection. As Gilligan (1993) observes, adolescents have a tremendous desire to bring their own inner world of thoughts and feelings into relationship with the thoughts and feelings of others. Maher and Tetreault concur, suggesting the need for teachers to view voice as a relational and evolving process. Thus, teachers need to avoid instructional models in which the flow of information is unidirectional. As Delpit argues, authoritarian teaching styles in which teachers display their power in the classroom and focus primarily on skills learning rob students of the opportunity to express their own ideas and creativity. For Delpit, the teacher cannot be the only expert in the classroom, since to deny students their own expert knowledge is to disempower them. As Bartolome (1994) also observes, a humanizing pedagogy in which teachers build upon the life experiences of students, rather than upon rigid adherence to particular techniques and academic content, will lead students to become more engaged in the learning process.

Listening to others is a powerful form of validation, although not always high on teachers' lists of educational priorities. Increasingly, with accountability criteria and the importance of scores on standardized tests, teachers are more likely to see their mission as ensuring that students are mastering those skills and memorizing the content of school subjects on which they will be evaluated. Nor, given economic cutbacks leading to larger numbers of students per classroom, are class sizes and physical configurations conducive to discussions in which student voices can be expressed, clarified, and respectfully heard by teachers as well as other students. As educational researchers (see Lee, Bryk, & Smith, 1993) have argued, schools need thoughtfully to reconsider such values and the consequences that emerge as a result. Moreover, schools need to restructure programs such that they do not continue to foster negative or debilitating gender stereotypes about abilities and social roles (Brophy, 1985; Humberstone, 1990).

As important as it is to have validation from teachers, adolescents need validation from peers. A major challenge in this regard is to create an atmosphere in which male students will seriously listen to the opinions of females. As we have seen, beginning at an early age, boys either ignore or devalue what females have to say. With adolescence, feminine girls are particularly at risk, since males are more likely to focus on the *outer* selves of such girls, their physical appearance, rather than support them for those personal qualities that comprise their *inner* selves and are primarily expressed through language. Thus, we need educational interventions that will help male students better appreciate what female students can meaningfully contribute, rather than merely allowing patterns in which males ignore or devalue girls' voices to persist. The continuation of such patterns into adulthood undoubtedly contributes to gender inequities in heterosexual relationships, within the workplace, and in society as a whole.

Finally, we need to guard against a singular focus on enhancing *girls'* voices. There are also boys in the silent ghetto of the classroom, as our findings have documented. *Reviving Ophelia* (Pipher, 1994) is certainly a worthy goal. However, Hamlet also displayed serious problems of indecision and lack of voice. Thus, efforts to encourage adolescents of both genders to express themselves in ways that will be respectfully heard are challenges that educators must face if we genuinely want to support the development of students' authentic selves.

The Effects of Child Abuse
on I-Self and Me-Self Processes

The preceding chapters have focused primarily on normative developmental changes in the I-self and the Me-self, as well as how the caregiving practices of socializing agents produce individual differences in the content and valence of children's self-evaluations. This chapter builds upon themes that have been discussed in previous chapters, in describing how certain cognitive-developmental structures in childhood conspire with abusive treatment by significant others to produce a constellation of negative outcomes. The focus is on the deleterious effects of multiple victimization (namely, the combination of severe sexual, physical, and psychological abuse from an early age) on the development of both I-self and Me-self functions. Attention first turns to how such severe and chronic abuse will seriously interfere with those I-self functions initially identified by James, including (1) an awareness of one's sense of *agency*, (2) an appreciation for one's sense of personal *continuity* over time, and (3) the awareness of awareness, namely, introspective attention to internal states, needs, and thoughts. Stern (1985) adds another feature, namely, *self-coherence*, a sense of self as a single, integrated entity. Stern cogently argues that these dimensions of the I-self have their developmental roots in infancy and emerge within appropriate (i.e., relatively consistent and positive) interpersonal interactions with caregivers. As becomes evident, each of these I-self functions undergoes disruption and disturbance given repeated, severe trauma in childhood.

Trauma, in the form of abuse, also results in serious disturbances in the Me-self. Victims of chronic abuse report negative domain-specific evaluations as well as low global self-worth. These self-perceptions extend to a sense of profound inner badness, namely, that one is "rotten to the core," and are accompanied by excessive self-blame and the belief that one is responsible for the abuse; therefore, it is deserved. Moreover, abuse leads to negative self-affects that are crippling, results in life-threatening forms of intropunitive or self-injurious behaviors, and promotes excessive false-self behavior. The processes leading to these deleterious outcomes are explored, with illustrations from case examples after an initial discussion of dynamics of child abuse.

FORMS OF CARETAKER ABUSE

There is considerable agreement that many aspects of the abusive family environment are clearly dysfunctional. Thus, effects attributed to abuse may be more appropriately interpreted within the context of a pathological family system (Briere, 1992; Bukowsky, 1992; Cicchetti, 1989; Erickson, Egeland, & Pianta, 1989; Finkelhor, 1979; 1984; Herman, 1992; Westen, 1993; Wolfe, 1989). Cicchetti conceives of child maltreatment as "relational psychopathology," namely, dysfunction in the parent–child–environment transactional system (see also Crittenden, 1981, 1988; Crittenden & Ainsworth, 1989). Erikson et al. (1989) concur, citing the difficulty of separating "maltreatment" from "family dysfunction," particularly if one adopts Newberger's (1973) view of maltreatment as an inability of the parents to nurture their offspring.

Although sexual abuse has received, to date, major attention in the literature, Briere (1992) observes that it is difficult to conceive of sexual molestation as the only form of abuse experienced by the child. The child who is sexually abused is also highly likely to experience psychological abuse (e.g., betrayal, threats, stigmatization) as well as physical maltreatment. In addition to physical damage due to sexually abusive acts themselves (tissue damage due to penetration), the child will invariably be subjected to other violent contact (e.g., physical beatings to ensure compliance). There are certainly cases in which only one form of abuse may be experienced. However, this chapter focuses primarily on *multiple* victimization (see Rossman & Rosenberg, 1998), since the combination of chronic sexual, physical, and emotional abuse from an early age has the most observable effects upon self-development.

Westen (1993) concurs, noting that we have paid far less attention to the continuous, pathogenic experiences that are associated with sexual abuse, namely, neglect, indifference, and empathic failures on the part of parents. He cogently observes that these other forms of maltreatment do not as readily elicit the horror or indignation we feel about sexual molestation. However, those who have carefully described their sampling procedures and populations note that the majority of maltreated children suffer from more than one form of abuse, including sexual molestation, physical abuse, neglect, and emotional abuse (Cicchetti, Beeghly, Carlson, & Toth, 1990). In addition, the child may also be a witness to domestic violence. Given this constellation of potentially abusive practices, it is difficult to isolate the effects of one from another, as well as from other dysfunctional features of family interactions (Wolfe, 1989).

Briere (1992) summarizes the major forms of parental or caretaker psychological abuse, drawing upon the work of Hart, Germain, and Brassard (1987), Navarre (1987), and Garbarino, Guttman, and Seeley (1986). These include (1) rejection, causing the child to feel unworthy or unacceptable; (2) degradation, criticism, stigmatization, humiliation, and deprivation of dignity, leading to feelings of inferiority; (3) terrorization, in which the child is verbally assaulted, frightened, and threatened with physical or psychological harm; (4) isolation, in which the child is deprived of social contacts outside of the family; (5) corruption, in which the child is encouraged to engage in antisocial behaviors; (6) lack of emotional responsiveness or availability, in which the child is deprived of loving, sensitive caregiving, or is ignored and neglected; and (7) unreliable or inconsistent parenting, in which contradictory demands are placed on the child. Many of these features represent extreme forms of what Baumrind (1966, 1971) has labeled "authoritarian" parenting practices.

Bukowsky (1992) echos these themes from the perspective of our knowledge of those positive parental practices (the "authoritative pattern") that result in feelings that one is capable, worthy, lovable, and able to engage in gratifying relationships with others (Baumrind, 1966, 1971; Coopersmith, 1967), practices that he notes are decidedly absent in abusive families. These include consistent expectations for responsible behavior, firm but sensitive enforcement of developmentally appropriate standards of behavior, encouragement of independence and individuality, the value of open communication, the provision of support and emotional warmth, and the recognition that children have rights, responsibilities, and legitimate points of view. The absence of these parenting behaviors, therefore, contributes greatly to the effects that are associated with child maltreatment and abuse.

Complementing this perspective are contributions from attachment theory. There is considerable consensus that the vast majority of maltreated children form insecure attachments with their primary caregivers (Cicchetti et al., 1990; Crittenden & Ainsworth, 1989; Erickson et al., 1989; Schneider-Rosen, Braunwald, Carlson, & Cicchetti, 1985; Westen, 1993). Thus, the effects of early sexual and/or physical abuse, coupled with other forms of parental insensitivity, disrupt the attachment bond, which in turn interferes with the development of positive working models of self and others. The foundation of attachment theory rests on the premise that if the caregiver has fairly consistently responded to the infant's needs and signals, and has respected the infant's need for independent exploration of the environment, the child will develop an internal working model of self as valued, compe-tent, and self-reliant. Conversely, if the parent is insensitive to the infant's needs and signals, inconsistent, and rejecting of the infant's bid for comfort and exploration, the child will develop an internal working model of the self as unworthy, ineffective, and incompetent (Ainsworth, 1979; Bowlby, 1973; Bretherton, 1991, 1993; Crittenden & Ainsworth, 1989; Sroufe & Fleeson, 1986). Clearly, the parental practices that have been associated with child abuse represent precisely the kind of treatment that would lead chil-dren to develop insecure attachments, as well as an internal model of self as inadequate and unworthy.

Of particular interest is the specific type of insecure attachment that children of abuse appear to manifest. A high percentage of such children display the *disorganized/disoriented* (D) style identified by Main and Solomon (1990; see discussions by Cicchetti, 1989; Crittenden & Ainsworth, 1989). Such children perform contradictory behaviors, for example, they vacillate between approaching and avoiding the caregiver. There are also signs of disorientation, such as stereotyped rocking and dazed facial expressions. It has been hypothesized that a history of severe negative and inconsistent parent–child interactions would produce such an attachment style. It is of interest that Crittenden (1985) takes exception to the interpretation that such children are disorganized and disoriented. Her observations suggest that such children are actually displaying a combination of avoidant (A) and ambivalent (C) attachment styles, organized around the attempt to resolve the conflict between the child's need for proximity to the caregiver and his/her expectations of aversive treatment at the hands of parents.

DISSOCIATIVE REACTIONS TO SEVERE AND PROLONGED ABUSE

As experts on maltreatment have pointed out (see Briere, 1992; Cicchetti, 1989; Herman, 1992; Marold, 1998; McCann & Pearlman, 1992; Putnam, 1989, 1990, 1991, 1993; Terr, 1990, 1991; Westen, 1993), abuse presents formidable challenges, because it thwarts so many basic, develop-mental needs. The child must attempt to cope with a situation that is un-safe, as well as try to find a way to preserve trust in those who have violated that trust. He/she must find a way to remain connected to caregivers whose behavior has seriously threatened a sense of secure attachment and connec-tion. The child is also prevented from successfully exerting some sense of autonomy and control given unpredictable situations in which he/she feels helpless. Disturbances in *identity* formation are also common among abuse victims when they reach adolescence (see Marold, 1998, who has adopted

Erikson's developmental model as the framework for her treatment approach).

The major strategy for coping with these formidable obstacles is to activate a complex system of psychological defenses, which relies heavily on *dissociative* reactions. Dissociative processes are generally conceptualized as the most adaptive defensive response to overwhelming trauma (see Herman, 1992; Putnam, 1989, 1991, 1993; Terr, 1991; van der Kolk, 1987). Terr makes reference to Type II trauma, which involves chronic exposure to external events that are severely damaging to the self (in contrast to Type I trauma, which involves a single event). If such abuse occurs in childhood, it conspires with the natural penchant for dissociation, splitting, or fragmentation. As noted in Chapter 2, dissociation in childhood, what Fischer and colleagues refer to as normative affective splitting, represents the typical organization of childhood cognitive structures (Fischer, & Ayoub, 1994; Fischer & Pipp, 1984). Thus, the mind of the young child naturally fractionates by virtue of its cognitive-developmental limitations (see also Harter, 1998b; Harter & Buddin, 1987; Harter & Whitesell, 1989; Putnam, 1991), compartmentalizing content into positive versus negative, good versus bad. Fischer and his colleagues refer to this natural tendency as "passive dissociation." Dissociative processes, as normative developmental phenomena, continue into adolescence and adulthood in forms that are increasingly complex and often quite adaptive.

Trauma caused by chronic abuse, however, leads to active, highly motivated (in Fischer's terminology) dissociative symptoms that represent massive attempts to protect the psyche by attempts to eliminate the event from consciousness. As such, they represent not only a defensive adaptation but a fundamental reorganization of one's personality (Herman, 1992; Terr, 1991; Putnam, 1991). More specifically, dissociation serves multiple purposes, namely to allow the abuse victim to escape from the punishing constraints of reality, to contain traumatic memories and affects outside of normal conscious awareness, to detach the self from the traumatic event such that it appears to happen to someone else, and to serve as an analgesic, numbing the physical and psychic pain that is being inflicted (Putnam, 1989). Thus, fully integrated functioning is seriously compromised as the abuse victim attempts to lessen the pain and anxiety associated with total awareness of the traumatic events (Briere, 1992).

Dissociative symptoms, which represent altered states of consciousness, take several forms. Perhaps the most dramatic is psychogenic amnesia for the abuse itself. Entire segments of one's childhood are lost, repressed, denied (see Briere, 1992; Herman, 1992; Putnam, 1989, 1991, 1993; Terr, 1991). These theorists also identify a number of other mechanisms, including attempts at detachment and numbing, invoked to attenuate the intensity of negative affects surrounding abusive assaults. Depersonalization represents another dissociative strategy in which one experiences the self as observing (rather than participating in) the abusive event. Various forms of self-hypnosis, prompted by the desire to become invisible, also add to the dissociative repertoire. In the extreme, dissociative symptomatology leads to a dissociative identity disorder (formerly labeled multiple personality disorder) in which the self becomes so fragmented that different alters, now termed ego states, are created to bear the burden of contradictory events that defy integration.

A 30-year-old client diagnosed with dissociative identity disorder exemplifies a number of these symptoms. In childhood, she had been sexually abused by an uncle who would first tie her to the bed. During adolescence and adulthood, she developed an intense and defensive desire to make herself invisible to others. In addition, she developed pervasive amnesia for the abusive events. It was not until age 30 that she recalled these episodes, not uncommon among victims of severe and chronic childhood abuse. When she did retrieve certain memories, she described the process of depersonalization in that she experienced herself hovering in space over the bed, as if she were a detached observer of the uncle's assaults. One alter, a protector, held most of the memories about the abuse, whereas other alters did not have conscious access to memories of the childhood sexual assaults. However, the client herself was unable to speak about these experiences given her wish to be invisible to others. Her efforts to remain in psychological hiding were also reflected in the fact that she always wore black clothing given her belief that colorful clothing would attract the attention of others. Black also symbolized her grief, as well as her sense of inner badness. In therapy, although she continued to have great difficulty talking about the abuse, she was able to make some progress by writing about her early experiences in a journal.

The preceding discussion has emphasized the causes of abuse as well as its pathological manifestations. It should be noted that the dissociative manifestations, including the construction of alters or multiple personalities, are qualitatively different from those more normative dissociative processes and from the adaptive emergence of multiple selves in different interpersonal contexts during adolescence (see Chapter 3). In the next sections, the focus shifts to a more specific analysis of how chronic abuse in childhood disrupts both I-self and Me-self functions, illustrating many of these disruptions through case examples. Table 10.1 summarizes the deleterious effects of such abuse on the self-system. It is beyond the scope of this chapter to deal with issues of treatment and remediation. For excellent discussions of treatment approaches, see chapters by Culbertson and Willis, Shirk and Eltz, and Marold in Rossman and Rosenberg (1998).

TABLE 10.1. Deleterious Effects of Child Abuse on the Self-System

Disturbances in the I-self functions
1. Reduced self-awareness, introspection, attention to internal states, needs, thoughts, emotions
2. Impaired sense of agency, volition, control over one's actions
3. Disruptions in sense of self-continuity, the sense that one is the same person over time
4. Lack of a sense of self-coherence, the sense that oneself is integrated or unified

Disturbances in the Me-self
1. Negative domain-specific self-evaluations and low global self-worth
2. Profound sense of inner badness, malevolent core self
3. Excessive self-blame, belief that abuse is one's fault and therefore deserved

Negative self-affects
1. Severe guilt and shame over participation in abuse
2. Depressive affect, anger toward self

Intropunitive behaviors
1. Suicidal ideation, suicide attempts as escape from the self
2. Self-destructive behavior, self-injury, self-mutilation

Excessive false-self behavior
1. Suppression, loss of one's true or authentic self
2. Development of a socially acceptable self that conforms to demands and desires of others

SPECIFIC EFFECTS OF ABUSE ON THE I-SELF

Self-Awareness

As James (1892) observed, self-awareness is one of the basic functions of the I-self. However, as described by the scholars cited earlier, the very mechanisms of dissociation, including psychogenic amnesia, render abuse victim unaware of events and self-representations that have become inaccessible to consciousness because the content is too terrifying or painful. Westen (1993) refers to a "metacognitive shutdown." Thus, one does not observe the typical processes of introspection, namely, the ability to think about one's thoughts and actions, which becomes particularly rampant during adolescence. The cognitive constriction associated with the dissociative symptomatology precludes this type of self-awareness.

Briere (1992) points to another feature of abusive relationships that interfere with the victim's lack of awareness of self. The fact that the child must direct sustained attention to external threats draws energy and focus away from the developmental task of self-awareness. Thus, the hypervigilance to others' reactions, what Briere (1989) terms "otherdirectedness," interferes with the ability to attend to one's own needs, thoughts, and desires.

This analysis is consistent with the formulation of Miller (1986), who addresses the impact of the stance that subordinates (e.g., children, as well as women in a patriarchal society) must adopt toward dominants. They must attend to the needs and desires of the dominants, and in so doing, they become alienated from, and unaware of, their own needs, thoughts, and emotions. Moreover, the fact that, as children, abuse victims do not share their experiences with others, due to parental prohibitions and codes of secrecy, also contributes to the defensive exclusion of certain experiences from awareness.

Recent research findings with children support these contentions. Cicchetti (1989) and colleagues (Cicchetti et al., 1990) found that maltreated children (ages 30–36 months) report less internal-state language than do their nonmaltreated, securely attached counterparts. Similar findings have been reported by Beeghly, Carlson, and Cicchetti (1986). Coster, Gersten, Beeghly, and Cicchetti (1989) have also reported that maltreated toddlers use less descriptive speech, particularly about their own feelings and actions. Gralinsky, Feshbach, Powell, and Derrington (1993) have also observed that older, maltreated children report fewer descriptions of inner states and feelings than children with no known history of abuse. Thus, there is a growing body of evidence that the defensive processes that are mobilized by maltreated children interfere with one of the primary tasks of the I-self, namely, awareness of inner thoughts and feelings.

Sense of Agency

As James (1892) and later Stern (1985) have observed, self-agency involves the sense that one has authorship over one's actions, thoughts, and emotional experiences, that one has volition and control over one's behaviors, that one is the architect of one's intentions and plans. However, the defenses structures driven by abuse will compromise the victim's sense of agency (Briere, 1989; Putnam, 1993). The very fact that abuse victims manifest less self-awareness and attention to internal processes, motives, and intentions will interfere with a sense of agency (Westen, 1993).

Putnam (1993) describes how significant levels of dissociation will interfere with the development of perceptions of agency on several levels. The person's sense of volition is undermined by "passive influence experiences" in which certain actions, thoughts, and affects are experienced as if a powerful force outside of the individual's conscious awareness or control is coercing the person to do something against his/her will. "Automatic writing" represents on such manifestation in that the person finds himself/herself writing words that are not linked to conscious thoughts. Depersonalization, in which the person feels that he/she is observing the self from a detached perspective, also contributes to a lack of a sense of agency. The very fact that one cannot remember, or account for, various actions he/she has performed also robs the abuse victim of a sense of control.

In the adult survivor of abuse, Westen also describes how there is a distortion in his/her sense of agency due to the splitting off of sexual impulses that cannot be owned. In addition, the tendency to experience overwhelming affects can also prevent a sense of agency, since impulsive, emotion-driven behaviors (e.g., suicidal gestures) may appear to come out of the blue. Westen presents one adult patient who described herself as a sailing ship with no one at the helm. Other theorists (see Briere, 1992; McCann & Pearlman, 1992; van der Kolk, 1987; Wolfe, 1989) similarly describe how abuse victims lack feelings of efficacy, independence, and control; helplessness and external attributions of control are more common, further eroding their sense of agency.

Another clinical case example illustrates many of these processes in combination. This middle-aged male client had suffered repeated childhood sexual molestation by an older sister, who, during the abusive episodes, forced him to dress up in girls' clothing and wear lipstick. As an adult, he became a husband and father, and was greatly respected in the community, as reflected in the fact that he was a high-ranking elected official in the town in which he lived. He was, as an adult, very religious, as well as politically conservative. However, another persona would often emerge unexpectantly in that he would find himself in all-night bars in a neighboring big city, where he would allow himself to be picked up and sexually used by men and women. He would later hate himself for engaging in these sordid acts, which he viewed as despicable and very ego-dystonic, given his value system. However, he could not contain his sexual impulses and felt he had no choice given that he did not feel in control of his actions. "Something just comes over me," he would lament, in expressing his perceived lack of agency over these behaviors.

Cicchetti (1989) brings another perspective to the origins of a sense of agency, integrating attachment and Eriksonian perspectives. He notes that autonomy and mastery must build upon a sense of trust in the caregiver's accessibility, one feature of a secure attachment. However, given the interpersonal dynamics in abusive families that lead to insecure attachment, the maltreated child may well not develop the sense of agency that permits him/her to explore and master the environment with confidence. Bukowsky (1992) cites another family interactive theme that impacts sense of self as agent among child victims of sexual abuse. The fact that the child is forced to be a passive participant in an activity that brings the victim little or no satisfaction is antithetical to the development of a sense of self based upon will and agency.

Sense of Self-Continuity

Contemporary self-theorists, particularly Stern (1985), have built upon James' (1982) contention that a critical "I-self" function is the maintenance of a sense of self-continuity over time, over one's own history. There is now considerable agreement that *autobiographical memory* is a key source of a sense of continuity, the sense that one is the same person over time (see Eder, Gerlach, & Perlmutter, 1987; Rubin, 1985; Stern, 1985). However, traumatically induced dissociative states and amnesic gaps contribute to a temporally discontinuous sense of self (Herman, 1992; McCann & Pearlman, 1992; Putnam, 1990, 1991; Westen, 1993); that is, the loss of significant childhood and adolescent memories typically encountered with incest victims in particular (Herman, 1992), deprive the individual of the autobiographical memory upon which the sense of self hinges. Building upon Tulving's (1972) distinction between autobiographical or episodic memory and semantic memory, Bowlby (1980) was one of the first theorists to suggest that child abuse victims repress their autobiographical memory for the traumatic events. Bowbly suggested that they may retain conscious access only to parental interpretations stored in semantic memory (see also Bretherton, 1993).

As Putnam (1993) describes, difficulty in determining whether a memory actually happened to oneself or was "incorporated" into memory from other sources degrades the important self-referential qualities of memory and creates doubt about the reality of what one remembers as his/her life. In addition, among those with dissociative identity disorder, amnesia, loss of time and memory for the significant events that occurred during such a lost period of time, coupled with more severe dissociative symptoms in the form of fugue states and switching from one personality to another, seriously disrupt self-continuity.

Finally, it has been argued that the very ability to create autobiographical memories hinges upon the early development of a sense of self-agency and self-recognition (Howe & Courage, 1993). As noted earlier, early onset of abuse has been shown to interfere with a sense of self as causal agent. Moreover, Cicchetti et al. (1990) have demonstrated that early maltreatment interferes with the normative process of self-recognition among toddlers. Thus, a constellation of factors conspire to interfere with the abuse victim's sense of self-history, including the continuity of who one is as a person, over time.

Adult clients diagnosed with dissociative identity disorder often struggle with the amnesic gaps that prevent them from reconstructing their abusive childhood. One such client, who as a child had been sexually abused by her mother and physically abused by a grandparent, could not remember large blocks of her childhood. With the help of feedback from other supportive family members and friends, she was able partially to reconstruct her past by putting together a scrapbook of memorabilia and pictures that served to provide an autobiographical account of her childhood. As a child, she had attempted to soothe herself by repeatedly listening to certain songs that she found comforting. Her first memories in therapy were of these childhood songs, which were easier to recall than the abusive episodes. As an adult, she went to great lengths to find recordings of these songs, which was often difficult. However, her goal was to make an audiotape to accompany pictures of the more positive experiences of her childhood in order to recover her memories, against the backdrop of the abusive episodes, which she also attempted to retrieve.

Self-Coherence and Sense of Unity

Another I-self function, namely, the maintenance of the sense of a co-herent, integrated self (Stern, 1985), is also compromised among victims of abuse. As noted in an earlier section, from a developmental perspective, the self is naturally fragmented, particularly along attributes that can be catego-rized as either positive or negative, good or bad. The natural dissociative tendencies of childhood and early adolescence preclude an integrated self-structure (Fischer, 1980; Fischer & Pipp, 1984). However, developing cogni-tive capabilities that emerge toward the end of adolescence provide the nec-essary psychological tools whereby one can craft a more integrated, coherent self (see also Harter & Monsour, 1992).

However, the dissociative symptomatology defensively mobilized by the abuse victim seriously interferes with the consolidation of features of one-self that would be experienced as integrated (see Briere, 1992; Fischer & Ayoub, 1994; Putnam, 1990, 1991, 1993; Westen, 1993). Splitting, fragmen-tation, compartmentalization, the staples in the abuse victim's dissociative armamentarium, all, by definition, preclude a sense of the coherence of the self. As Putnam (1993) observes, depersonalization and passive-influence experiences also undermine the individual's sense of a unified self.

These tendencies are further exacerbated among those with dissocia-tive identity or multiple personality disorder victims of severe and chronic sexual abuse (Putnam, 1989, 1990, 1993). Multiple identities are created to compartmentalize traumatic memories and affects, and these dissociated alters or personality states function as separate entities capable of indepen-dent volitional activities. By necessity, they will lead to a fragmented and incoherent self-portrait. Not only do clients with dissociative identity disor-ders (or multiple personality disorders) represent the self as a disjointed collection of autonomous agents, but often the alters (or different ego states) will be in diametric conflict with each other. For example, a sexually promis-cuous alter will be countered by another, morally upstanding personality; a self-destructive or persecuting alter will coexist along with a protective alter. Dissociative symptomatology represents a continuum of severity. Level of severity, in turn, will affect the degree to which the self lacks unity and coherence.

A 30-year-old mother diagnosed with dissociative identity disorder il-lustrates the creation of multiple personalities, each of which serves a par-ticular function. As a child, she suffered severe sexual and physical abuse at the hands of multiple perpetrators, including her father and his male friends. At age 13, she gave birth to her father's child. The family was constantly on the move, living in a traveling van and in a series of cheap hotels, which served to enhance the unpredictability in her life, particularly with regard to who the next perpetrator might be and when she would be assaulted. In order to cope with these experiences, she gradually developed a very com-plex and functional system of alters or ego states to manage her very pain-fully intense emotions and to assist her in dealing with an exceedingly hos-tile world. For example, Rocky, one personality, had the streets smarts to help her negotiate the challenges and threats posed by city life. Little Mama, another personality, was the nurturer who helped her to care for her own children. Flame was an alter that helped her to contain her rage, and finally, Nojoy held her intense grief.

DISTURBANCES IN THE ME-SELF

Negative Domain-Specific Self-Evaluations and Low Global Self-Worth

In addition to disturbances in the functions of the I-self, the very con-tent of the Me-self is impacted by abuse, leading to a range of negative self-evaluations. There is a growing body of evidence that children experiencing serious forms of maltreatment and abuse describe themselves more nega-tively, report greater feelings of inadequacy and incompetence, and mani-fest lower self-esteem (see Briere, 1992; Browne & Finkelhor, 1986; Cicchetti & Carlson, 1989; Coons, 1984; Green, 1982; Herman, 1992; Jehu, 1988; Kaufman & Cicchetti, 1989; Kazdin, Moser, Colbus, & Bell, 1985; Kendall-Tackett, Williams, & Finkelhor, 1993; McCann & Pearlman, 1992; Navarre, 1987; Oates, Forrest, & Peacock, 1985; Putnam, 1989; Westen, 1993; Youngblade & Belsky, 1990). In an attempt to integrate the various mecha-nisms leading to negative self-evaluations, the original model of the causes of self-worth will serve as a framework. Recall that this model identified two broad antecedents, perceptions of competence or adequacy in domains where success was considered important (originally from James, 1892) and internalization of the opinions of significant others (originally from Cooley, 1902, and Mead, 1925, 1934).

Experts in abuse readily point to the sense of inadequacy that victims feel in a number of domains of their life. At the most basic level of the bodily self, abuse leaves many victims feeling fundamentally damaged (see Nash, Hulsey, Sexton, Harralson, & Lambert, 1993; Newberger, 1973; Putnam, 1990; Westen, 1993). Further contributing to their sense of inadequacy and incompetence are early experiences and messages from caregivers who communicate that they are generally flawed and ineffective (see Briere, 1992; Crittenden & Ainsworth, 1989; Navarre, 1987; McCann & Pearlman, 1992). As Navarre observes, the assault is not merely upon the physical body but upon the individual's perception of the self as competent and valuable. Cicchetti et al. (1990) report that beginning in middle childhood, maltreated children report that they are less competent and accepted than nonmaltreated peers of the same socioeconomic level.

In their efforts to attempt to avoid further abuse and to please punitive parents who set harsh and often unattainable standards, many child victims of abuse strive to do better, to be perfect. However, such a strategy may backfire as they develop overidealized images that they cannot attain (Putnam, 1990). Bleiberg (1984) also observes that abuse can put one at risk for what he terms "narcissistic vulnerability," in which there is a mismatch between the ideal and the real self. Such a mismatch results in part from parents setting conditional and unreachable ideals for their maltreated child. As noted earlier, it is the *discrepancy* between one's competence and the importance attached to success, between one's actual and one's ideal self-image, that contributes to feelings of low self-worth.

An example of this pattern can be observed in an adult female who was the firstborn and as a child experienced emotional and verbal abuse at the hands of parents, and sexual abuse by an uncle. When her parents learned that they were expecting their first child, they desperately wanted a boy; however, their wishes were not granted. They proceeded to give their daughter a boy's name, closely resembling that of the father. The daughter was athletically talented and attempted to make her mark in gymnastics, where she was exceedingly successful by objective standards. However, her performance was never good enough for her parents, whose conditional support led to the expectation that she would always excel, which by their definition meant coming in first, not second. She would be severely ostracized and shunned for days if she did not meet these high parental standards. As an adult, this woman became a surgeon and was the first female faculty member in a surgery department at a prestigious medical school. However, the damaging effects of emotional abuse at the hands of her parents, who also did not acknowledge and therefore protect her from sexual abuse by an uncle, led to severe psychological damage. In her own words, "I don't allow myself to get close to anyone because I am a nobody. No matter what I do, I know I will never be good enough at anything. I'm a loser." The pattern was established in childhood for this woman, namely, that she would never meet the ideals that were made clear by her parents and that she internalized, despite her successful professional accomplishments. She was not a male. As a result, despite her professional success, she experienced little approval from family members, which in turn took its toll on her overall sense of worth as a person.

Significant others, notably parents in the early years, not only set standards of performance and provide feedback in particular areas of competence but also communicate their opinions about one's overall worth as a person. As described in Chapter 7, these more generalized messages have been found to have a powerful impact on children's sense of self-worth (e.g., Harter, 1990a, 1993). In the previous discussion of the nature of parenting, it was observed that maltreating parents not only physically or sexually abuse their children but are also likely to engage in a variety of emotionally and psychologically abusive behaviors, including rejection, which causes the child to feel unworthy or unacceptable, as well as degradation, criticism, and stigmatization, which further contribute to feelings of inferiority and low self-worth.

As attachment theorists have informed us, these processes begin during the first year of life, within the context of insecure forms of attachment (see Cicchetti et al., 1990; Crittenden & Ainsworth, 1989; Erickson et al., 1989; Schneider-Rosen et al., 1985). Although very young children cannot verbalize their sense of low self-worth, they manifest it in their behavior (Haltiwanger & Harter, 1994). As Green (1982) observes, the preverbal infant who is repeatedly assaulted acquires an unpleasurable awareness of self that becomes transformed into a devalued self-concept with further cognitive development and the emergence of language. Such children ultimately internalize the contempt that their parents directed toward them, resulting in extreme, self-deprecatory ideation. Many of the clinical examples provided reveal the absence or lack of support from parents, which, when coupled with abuse, results in the constellation of symptoms that have been described.

In the earlier discussion of normative processes contributing to self-worth, it was noted that *peer* support becomes increasingly critical as one moves into later childhood and adolescence (Harter, 1990b). Unfortunately, there are a number of factors associated with child abuse that cause peer support to become problematic. A number of abuse experts point to the fact that maltreating parents often deprive the child of social contacts outside the family. Such social isolation removes opportunities for the development of social relationships, social skills, and the potentially buffering effects of peer relationships (Briere, 1992; Cicchetti, et al., 1990; Mueller & Silverman, 1990; Putnam, 1990; Wolfe, 1989). Moreover, these authors point to the fact that abused children typically develop one of two stances toward peers, either aggression or avoidance, which in turn alienates peers whose approval constitutes a vital source of self-worth. Many abuse victims provoke peer disapproval, which further contributes to the negative feelings of worth that were initially fostered at the hands of parents. Marold (1998) describes an abused, suicidal 17-year-old male, who, in addition to identity problems, had problems in establishing relations with peers. In his own words, he describes how "I just can't seem to make it in a relationship with anyone, male or female. I fall for someone and they walk out on me, just like my parents. I hurt so much inside, and the only thing that seems to help is a six-pack."

Given potential rejection by one's normative peer group, abused youth may well turn to other sources of support, joining a gang that may also serve as an outlet for their aggression. The support provided through gang membership may in turn provide an arena in which one can enhance one's status and self-worth. Such speculation, supported by the higher incidence of abused children and adolescents involved in delinquent behavior (Lewis, Mallouh, & Webb, 1989) as well as in gangs, underscores the importance of understanding the particular *motives* underlying gang membership. Thus, age-appropriate needs for approval, esteem, status, power, and outlets for the expression of aggression, needs that may be thwarted in one's family and school environment, can be met through gang-related activities.

The Abuse Victim's Sense of Inner Badness and Self-Blame

In discussing the negative self-evaluations of abuse victims, many experts point out that such negativity extends beyond mere low self-worth to include a profound sense of inner badness (see Briere, 1992; Fischer & Ayoub, 1994; Fine, 1990; Herman, 1992; McCann & Pearlman, 1992; Terr, 1990; van der Kolk, 1987; Westen, 1993; Wolfe, 1989). Thus, abuse victims see themselves as fundamentally and innately bad, as "malevolent" in Westen's terms. Moreover, this sense of pervasive badness includes their perceptions that they will bring trouble and grief to family members and that others who have contact with them will be harmed, contaminated, or doomed. Moreover, such victims blame themselves for their core or inner badness, making internal, global, and stable attributions about their character flaws.

For example, a sexually abused 17-year-old female African American adolescent, who was also regularly beaten, exclaimed, "I would rather die than remember anymore. I am evil and made all the bad things happen" (Marold, 1998, p. 255). Another of Marold's clients had a history of sexual, physical, and emotional abuse at the hands of her grandfather. However, she blamed herself for her victimizations, including a rape by a male teacher. She concluded, "I am rotten inside, no one will be able to love me, and I can never love anyone" (p. 258).

From a socialization perspective, the *stigmatization* of abuse victims by the abuser, family members, and society contribute to this self-perception (see Briere, 1992; Finkelhor & Browne, 1985; Kendall-Tackett, et al., 1993). Thus, the victim is given the message from the abuser and possibly family that "You deserved that," "You asked for it," "You are being punished for being bad" (Briere, 1992). As Briere also notes, our victim-blaming social system also condemns the victim after the fact ("You seduced him," "Why didn't you just say 'No'?" "What must you have done to deserve it?").

From a cognitive-developmental perspective, the young child who is abused will readily blame the self (Herman, 1992; Piaget, 1932; Watson & Fischer, 1993; Westen, 1993); that is, given young children's natural egocentrism, they will take responsibility for events they did not cause or cannot control. Moreover, as Piaget demonstrated, young children focus on the *deed* (e.g., the abusive act) rather than on the intention (e.g., the motives of the perpetrator). As Herman points out, the child must construct some version of reality that justifies continued abuse and therefore inevitably concludes that his/her innate badness is the cause.

Briere (1992) also provides an analysis of the sequential "logic" that governs the abused child's attempt to make meaning of his/her experiences. Given maltreatment at the hands of a parent or family member, the child first surmises that either "I am bad or my parents are bad." However, the assumption of young children that parents or adult authority figures are always right leads to the conclusion that parental maltreatment must be due to the fact that they were bad, that the act was their fault, and that therefore they deserve to be punished. When children are repeatedly assaulted, they come to conclude that they must be "very bad," contributing to the sense of fundamental badness at their core.

Paradoxically, many children opt for the attribution of *self*-blame (rather than blaming others), since it would seem to offer them some sense of hope and control (see Herman, 1992; Janoff-Bulman, 1992; Westen, 1993). Such a stance may offer some opportunity for atonement. If one has brought this abusive fate upon oneself by being bad, then perhaps one has the power to alter it, by trying to be good. This, in turn, may earn one's parents' forgiveness, as well as the care and protection that has been so desperately lacking.

Fischer and his colleagues (Calverley, Fischer, & Ayoub, 1994; Fischer & Ayoub, 1994) have provided an interesting documentation of the sense of profound negativity that female adolescent sexual abuse victims experience with regard to their core self. In their study, they compared two groups of adolescents, both of whom suffered from depressive/affective disorders; one group had documented sexual abuse as well as the diagnosis of post-traumatic stress disorder, while the second group did not. These investigators built upon the procedure developed by Harter and Monsour (1992), in which adolescents arranged spontaneously generated self-attributes into a self-portrait by identifying attributes that were the *most important* or central, *less important*, and *least important*. Adolescents in Harter and Monsour's normative sample placed the majority of positive attributes at the core of the self and relegated negative attributes to the periphery of their self-portrait, judging them to be their least important characteristics. Such findings corroborate the general positivity bias that has been documented among normative populations.

The findings of Fischer and colleagues revealed that adolescent girls with depressive disorders that were coupled with a history of sexual abuse not only reported significantly more negative self-attributes but also identified negative characteristics as far more *central* to their self-concepts, as far more important defining features of their core self. The comparison group, with depressive symptomatology but no known history of abuse, showed the positivity bias reported in normative samples. Thus, these findings provide clear research support for the argument that one of the sequelae of abuse is a sense of the core badness of the self.

Guilt and Shame

Closely linked to abuse victims' perceptions of low self-esteem, self-blame, and a sense of inner badness are *emotional* reactions of guilt and shame (see Briere, 1992; Herman, 1992; Kendall-Tackett et al., 1993; McCann & Pearlman, 1992; Terr, 1990; Westen, 1993; Wolfe, 1989). Normatively, such self-affects are intimately related to evaluative self-perceptions, both of which result from the internalization of the opinions of significant others (Cooley, 1902; Harter, 1998a). Thus, the blame, stigmatization, condemnation, and ostracism that parents, family, and society express toward the abuse victim are incorporated not only into attributions of self-blame but also result in powerful negative affects directed toward the self. The sexual abuse victim is made to feel humiliated for his/her role in shameful acts. Moreover, guilt and shame are also fueled by the perception that one's badness *led* to the abuse, rather than the abuse was the cause of one's negative self-views. In the clinical examples already provided, the clients' affective reactions to their inner badness invariably were associated with personal condemnations that included either guilt or shame.

Depression, Suicide, and Self-Destructive Behaviors

As noted in Chapter 8, negative self-perceptions and low global self-worth are highly linked to depressive symptomatology. Abusive treatment by significant adults, coupled with the forms of psychological abuse that have been documented, not only provoke a range of self-deprecatory ideation but also depression associated with both the loss of a caring significant other and loss of the self. This pattern is common among abuse victims who typically manifest a range of depressive reactions, including suicidal behavior (Bagley & McDonald, 1984; Briere & Runtz, 1988; Briere & Woo, 1991; Browne & Finkelhor, 1986; Elliot & Briere, 1992; Herman, Russell, & Trocki, 1986; Kazdin et al., 1985; Kendall-Tackett et al., 1993; Lipovsky, Saunders, & Murphy, 1989; Putnam, 1989, 1991; Wolfe, 1989). Moreover, the single most common presenting symptom in dissociative identity disorder patients who have severe history of sexual abuse is depression (see Putnam, 1989). Many not only report depressive symptoms but would appear to be at risk for a major affective disorder as well as suicidal behaviors.

Suicidal behaviors among abuse victims typically represent the ultimate avoidance strategy (Briere, 1992). Thus, suicide represents the final out, providing an escape from extreme psychic pain, including intolerable memories, depression, and hopelessness (Schneidman, 1991) in the face of other strategies that did not provide relief. As Baumeister (1990) observes, suicide can also be conceptualized as "escape from the self," given a history of events leading the individual to extremely negative self-evaluations and profound depression. These dynamics can be particularly observable in clients who have been chronically abused. A 13-year-old who came to our attention was referred for therapy given low self-esteem, depressed affect, and suicidal thinking, accompanying an eating disorder. She had been sexually abused as a child and came to feel unloved and not valued. She felt that she was overweight, and her negative perceptions of her appearance were not contradicted by her parents. She felt sullied by the abuse, all of which led to her desire to escape the pain of the very unfavorable views that she held of herself.

Self-injury, in the form of carving or burning parts of the body, is also common among victims of severe sexual abuse. However, abuse experts note that such behaviors are not to be confused with suicidal gestures (see Briere, 1992; Herman, 1992; Putnam, 1989). Rather, self-mutilation strategies serve to allow the abuse victim to regulate autonomic arousal and therefore certain internal states. Moreover, the pain functions to allow the individual to reconnect with his/her physical body. For example, one abused youth in our sample who was carving on her arms reported that "I do this just to know I am alive." Such behaviors also temporarily reduce the psychic tension associated with negative affect, self-deprecatory ideation, guilt, and painfully fragmented thought processes, states that are inevitable for abuse victims (see Briere, 1992). For example, another female adolescent client who had been sexually and physically abused from an early age was found to cut her arms with a razor blade in an attempt to ease the tension she experienced and to punish herself for being bad. However, such self-injurious strategies provide only temporary relief.

For some victims, self-mutilating behaviors occur during periods of profound dissociation and depersonalization, which is often accompanied by profound agitation and a desire to attack the body (Herman, 1992). The mutilating act itself produces feelings of calm and relief, since physical pain is preferable to the severe emotional pain that abuse victims experience. In abuse victims suffering from dissociative identity disorders, self-mutilation may also reflect one persecutor personality who is punishing another alter or the host personality, herself (Putnam, 1989). Thus, self-mutilation serves a variety of functions, each of which represents a defensive strategy to find relief from other symptoms associated with abuse.

False-Self Behavior

Abuse puts one at risk for suppressing one's true self and displaying various forms of inauthentic or false-self behavior. Such a process has its origins in childhood, given the very forms of parenting that constitute psychological abuse. As described in Chapter 9, parenting practices that represent lack of attunement to the child's needs, empathic failure, lack of validation, threats of harm, coercion, and enforced compliance all cause the true self to go underground (Bleiberg, 1984; Stern, 1985; Winnicott, 1958, 1965) and lead to what Sullivan (1953) labeled "not me" experiences.

Moreover, it was also observed in Chapter 9 that the ability to express oneself verbally allows one to falsify what is shared with others. In the maltreated child, secrecy pacts around sexually abusive interactions further provokes the child defensively to exclude such episodic memories from awareness (see also Bretherton, 1993). Thus, sexual and physical abuse cause the child to split off experiences, either consciously or unconsciously, relegating them to either a private or inaccessible part of the self. The very disavowal, repression, or dissociation of one's experiences, coupled with psychogenic amnesia and numbing as defensive reactions to abuse, therefore, set the stage for loss of one's true self.

Herman (1992) introduces other dynamics that represent barriers to authenticity among victims of abuse. She notes that the malignant sense of inner badness is often camouflaged by the abused child's persistent attempts to be good. In adopting different roles designed to please the parent, to be the perfect child, one comes to experience one's behavior as false or inauthentic (see also Miller, 1990). Thus, one develops a socially acceptable false self that conforms to the demands and desires of others in an attempt to obtain their approval (see Harter, Marold, et al., 1996). If one's true self, corroded with inner badness, were to be revealed, it would be met with scorn and contempt. Therefore, it must be concealed at all costs.

Moreover, as our own findings reveal, lack of parental validation or support, coupled with *conditionality* in which approval is contingent upon meeting very high and often unrealistic standards, lead to a constellation of negative outcomes. These include high levels of false-self behavior, lack of knowledge about one's true self, as well as depression, low self-esteem, and hopelessness. These dynamics would appear to be even more exaggerated among victims of abuse, compromising their sense of authenticity.

CONCLUSION

Against a backdrop of normative-developmental phenomena, this chapter has attempted to demonstrate how traumatic abuse in the form of multiple victimization during childhood can lead to profound disturbances in the self. In addition to abusive acts themselves, accompanying psychological abuse at the hands of parents, coupled with dissociative defensive reactions, conspire to disrupt the self-system. With regard to I-self functions, one can observe impairments in self-awareness, sense of agency, sense of self-continuity over time, and sense of a unified self. Disturbances in the Me-self include feelings of incompetence, low self-worth, a profound sense of inner badness, self-blame, guilt and shame, depression, suicide, and other self-destructive behaviors, as well as a sense that the self that one presents to the world is false or inauthentic. The mandate of this chapter was to describe and document these painful sequelae of abuse. The larger mandate for the field and for society is to develop our skills in understanding and treating these disorders, as well as, ultimately, to prevent their occurrence.

Autonomy and Connectedness as Dimensions of the Self

Much of the content of this volume has reflected a very Western view of the self. Constructs such as self-concept, self-worth, self-enhancement, and so on, all make reference to goals that involve the maintenance of positive self-evaluations for the *individual*. As many have observed (e.g., Emde, 1994; Guisinger & Blatt, 1993; Jordan, 1991; Kim & Berry, 1993; Markus & Kityama, 1991; Sampson, 1988), the Western view of self emphasizes separateness, autonomy, independence, individualism, and distinctness. From a developmental perspective, therefore, the role of socializing agents is to ensure that their child-rearing practices encourage these characteristics. Western conceptions of the ideal adult self have also been labeled "self-reliant" (Spence, 1985) and "self-contained," if not "egocentric" (Shweder & Bourne, 1982). In contrast, most non-Western societies have adopted a more sociocentric or collectivist ideal in which self-definition is deeply embedded in the matrix of social relationships and obligations.

However, the field is beginning to witness a shift away from the dichotomous characterization of entire cultures given that it has been demonstrated to be too simplistic. Although one can broadly describe particular features of a given culture that appear on the surface to be relatively more individualistic versus collectivistic, certain contemporary theorists argue that features of both individualism and collectivism can be observed within a given culture. Among developmentalists, there has also been a change of focus with regard to the goals of development. Whereas previous formulations emphasized the importance of fostering autonomy and independence, we now see the focus shifting to a combination of autonomy and connectedness as the more appropriate pathway to healthy outcomes. This emphasis can be observed in the infancy, child, adolescent, and adult literature. Moreover, although the earlier gender literature portrayed males as autonomous and females as connected, this polarization has been found wanting.

In this chapter, the arguments for reconceptualizing culture, develop-ment, and gender to reflect the combination of autonomy and connected-ness are first reviewed. Attention then shifts to a description of our own efforts to move beyond the typical dichotomy by developing a trichotomy of styles that define the self within a relationship with spouse or partner. We have labeled these three styles as self-focused autonomy, other-focused con-nectedness, and mutuality (which reflects a balance of healthy autonomy and connectedness). Our focus has been the demonstration of individual differences within each gender. These orientations have important implica-tions for constructs heretofore discussed, namely, the ability to be one's authentic self, level of self-worth, and depressed affect. As will become evi-dent, the two extreme styles, namely, self-focused autonomy and other-focused connection, particularly in combination with the style of one's spouse or partner, can more seriously compromise the self for both men and women.

WESTERN VERSUS EASTERN VIEWS OF THE SELF

A number of scholars have argued that Western and Eastern cultures have adopted different prototypes of self and that individuals are socialized to meet a particular cultural ideal. After presenting this perspective, it will be argued that such dichotomous conceptualizations are too simplistic and do not take into account the complexities of most cultures. For those mak-ing the general distinction between Western and Eastern cultures' conceptualization of the self, the core feature of individualistic cultures is that individuals are primarily motivated to obtain personal goals. Thus, people are primarily concerned with displays of self-sufficiency, self-reliance, and autonomy. Moreover, the individual person is the defining feature of social life, in that one is not only respected for one's independence but also is ideally detached from others and protected from interference by society. In contrast, within collectivistic cultures, value is placed upon the network of social relationships (family, community, the larger society) that transcends the individual; that is, the individual is subordinated to the social system. Tradition, duty to others, hierarchy, and respect for authority are paramount. The group is the defining feature of social life, which implies that individu-als are not distinguished from the social status roles that they occupy. Indi-viduals come to view themselves as extensions of the collective, where their own welfare is subordinate to the needs of the larger social group.

Shweder and colleagues (Shweder, 1991; Shweder & Bourne, 1982; Shweder & Miller, 1991) label these two orientations as *egocentric* versus *sociocentric* and give the United States and India as respective examples of each. The Western self emerges in a context that values the privacy, autonomy, and the freedom of the individual, and in which personhood is more abstract. In contrast, in societies such as India, the person is regulated by strict rules of interdependence that are context-specific and particularistic. Findings reveal that these cultural differences are associated with differences in the nature of self-descriptions (Shweder & Miller, 1991). In India, such descriptions focus on behavioral acts that are context-dependent, namely, situated in time and place (e.g., "I bring cakes to my family on festival days"). Americans, however, emphasize situation-free personality traits and dispositional factors (e.g., "I am friendly").

Triandis (1989a, 1989b), in describing the distinction between *individualistic* and *collectivistic* cultures (as introduced by Hsu, 1983), discusses implications for the salience of private versus public selves. Triandis builds upon the assumptions that in individualistic cultures, the individual is the basic unit of society, personal goals are valued over group goals, and there is an emphasis on privacy and autonomy. However, in collectivist societies such as Japan and China, priority is given to the goals of the in-group whose belief systems one shares; within this in-group, obedience and harmony are demanded. Triandis observes that in individualistic cultures the private self is more salient than the public self; however, there is greater overlap between these two selves given the values of frankness and honesty. In collectivist cultures, the public self is more likely to be on display, and there is a greater disparity between public and private selves, since the individual presents socially desirable attributes that may be very different from his/her "true" self, behind the mask (Doi, 1986). Hart and Edlestein (1992) have provided similar cross-cultural analyses.

In focusing more specifically on how the self is construed in such cultures, Markus and Kityama (1991) have distinguished between *independent* and *interdependent* conceptions of self. The former, which characterizes the Western self, locates crucial self-representations *within* the individual, such that salient identities are quite distinct from those of others. Thus, there are clear psychological boundaries that are established between self and other. In an interdependent self-system (e.g., among the Japanese), individuals are not defined by their uniqueness but by their social connectedness to others (see also Cousins, 1989). Markus and Kityama's analysis extends to the cognitive, emotional, and motivational consequences of the culturally dependent construal of self. For example, they review findings revealing that, unlike English, the Japanese language contains *emotion* concepts that refer specifically to relational issues (Doi, 1973). Emde (1994) and colleagues have found that such terms are employed by mothers in describing the emotional expressions of their infants. Mothers report terms for "loneliness" and "seeking a person" (in Japanese, *amae*). Shaver and colleagues (Shaver, Wu, & Schwartz, 1992), in their cross-cultural studies of emotion terminology in the Chinese language, also underscore the vast number of words that refer to different dimensions of social shame. The work of Fischer, Wang, Kennedy, and Cheng (in press) reveals that there are 113 words or common phrases that native Chinese identify as strong reflections of shame and associated states.

Although such cultural differences have clearly been demonstrated, certain contemporary theorists and investigators (see Neff, 1998; Turiel & Wainryb, in press) argue that these cultural construals of self are one-sided stereotypes that fail to take into account the heterogeneity that can be observed within a given culture. Their empirical efforts reveal that cultures have more than one agenda with regard to morality and social convention. For example, these investigators take issue with the assumption that in collectivistic cultures, there is little concern with personal agency and entitlements. Many so-called collectivistic societies are very hierarchical with regard to positions of status and power. There are duties and roles within these social hierarchies, and those afforded privileged status maintain positions of dominance over subordinates that carry with them a strong sense of agency, individualism, and personal entitlement.

Their findings also reveal that in cultures labeled as collectivistic, judgments about social convention and fairness are very context-dependent. To take but one example, within the Druze culture, Turiel and Wainryb (in press) report that husbands in this traditional culture display considerable power over their wives, as do fathers in relation to their daughters. However, members of this culture do not attribute the same authority to the father in relation to a son. These distinctions can be illustrated in several domains, one being occupational choice. Thus, fathers should make such decisions for wives and daughters but not for sons, who have a right to exercise their personal choice and rights. The point of these analyses is to demonstrate those conditions and situations under which displays of behaviors more typically thought of as individualistic can be observed in collectivist cultures.

Turiel and Wainryb (in press) also perform similar analyses within Western cultures demonstrating those conditions under which individuals act in ways that support group, rather than personal, goals. Moreover, subordinates within Western societies are also compelled to define themselves in ways that reflect a more collectivist orientation given that their role within the hierarchy demands that they meet the needs of the dominants. These theorists would argue, therefore, that individualistic and collectivistics stances should not be viewed as competing orientations. Rather, both exist within a given culture, although they may be defined somewhat differently across cultures. Therefore, our task is to understand the complex social dynamics underlying the combination of styles that govern human interaction.

AUTONOMY AND CONNECTEDNESS IN WESTERN THEORIES OF DEVELOPMENT

Similar issues have emerged within the developmental literature for every stage of the life span, beginning with the period of infancy. As Jordan (1991) cogently observes, in American culture, it is imperative to transform the "helpless" and "dependent" infant into an individual who is self-sufficient and independent. She notes that these biases are so ingrained that it is difficult for us to realize that in many non-Western cultures, the newborn is considered be independent and in need of socialization toward dependency. Earlier Western theories of infant development document such assumptions. For example, in Mahler's (1968) theory, particular attention is paid to the process of differentiation or separation (from others) and individuation (of self).

Mahler built upon psychoanalytic theory, as introduced by Freud (1952), who initially discussed the general process by which the infant must come to recognize that the self is separate from mother. Mahler went on to document the sequence of stages through which the infant acquired a sense of separation and individuation. This process involves a "rapprochement crisis" in which realization of separateness is acute and provokes both anxiety and anger, given that the infant feels helpless to control the mother as well as ambivalent, given some desire to remain connected. However, during the final stage of "consolidation," the toddler is able to withstand separations from the mother and derives security from the ability to call forth a comforting image of the mother in her absence. This security, in turn, enables the older infant to pursue independent interests and to begin to acquire a distinct sense of his/her own individuality. Thus, given Mahler's focus on autonomy as a goal of development, little attention is devoted to the infant's need and desire to remain connected to significant caregivers, nor to the developmental advantages such connection might confer.

This Western perspective can also be observed in the self studies of those cognitive developmentalists (Bertenthal & Fischer, 1978; Lewis & Brooks-Gunn, 1979) who sought to document the stages of infant self-development. These investigators made inferences about this developmental trajectory on the basis of tasks that tapped infants' reactions to their image in mirrors. The first three stages chronicle the emergence of the I-self as independent agent, along with increasing differentiation of self and other. Thus, the infant comes to learn that his/her actions are independent of others, affording him/her a sense of both agency and autonomy. This knowledge, in turn, serves as a prerequisite to the development of an understanding of the Me-self as a separate *object*, with recognizable features and specific attributes that distinguish one from others. This account, therefore, empha-sizes the initial normative-developmental pathways toward independence and distinctness that have been heralded by others as the accomplishments of the Western self.

Although these accounts greatly enhance our understanding of infant development, there has been increasing dissatisfaction with formulations that have touted autonomy as the major developmental goal of the first 2 years of life, to the exclusion of connectedness. In contrast, attachment theo-rists have emphasized the importance of forming secure bonds with caregivers, as exemplified by such constructs as the "goal-corrected partnership" (Ainsworth, 1974) formed between the toddler and caregiver. In contrast to Mahler, for Ainsworth, an important goal for the toddler to achieve at 2 to 3 years of age is a greater understanding of those factors that influence the mother's behavior, allowing the child to participate in the negotiation of compromises if mother and child do not share the same agenda.

From an attachment theory perspective, both individuation and con-nectedness are essential, in combination; that is, secure social attachments with caregivers facilitate the type of exploration in the absence of parents that contributes to a sense of healthy autonomy. However, exploratory for-ays that may create doubt or anxiety in situations that are experienced as unmanageable activate the child's retreat to the caregiver, whose comforting further solidifies a sense of connectedness. More contemporary attachment theorists (see Bretherton, 1991; Cassidy, 1990; Pipp, 1990; Sroufe, 1990) also contend that the first working model to be developed is not of the self per se, but of the *relationship* between self and other. Subsequently, separate working models of self and other emerge.

Other contemporary theorists have underscored the role of connected-ness in promoting healthy infant development. For example, Stern (1985) places considerable emphasis on how the subjective self emerges from the context of intersubjective relatedness. By this, Stern means that the infant and caregiver share important experience, and such sharing is often initi-ated by the child. For example, displays of *joint attention*, the gesture of point-ing and the act of following another's line of vision, are among the first overt acts that permit inferences about the sharing of perspectives. The shar-ing of *intentions* represents another such arena in that the infant utilizes protolinguistic forms of requesting. For example, if the mother is holding a cookie, the infant will reach out, palm upward, making grasping movements and imperative intonations. Case (1991) also describes the *infant's* efforts to share aspects of mutual toy transactions with mother. For Stern, the sharing of *affective* states can also be observed. A primary example involves displays of social referencing (Campos & Stenberg, 1980; Emde, 1988). In situations of uncertainty, the infant looks to the mother to detect and utilize her affect as a guide to his/her own behavioral and affective reactions. Current theorists contend that feedback from other people as *social* mirrors is far more critical to self-development than feedback from physical mirrors (see Meltzoff, 1990). Each of these processes represents important, rudimentary forms of connectedness during infancy.

These various descriptions of mutuality converge with Emde's (1988) concept of the *we-self* that emerges in infancy. According to Emde, through reciprocal interactions with the caregiver, leading to shared meaning, a sense of "we" emerges, in addition to a sense of the I-self. The internalization of this executive we-self serves to empower the infant, to give him/her an added sense of control and to aid in self-regulation, particularly in situations in which the mother is not present. This process has features in common with the formation of an initial working model of the relationship, as described by contemporary attachment theorists. Emde's we-self, therefore, highlights the role of connectedness in combination with the autonomy that is provided through the emergence of the I-self as an active, independent agent.

The field has witnessed a similar shift in emphasis for the period of *childhood*. For example, themes of independence are paramount in Erikson's (1950, 1968) psychosocial theory of development. The establishment of trust is a goal of infancy. However, in the subsequent stages during childhood, Erikson touts the goals of *autonomy* (vs. shame), *initiative* (vs. guilt), and *industry* (vs. inferiority), all goals that focus on the independence of the individual. In his treatment of adolescence, the goal of *identity* (vs. role confusion) continues this theme as the individual searches to define "Who am I?" (not "Who are we?"). It is only at his sixth stage, during early adulthood, that themes of connectedness occur, where the developmental task is the establishment of *intimacy* (vs. isolation). However, such interrelatedness must await years of development during which one's sense of self as an independent agent is first solidified.

More recent treatments of childhood have emphasized connectedness with both peers and parents. For example, building upon Sullivan's (1953) observations of the importance of the establishment of "chumships," contemporary theorists and investigators have emphasized the importance of the close, personal friendships that are fostered during middle to later childhood (Brown, 1990; Furman & Bierman, 1984; Savin-Williams & Berndt, 1990). Such friendships are based upon the principles of loyalty and trust, emotional support, mutual understanding, and conflict resolution skills, as well as the sharing and clarification of thoughts and feelings. The focus on such forms of connectedness does not supplant the development of autonomy. Rather, they develop in tandem, in that connectedness not only cements personal bonds with others, but also provides a context in which one can learn about oneself as an individual (see also Selman & Shultz, 1990).

A number of scholars who have focused on *adolescence* have also argued that concepts such as autonomy and connectedness should not be polarized. For example, Cooper, Grotevant, and colleagues (Cooper et al., 1983; Grotevant & Cooper, 1983, 1986) emphasize that while one task of adolescence is to individuate from parents, another goal is to remain psychologically connected to the family in the process (see also Collins, 1990; Hill & Holmbeck, 1986; Moore, 1987; Steinberg, 1990). These authors contend that the developmental tasks of adolescents are made more challenging by the fact that the adolescent experiences some tension between these potentially competing goals. Cooper and Grotevant have identified particular features of individuality and connectedness in the *parents* of adolescents and then assessed their effects upon the adolescent children. They have identified two dimensions of individuality: *self-assertion*, the ability to have and communicate a point of view, and *separateness*, the use of communication patterns that express how one is different from others. They reason that it is not sufficient to possess a point of view but to actively communicate how it may be different from the position held by the adolescent, in order to serve as a role model to foster individuality.

They have also identified two dimensions of connectedness: *permeability*, openness to the views of others, and *mutuality*, the respect and support of other's opinions. Cooper and Grotevant contend that merely serving as a role model is not enough. Rather, parents must communicate their respect for their adolescent's opinions, even if they do not agree. These investigators have studied such processes in the context of actual family interaction patterns, as they affect identity formation, namely, the exploration and active consideration of alternative possibilities, sense of commitment, and faith in one's decisions. Their findings reveal that the adolescent's identity formation is facilitated by family relationships characterized by the combination of parental individuation and connectedness, which together offer a model for the construction of goals, give the adolescent permission to develop his/her own point of view, and provide a secure base from which to explore options outside the family.

In a similar vein, Allen, Hauser, Bell, and O'Connor (1994) have stressed the importance of those processes through which the adolescent can achieve autonomy while maintaining a positive relationship with parents. Behaviors reflecting autonomy have included differentiation from others, independence of thought, and self-determination in social interactions. Behaviors reflecting relatedness included interest, involvement, and validation of another person's thoughts and feelings. Their findings reveal that parental displays of autonomy and relatedness positively impact these same characteristics in the adolescent. Moreover, adolescents' displays of autonomy and relatedness, in turn, positively influence their self-esteem and their level of ego development. Deci and Ryan (1995) also observe that too often, autonomy and relatedness are viewed as competing orientations. They argue that individuation during adolescence is facilitated not by detachment from parents but rather by continued emotional attachment.

In a recent study from our own laboratory (Buddin, 1998), we built upon the model of Cooper and Grotevant, explicitly, in exploring the implications of the dimensions of parental individuation and connectedness for adolescent expression of *voice,* namely, the ability to share one's opinions with others (as described earlier in Chapter 9). We reasoned that parents who both express their own opinions clearly and are open to, as well as respectful and supportive of their teenagers' opinions, should facilitate adolescent voice. Thus, we predicted that both parental displays of individuality and connectedness would foster the highest levels of voice, and we obtained clear evidence for such an additive model. Those adolescents with parents who both modeled the clear expression of their own opinions *and* provided support for the expression of their adolescents' views, reported the highest level of voice (3.52 on a 4-point scale). In contrast, those adolescents at the other extreme, with parents who neither modeled the expression of their own opinions nor reinforced their adolescents' viewpoints, reported the lowest levels of voice (2.23). Levels of voice for the other two combinations, parental modeling without support (2.63) and parental support without modeling (3.29) fell in between. We found no evidence of significant gender differences. Rather, as in our earlier studies reported in Chapter 9, individual differences in parenting styles contributed equally to individual differences in adolescent voice for both males and females. Overall, the pattern of findings supports the importance of the combination of both models of autonomy and connectedness in fostering the healthy displays of one's opinions.

Blatt and colleagues (Blatt, 1990; Guisinger & Blatt, 1993) make a similar argument that can be applied to *adulthood.* They contend that both individuality and relatedness to others develop throughout the life span as a dialectical process. They review analyses that point to how our overemphasis on individualistic values has led to a number of liabilities, including alienation from others, narcissism, violence, and the devaluation of women. Blatt (1995) has also argued that an exaggeration of either relatedness or isolation of the self distinguishes different types of psychopathology. A distorted preoccupation with issues of interpersonal relatedness leads to what Blatt terms "anaclitic" disorders, whereas a preoccupation with issues involving isolation of the self leads to "introjective" disorders. Moreover, Blatt observes correspondences between these two orientations and the two types of insecure attachment, preoccupied and avoidant, respectively.

A similar perspective has been advanced by members of the Stone Center at Wellesley College (Jordan, 1991; Jordan et al., 1991; Miller, 1986). Their concept of "self-in-relation" makes reference to their conviction that the deepest sense of oneself is continuously formed in connection with others and is inextricably tied to growth within the relationship. While there is still a "felt sense of self," it is a "self inseparable from a dynamic interaction" (Miller, 1986). Mutual empathy is a cornerstone of this perspective. Empathy is defined as the dynamic process, involving both cognitive and affective features, of joining with and understanding another person's subjective experience. According to Jordan, mutual empathy, characterized by the flow of empathic attunement between people, alters the traditional boundaries between subject and object and thus experientially alters the sense of a separate sense, profoundly. As Jordan observes, "In true empathic exchange, each is both object and subject, mutually engaged in affecting and being affected, knowing and being known" (1991, p. 141). It is argued that one does not lose one's sense of self in such interactions. Rather, relatedness with others brings clarity and reality to the self. A major contribution of this formulation is the spotlight that it shines on connectedness. Less attention is devoted to the role of autonomy, although it is implied that mutuality represents a balance between healthy forms of autonomy and connectedness, an issue to which I return in describing our own research on adult relationship styles.

Gender Issues

The distinction between individuality or autonomy versus connectedness or relatedness has also been applied to differences in the self-system of men and women. However, as will become apparent, generalizations to the effect that men are autonomous, whereas as women are connected do not capture the complexity of these dimensions in interaction. By way of background, within the gender literature, a number of women theorists have challenged the individualistic conceptualizations of development and adaptation, models that were put forth by men and were primarily applicable to men (Chodorow, 1989; Gilligan, 1982; Miller, 1986). As Miller observes, the notion of the "self" that we inherited does not appear to characterize many women's experience. For Gilligan, issues involving interpersonal connection and the ethics of caregiving were conspicuously absent in the traditional male-dominated psychological models. These and other writers have pointed to gender differences in self-definition. Men's sense of worth is closely linked to autonomy and the sense of personal accomplishment, whereas women emphasize connectedness and sensitivity to others (Eagly, 1987; Josephs, Markus, & Tafarodi, 1992; Miller, 1986; Oyserman & Markus, 1993). Gilligan and colleagues (Gilligan et al., 1989) as well as Rubin (1985), further describe the liabilities of the different orientations adopted by women and men. Given the importance of connectedness to women, they are threatened by separation and have difficulty with individuation. In contrast, men are less likely to form close relationships and are threatened by intimacy and connectedness.

Chodorow has offered a developmental perspective on the origins of such gender differences. She observes that in families where the mother is still the primary caregiver, both male and female infants initially identify with the mother. Connection, she contends, is more difficult for boys, since they must *shift* their identification from mother to male role models, be they the father or masculine images in the culture; that is, boys must actively reject a definition of self that involves the incorporation of feminine attributes. This process fosters *differentiation* from mother, a task that is required of boys. Thus, the greater individuality of males stems from the fact that the young boy is driven to create boundaries between himself and his mother upon discovering that he is of a different gender and therefore must relinquish his earlier identification with the mother. Females, in contrast, are not impelled to reject their identification with their mothers. Rather, such identification is typically actively rewarded. Thus, connection is an easier developmental task. What is more difficult for girls, according to Chodorow's analysis, is differentiation from others based upon the fact that they were not impelled to do so during childhood. Thus, this differential pattern leads females to be more connected and males more individuated. In addition to this analysis of family dynamics, a growing literature points to differences in the socialization of girls and boys, noting that girls are socialized to be cooperative, friendly, empathic, and obedient, whereas boys are socialized to be assertive, creative, confident, and independent (see Basow, 1992; Beale, 1994; Eisenberg et al., 1996; Ruble, 1998).

Certain researchers have directly identified the links between such gender differences and self-esteem. For example, Block and Robins (1993) report that the ability to relate to others in an interpersonally positive manner promotes self-esteem in females, whereas lack of emotion, independence, and personal uninvolvement are more highly related to self-esteem in males. In their longitudinal study (ages 14 to 23), they find that males and females come to be more similar to one another over time (see also Block, 1983; Pratt, Pancer, Hunsberger, & Manchester, 1990); however, the long-recognized basic interpersonal asymmetry is still observed. Block and Robins (1993) observe that females are still socialized to "get along," whereas males are socialized to "get ahead." In this same sample, Thorne and Michaelieu (1994) examined the memories of males and females with both low and high self-esteem at age 23. High-self-esteem males recounted experiences in which they had successfully asserted themselves, whereas high self-esteem women recalled memories of wanting to help female friends. The memories of low-self-esteem men focused on failures to avoid conflict or to establish intimate relationships with girlfriends, whereas low-self-esteem women were concerned with failures to obtain approval or validation from friends.

Despite such findings, it would appear that the constructs of autonomy and connectedness have been dichotomized too sharply and have been too readily generalized to characterize the styles of men and women, respectively. Views of development that have focused solely on growth toward self-focused autonomy *or* the primacy of other-focused connection have each contributed to distortions about what constitutes healthy development. Thus, it is refreshing to observe the recent emphasis on healthy adaptation as an integration of autonomy and connectedness that has been observed within the developmental literature. As discussed earlier, there are increasing numbers of theorists and investigators who argue that a continuing developmental task involves individuation that is best achieved in a context of connectedness and ongoing transformations in relationships with significant others. However, this perspective has not been adequately applied within the gender-difference literature, where it is still commonly asserted that women are primarily connected, whereas men are primarily autonomous. Thus, we have addressed this concern in our own work to be reported here.

Autonomy and Connectedness as Self-Defining Dimensions of Adult Relationship Styles

Consistent with more contemporary frameworks, we have adopted the perspective that healthy adaptation best represents an integration of autonomy or individuality and connectedness, applying this framework to the context of one's relationship with a spouse or partner (Harter, Waters, Pettit, et al., 1997). This perspective has not been central to most treatments of the adult self, particularly where gender differences have been the focus. Rather, as the previous section revealed, there has typically been a sharp dichotomy between orientations that are *self-focused* (the more individuated style), typically associated with males, versus *other-focused* (a more connected style), usually attributed to females. According to these typologies, the self-focused individual is characterized as overly autonomous, independent, and dominating, with sharply defined boundaries between the self and others. These individuals experience discomfort with intimacy and acknowledge greater clarity about their own needs and feelings than about their partner's. In contrast, the other-focused individual is oriented toward caring and concern for others, as well as compliance, typically subordinating his/her own needs to those of the partner. As a result, there is often greater attentiveness to, and therefore, clarity about, one's partner's feelings than about one's own (Miller, 1986).

We found such a framework wanting because it defines two extreme styles, each of which would appear to have liabilities, and fails to acknowledge the possibility that healthier forms of autonomy and connectedness can be integrated in a style that is more adaptive for men as well as women. To the initial dichotomy, therefore, we have added a third style, labeled "mutuality," which we predicted would result in the most positive outcomes. Specifically, we contrasted mutuality to the two styles considered less adaptive, one in which autonomy is excessive (self-focused autonomy), and the other in which there is a distortion of connectedness (other-focused connection). It is important to appreciate the fact that mutuality is *not* the combination of the two extreme styles. Rather, it is a qualitatively different style in which much less extreme forms of autonomy and connectedness are actively balanced.

The larger goal of this research was to determine whether there were liabilities of adopting the two extreme styles. Moreover, we examined whether particular partner combinations led to better or worse correlates or outcomes. The outcomes we selected emerged from our earlier work. We were particularly interested in the ability to be one's authentic versus false self within a relationship. Given that displays of false-self behavior are typically accompanied by low self-worth and depressed affect, we included these correlates as well. Consistent with our earlier efforts, we predicted that adults would be more likely to demonstrate authentic-self behavior if they were *validated* within the partner relationship. As a general prediction, we anticipated that those displaying the *mutual* style would report greater validation from their partners, compared to those manifesting either self-focused autonomy or other-focused connection. Greater perceived validation, in turn, was predicted to result in the ability to be one's *authentic self* within the relationship and result in higher levels of self-worth and lower levels of depressed affect.

Six theoretically derived dimensions define each style (see Table 11.1), drawing heavily upon the theorizing of Miller (1986) as well as Jordan (1991; Jordan et al., 1991), who played a central role in identifying and defining these dimensions. Our perspective is consistent with that of Fitzpatrick (1988), who urges that (1) we need alternative descriptive approaches that categorize marriages on more than one or two dimensions, and that (2) the variables that define the dimensions of a marital typology must be of central theoretical importance.

Our first dimension is *dominance versus submission*. The self-focused autonomous individual feels he/she has the right to dominate the partner, assertively making decisions for both. In contrast, the other-focused, connected individual defers to the partner, adopting a subordinate stance. Those displaying mutuality neither dominate nor submit, but strive for balance, although the decision-making process may involve disagreement and com-

TABLE 11.1. Dimensions of Autonomy and Connectedness

Dimension	Self-focused autonomy	Other-focused connection	Mutuality
Dominance–submission	Dominates partner; makes decisions for both	Lets partner take the lead and make decisions for self	Discusses decisions, may disagree; seeks compromise
Needs met	Gets own needs met; feels entitled to get needs met	Puts partner's needs ahead of own; cares for others first	Tries to balance own needs with those of partner
Sensitivity	Not very attuned to partner's needs and feelings	Very sensitive; empathetic to partner's needs and feelings, but not to own	Strives to be clear about own feelings and those of partner
Clarity of feelings	Feels clearer about own needs and feelings than partner's	Uncertain, often confused about own feelings; clearer about partner's feelings	Strives to empathize with partner's feelings as well as own
Boundaries	Needs to be separate from partner; intimacy is uncomfortable	Prefers intimacy to point of being "one" with partner	Wants closeness but also separateness from one's partner
Concern with the relationship	Not concerned with relationship issues; little interest	Concerned with relationship issues	Interest in relating is balanced with other concerns

promise. Closely related is the dimension of *meeting needs*. Self-focused, autonomous individuals feel entitled to have their needs met. In contrast, other-focused, connected individuals put the needs of the partner ahead of their own. Those with a mutual style place a premium on balancing their own needs with those of the partner.

The third dimension is *sensitivity to needs and feelings*. Self-focused individuals, given their emphasis on meeting their own needs, are not that attuned to their partner's needs and feelings. In contrast, other-focused individuals are extremely sensitive to the needs of their partner, at the expense of often ignoring their own. Those displaying mutuality strive to empathize with their partner's needs and feelings, while remaining sensitive to their own. The fourth, related, dimension involves *clarity of feelings*. The self-focused individual will report greater clarity about his/her own emotions than those of the partner. Interestingly, because the other-focused individual is so attentive to the partner, he/she will be clearer about the partner's needs and feelings than about his/her own (Miller, 1986). Those displaying mutuality attempt to be clear about the partner's feelings as well as their own.

A fifth defining dimension involves the *boundaries* between self and other. The self-focused, autonomous individual needs to be psychologically separate from the partner, since emotional intimacy is experienced as uncomfortable. In contrast, those who display other-focused connection seek to weaken boundaries between the self and other, preferring intimacy to the point of being "one" with the partner. Mutual individuals maintain flexible boundaries between themselves and their partners. A closely related sixth dimension is *concern with the relationship*. The self-focused, autonomous individual shows little interest in relationship issues. In contrast, the other-focused individual dwells upon emotional aspects of the relationship. Such individuals fear abandonment by the partner and believe that by focusing intensely on the relationship, they can prevent its dissolution (Miller, 1986). Those manifesting mutuality show a healthy interest in the relationship, balanced by their investment in concerns outside of the relationship.

It should be noted that other typologies have been proposed within the marital literature. These include Burgess and Locke's (1948) distinction between institutional and companionate marriages; Snyder and Smith's (1986) empirically derived typology based upon marital satisfaction versus distress; Olson's (1981) system based upon three dimensions of communicative interaction—conflict, task leadership, and affect; Hendrick and Hendrick's (1993) typology of love styles; and Hazan and Shaver's (1987) categorization system based on attachment theory. Fitzpatrick (1988) has been critical of the majority of such typologies for several reasons. They are based upon too few dimensions, they are too intuitively derived, without specifying reliable empirical procedures for classification, they yield too many possible marital groupings, the types are not mutually exclusive, and investigators do not give sufficient attention to outcomes. Fitzpatrick has attempted to rectify many of these concerns in her own work and has developed a typology that contains several dimension in common with our own. However, her conceptual and data-analytic strategies have a very different starting point from our own. Moreover, her identification of a "traditional male style" (dominant, assertive, task-oriented) and her "traditional female style" (nurturant, sensitive, understanding) did not serve us well given that we were trying to avoid a gender-stereotyped perspective.

Thus, we developed our own methodology, building upon the theoretically derived dimensions described earlier. Our goal was to develop cameos of each of our three styles—self-focused autonomy, other-focused connectedness, and mutuality—that included each of the six dimensions defining each partner style. At the time we were developing these cameos, we were approached by a major newspaper in the Denver area that invited us to develop a survey to assess attitudes about backlash against the women's movement, as identified by Susan Faludi (1991) in her book *Backlash: The Undeclared War against Women*. They were interested in having readers respond to such a survey in order to gauge the strength of these attitudes among residents in the Denver and surrounding areas. We suggested that our relationship styles might well be related to the types of attitudes that individuals held, and as a result, we were invited to include brief versions of our cameos, as well as outcome measures in a newspaper survey to which subscribers would hope-fully respond. (I return later to the issue of the link between our relation-ship styles and backlash attitudes.)

These cameos are presented in Table 11.2. Similar procedures have been successfully employed by those investigators identifying adult attachment styles (e.g., Hazan & Shaver, 1987; Shaver & Rubenstein, 1983). With re-gard to subjects, 3,282 returned the survey. Of these, we focused initially on those (2,527) who indicated that they were currently in heterosexual rela-tionships. While an individual's perceived relationship style, were he/she not currently in a relationship, is of some interest, our primary focus was how outcomes were contingent upon the combination of styles within a relationship; that is, what combinations of partner pairings are most preva-lent, and how do these relate to outcomes? To determine these combina-tions, we asked respondents not only to identify their own style but also their partner's style.

First, we predicted that the most common pairings would be men and women who indicated that they displayed mutuality and reported that their partners also displayed the mutual style. Those seeking balance between individuality and connectedness in a relationship should ideally select part-ners who share this value. Second, we predicted that the majority of other-focused women would be paired with self-focused men. There is an initial complementary fit between such styles in that a submissive woman may well seek a dominant man or, when paired with such a male partner, she may become more submissive. Similarly, a female oriented toward putting the needs of the partner first may well attract a male who feels entitled to have his needs met, or, when paired with such a male partner, may shift toward a focus on the needs of the partner at the expense of meeting her own.

Implications for the Self

As described earlier, we have initially been interested in two correlates, *authentic-self behavior* and *perceived validation* by one's partner. The first is the ability to express what is experienced as the "real me" with one's partner. Based upon earlier work (Harter, Marold, et al., 1996; Jordan, 1991; Miller, 1986), we hypothesized that the ability to be one's authentic self within the relationship would be directly related to whether one experienced *validation* by one's partner. We advanced hypotheses about the level of perceived vali-dation and authentic-self behavior for particular partner *combinations* that

TABLE 11.2. Cameo Descriptions That Define the Three Relationship Styles:
Self-Focused Autonomy, Other-Focused Connection, and Mutuality

Relationship style	Cameo description
Self-focused autonomy	I am able to get what I want in this relationship and feel that I have the right to do so. I assume that my partner values me. It's pretty natural for me to make decisions in this relationship, and I express my opinions forcefully. I don't feel the need to talk that much about my relationship. In fact, emotional closeness can sometimes make me feel uncomfortable. Sometimes it's hard for me to understand my partner's emotions, but I'm usually clear about what I think and feel.
Other-focused connection	I see myself as a caring and sensitive person, and tend to ensure that my partner's needs are met first. I usually go along with decisions that my partner makes, although this means that sometimes I feel like my point of view isn't valued. I think a lot about my relationship with my partner, because it's important to me. I thrive on intimacy and feeling emotionally close. At times, I pay more attention to my partner's thoughts and needs than I do to my own.
Mutuality	I work to balance my own needs with those of my partner. When it comes to making decisions, I try to discuss options with my partner, which means that we sometimes disagree. However, I generally feel valued in my relationship in the same way that I value my partner. It's important that I feel connected to my partner, so I work to be as clear about my partner's feelings as I am about my own. Although it is sometimes a challenge to consider both of our needs, it is worth it.

were of theoretical interest and that we anticipated would be relatively common. We predicted that other-focused women who perceived their partners to be self-focused men would feel least validated and therefore would report the lowest level of true-self behavior compared to females in any other combination of partner styles. Such women are paired with dominating men who, by definition, strive to meet their *own* needs and are less sensitive to their partner's needs and feelings, characteristics that preclude validation. Moreover, other-focused women paired with self-focused men adopt a submissive stance that may not invite validation. This should contribute to their inability to be their authentic selves. As Miller (1986) cogently argues, subordination and authenticity are totally incompatible, since subordinate women compromise their own needs. We advanced this prediction for other-focused *women* paired with self-focused *men*. However, it was of empirical interest to determine if other-focused *men* paired with self-focused *women* would manifest the same pattern. If so, it would suggest that the interpersonal dynamics of these styles are critical determinants of these outcomes.

In contrast, we predicted that *mutual* individuals who reported that their partner also displayed the mutual style would report the *highest* levels of validation from their partners. Not only do such individuals have partners who are, by definition, attuned to their needs and feelings, but also they value these relationship goals and are therefore appropriately seeking validation as well as attempting to reciprocate. Such individuals should also report the highest levels of authentic-self behavior, to the extent that one's real self is being validated.

The pattern of correlates for those self-focused, autonomous men reporting other-focused female partners was more difficult to predict. The fact that self-focused men feel *entitled* to have their needs met, in reality, may well lead to expectations that cannot be fulfilled. Miller (1986) describes the eventual disappointment that both dominants and subordinates may experience in such relational pairings. To the extent that such men feel less validated, they should also report lower levels of authentic-self behavior. We expected that self-focused, autonomous *men* paired with other-focused, connected *women* would be a much more common pattern than self-focused, autonomous females paired with other-focused males. The former pairing is a more heavily scripted combination in our society. However, it was of interest to determine whether the predicted pattern for validation and authentic-self behavior would also be obtained for the latter, less traditional pairing. Finding a similar pattern would underscore the role of the *psychological* processes of validation and authentic-self behavior that may transcend gender itself.

Newspaper Survey

The three cameos presented in Table 11.2 appeared in one of the two major newspapers in Denver, the *Rocky Mountain News*. Approximately 4,000 people mailed the survey back to us. Readers were asked to endorse the cameo that best reflected their *own* relationship style. If they had a partner, they reported their perception of his/her style. Validation and authentic-self measures were adapted from existing instruments that we had developed to assess these constructs in adolescents and adults. Given the space limitations of a newspaper survey, we selected the two items that contributed the most to the internal consistency of each subscale in previous research. This section of the survey was entitled "What I am Like." Questions were written in the structured alternative format we have designed to reduce the tendency to give socially desirable responses (Harter, 1982a). An example of a *validation* support item is "Some people feel that their partner values them for who they are as a person BUT Other people wish that their partner valued them a lot more than they do." The respondent first decides which of the two statements is *Most like you* and then indicates if this description is only *Sort of true* or *Really true*. Items are scored on a 4-point scale in which an endorsement of *Really true* for the more positive description would receive a score of 4, a *Sort of true* response for the more positive description would receive a score of 3, a *Sort of true* response for the more negative description would receive a 2, and *Really true* for the negative description would receive a 1. A sample item from the authentic-self subscale reads as follows: "Some people are able to be themselves with their partner BUT Other people find it difficult to be themselves with their partner." Scoring followed the same pattern. (The internal consistency reliabilities for these two-item subscales were .77 for perceived validation and .78 for the authentic-self behavior, quite acceptable given the very small number of items.)

Who Pairs with Whom?

Respondents were able to identify their own and their partner's relationship orientations, although it should be emphasized that we assessed *perceptions* of the partner's style. The finding that mutual individuals reported partners of the same style suggests that those seeking a balance between autonomy and connectedness select partners who also value such a combination. Alternatively, individuals reporting mutuality may encourage partners with a different relationship style to shift toward the more mutual orientation. The finding that other-focused, connected women were more likely to be paired with self-focused, autonomous men suggests that an other-focused woman, who is submissive and oriented toward meeting the needs of the partner, may well seek or attract a self-focused male who is dominating, and who feels entitled to have his needs met. Thus, the initial complementarity of these two patterns would appear to lead to such a match (see also Fitzpatrick, 1988). Another contributing factor may be that such individuals are drawn to each other, since the partner may display admirable characteristics that one feels are lacking in oneself (Lerner, 1989). It should be noted that this traditional, scripted pairing was more common than the mirror image (i.e., other-focused men with self-focused women). Thus, we found some support for stereotypical gender patterns in relationships. Our findings may well represent an underestimation of more societally scripted gender roles, however, given that the sample was not random.

Despite finding fewer other-focused men than women, 50.5% of such men reported having self-focused women partners, suggesting that we should not overgeneralize and identify a given style with a particular gender. Moreover, the less stereotypical pairing reveals that irrespective of gender, many individuals who are other-focused are attracted to self-focused individuals as partners. Therefore, it seems that dominants and subordinates (male or female) will be attracted to each other. An exception to this pattern was that self-focused *women* were not likely to report other-focused male partners. Approximately 60% of such women reported that their male partners were also self-focused. Thus, rather than seeking completion through association with a male partner whose characteristics complement their own, self-focused women appear to favor partners who share their attributes, and who can perhaps support their pursuit of a style that challenges traditional female-gender stereotypes.

How Partner Support Influences the Ability to Be Oneself

Findings confirmed our hypothesis that *other-focused* individuals with self-focused partners would feel *least* validated and would therefore also report the lowest levels of authentic-self behavior, (as can be seen in Figure 11.1). Not only should the self-focused partner's attributes contribute to lack of validation, but also the submissive stance of other-focused individuals may not invite validation. Therefore, the evidence supports Miller's (1986) claim that transforming one's own needs in the service of pleasing a partner necessarily involves the suppression of one's authentic self within that relationship.

Why should other-focused individuals remain in a relationship with little validation or opportunity to be one's authentic self? There is increasing evidence (see Gilligan et al., 1989; Jordan et al., 1991; Lerner, 1993; Miller, 1986; Stiver & Miller, 1988) that other-focused *women* are fearful that to act on their own needs and desires would cause conflict and threaten the relationship, leading to abandonment, in the extreme. Gilligan finds this to be a particularly compelling motive leading certain females, beginning in adolescence, to "silence their voices," one powerful manifestation of suppression of the authentic self. Other-focused women may also remain with self-focused male partners, because to do otherwise would disrupt the *balance* in the relationship, which may ultimately lead to its dissolution, an intolerable threat for other-focused, connected women (Lerner, 1989). Paradoxically, the other-focused style actually reflects *disconnection*, since one sacrifices genuine connection with one's partner, as well as with one's self, in order to preserve the relationship, albeit in a less than adaptive form. Such individuals are "being *for* others" rather than being *with* others in the relationship (Miller, 1986).

Findings also supported the prediction that partners who both identify with the mutuality style would report the highest levels of perceived validation and authentic-self behavior. Such individuals have, as one relationship goal, mutual validation, which in turn would appear to allow them to be

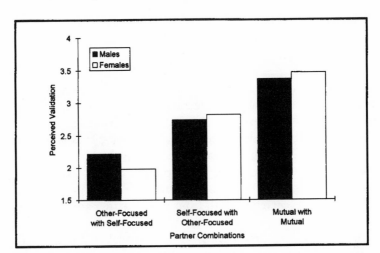

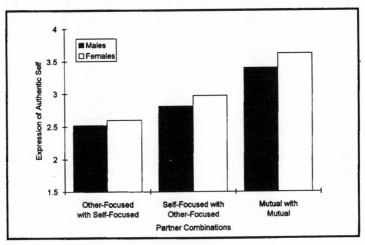

FIGURE 11.1. Perceived validation and authentic-self behavior as a function of relationship style.

their authentic self within the relationship. The results also supported the expectation that self-focused, autonomous men with other-focused, connected female partners would report less validation and authentic-self behavior than mutual individuals with mutual partners, but greater validation and authentic-self behavior than other-focused women with self-focused male partners. Although their partners seek to validate them, self-focused individuals' sense of entitlement may well lead to expectations that cannot be realistically fulfilled. Moreover, if the other-focused woman comes to realize that her self-focused male partner is not adequately meeting her needs, she may become less validating of her partner, leading him to feel unappreciated.

One's style may also influence the goals of the validation process. A self-focused male may desire support for *instrumental* accomplishments, which would be interpreted as validating. However, his other-focused female partner may encourage intimacy and the expression of emotions by her partner, which is not likely to be experienced as validating by self-focused men. Not only does the self-focused individual require boundaries *between* self and other but also he/she must create boundaries *within* the self that serve to suppress the expression of intimate emotions that are too threatening to experience or display. Thus, the self-focused relationship style also represents a form of *disconnection*, both from one's partner and from certain aspects of the self.

These dynamics may further contribute to relationship difficulties that preclude mutual validation, leading the woman to escalate her demands, which in turn causes the male to withdraw and become even more psychologically distant. As one female subject in such a relationship wrote, "My spouse is very closed-mouthed. He never seems to feel or express emotion. I press for more intimacy, try to get him to share thoughts and feelings, because I feel he is not *connecting*, is not *involved*, and this makes him even more distant! It's a no-win situation." This very pattern corroborates what has in the marriage literature been labeled as either the "demand–withdraw" or the "pursuit–withdraw" interactional pattern (Christensen, 1988; Christensen & Heavey, 1990; Floyd & Markman, 1983; Gottman & Krokoff, 1989; Heavey, Layne, & Christensen, 1993; Jacobson, 1989; Markman & Kraft, 1989). Such a pattern typically arises when women want greater intimacy and demand such a change, typically through complaints, whereas men want greater autonomy, which they attempt to achieve through withdrawal.

Not only did self-focused *males* with other-focused *female* partners report only moderate levels of validation and true-self behavior, but also the same pattern was obtained for self-focused *females* with other-focused *male* partners. These findings also highlight the need to consider the underlying psychological processes governing dyadic interactions, rather than viewing the outcomes as a product of gender differences per se. The importance of focusing on such dynamics can further be appreciated by examining the perceived validation and authentic-self scores of those other-focused individuals paired with either those displaying *mutuality* or the same *other-focused* style. In contrast to other-focused individuals with self-focused partners, such individuals report markedly higher levels of perceived validation and authentic-self behavior (see Harter, Waters, Pettitt, et al., 1997). Two other-focused partners, as well as an other-focused individual with a mutual partner, share common values about the primacy of the relationship and the importance of understanding and meeting the other's needs, all of which would contribute to a sense of validation and the permission to be one's authentic self.

Among the many interesting avenues to pursue is the issue of whether particular styles are attracted to one another or whether the particular style of an individual can *influence* the style of the partner (e.g., Do self-focused males select or transform females into other-focused partners?). More generally, what changes in styles are observed over time? In our pilot sample, 20% reported that their style had changed. One woman described the shift from other-focused to mutuality: "In the past I was definitely so concerned with his needs that I did not know my own needs. Now I work hard on staying 'healthy,' which has involved becoming much more aware of my needs and feelings *and* being true to them." A male subject wrote about his transformation from a self-focused style to mutuality. "Compromise and understanding do not require loss of self-image. Goal orientation can change to awareness of common needs and a new sense of common direction. Love and acceptance can result in some vulnerability, but it is worth it." Therefore, in future research, it will be of interest to study such shifts over time.

A related issues involves whether, at any given point in time, one's style is context specific. We do not view these styles as either categorically trait-like or situation-specific. For some individuals, their style may remain consistent across contexts, to the extent that the relational demands remain similar. For others, there may be variations across context. Waters (1993), for example, found that many individuals reported different styles in the workplace, compared to with their partner if their status as an equal, a dominant, or a subordinant within each context changed. For example, individuals who are dominating and self-focused with their partners may become more other-focused on the job if their work position is relatively low in the employment pecking order. Other-focused individuals with the partner relationship may become more mutual in the workplace if co-workers are relative equals. Thus, the relational dynamics within a given context will contribute to the stylistic attributes that one displays.

As noted at the outset, this research was made possible by the invitation of a prominent newspaper in the Denver area, the *Rocky Mountain News*, to develop a survey for their readership on backlash, as defined by Susan Faludi (1991). Faludi's basic argument is that a variety of societal factions have accused the women's movement of creating negative consequences for women, men, children and families, and society as a whole. For example, it has been claimed that the women's movement has been damaging to women's mental health, has caused them to compromise their femininity, and has led them to occupational choices that do not bode well for the upbringing of their children. Some backlash advocates have implied or asserted that women's greater contribution to the workforce, including entry into such professions as law, medicine, and business, has deprived men of the jobs that they rightfully deserve. Another argument is that the women's movement has weakened the moral fiber of the nation.

We wrote items to capture these sentiments and asked respondents to endorse their level of agreement. We anticipated that men and women displaying particular relationship styles would be more likely to endorse backlash attitudes. Specifically, we anticipated that self-focused men, who represent a more traditional stance about the role of men in this society, may be less sanguine about the emergence of women in the workplace and on the political scene. However, it is critical that one not place the onus of backlash just on men. There are women, we anticipated, who also hold backlash attitudes. We expected that women who may hold more traditional, stereotypical values about their role, namely, those endorsing the other-focused, connected style, may also have negative attitudes toward the women's movement and would therefore be more likely to want to turn the clock back to an era in which gender roles were more clearly defined.

The findings supported our expectations (Waters & Harter, 1998). Men who identified with the self-focused, autonomous style endorsed backlash attitudes, as did women who endorsed the other-focused style of connectedness. Men and women endorsing the mutual style were least likely to endorse backlash attitudes. Moreover, women who reported that they matched the self-focused, autonomous description also did not endorse backlash attitudes. Many of these women were quite successful at work and presumably supported the goals of the women's movement. Thus, while our styles are predictive of qualities within the relationship, as anticipated, they also have larger ramifications in terms of attitudes toward societal movements.

Links to Self-Worth and Depression

To address the link between validation and authentic-self behavior more directly, we put forth a process model in which we first postulated that across all individuals in the sample, perceived validation by one's partner would be correlated with the expression of authentic-self behavior within the relationship. Second, we predicted that authentic-self behavior in turn would mediate two other variables of interest, global self-worth and mood, along a dimension of *cheerful* to *depressed*. Contributing to the impact on self-worth should be the sense that if one's true characteristics are not appreciated, then one will assume that there is something wrong with the self (Eichenbaum & Orbach, 1983; Miller, 1986). As described in Chapter 9, our previous findings with adolescents have revealed that there is a strong relationship between authentic-self behavior with parents and peers and self-worth (Harter, Marold, et al., 1996). Those who feel that they can display their true selves in parent and peer relationships report high levels of self-esteem, whereas those driven, through lack of support, to engage in false-self behavior report low levels of self-worth.

The prediction that lack of validation and the inability to be one's authentic self should not only lead to low self-worth but to depressed affect was based on considerable research that demonstrates strong links between self-esteem and affect, as revealed in previous chapters. Among our normative samples (see Harter, 1990a, 1993; Harter, Marold, et al., 1992; Renouf & Harter, 1990), we have found that the correlation between self-reported depressed affect and self-esteem ranges from .70 to .80. These findings are consistent with the clinical literature in which self-deprecatory ideation has consistently been linked to depression (Beck, 1987; Bibring, 1953; Blatt, 1974; Kovaks & Beck, 1978; Seligman & Peterson, 1986). Theorists sharing the Stone Center perspective have also argued that lack of validation and the inability to be one's authentic self should not only result in devaluation of the self but also loss of self and accompanying feelings of depression (Jordan, 1991; Stiver & Miller, 1988).

Path-analytic findings (see Figure 11.2) provided strong support for such a model. In addition to direct paths from perceived validation by one's partner and authentic-self behavior, as well as from authentic-self behavior to self-esteem and mood, there were small, direct paths from validation to both self-worth and mood. The fact that the path from validation to authentic self was stronger than the paths from authentic self to either self-worth or

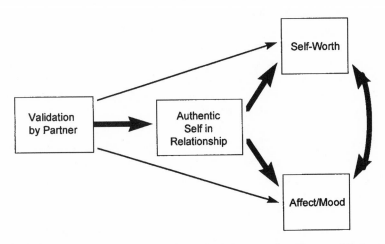

FIGURE 11.2. Process model of the effects of validation and authentic-self behavior on self-worth and affect/mood.

mood may well reflect how these constructs were operationalized; that is, both validation and authentic self were defined within the context of the relationship. Self-worth and mood, in contrast, were not defined contextually. Our research since this study on the construct of "relational self-worth" (as described in Chapter 7) has revealed that adolescents report different perceptions of their worth as a person in different interpersonal contexts. Thus, in future work with adults, it will be important to inquire into self-worth as well as mood *within the relationship*. We anticipate that validation and authenticity would be even more predictive of self-worth and mood defined within the context of the relationship with one's partner.

CONCLUSION

The Western view of self has typically held as an ideal the characteristics of autonomy, independence, separateness, individualism, and distinctiveness, in contrast to an Eastern self more deeply embedded in collectivist cultures that emphasize social roles within a hierarchy and subordination of the self to group goals. Within Western societies, socialization toward an autonomous, independent self have represented the predominant theme in developmental accounts of child rearing until recently. Many contemporary theorists argue that the healthiest pathway is one that fosters a combination of autonomy and connectedness to others. This chapter reviewed how such a perspective has been introduced for every period of the life span, namely, infancy, childhood, adolescence, and adulthood. Moreover, in the cross-cultural literature, it has been demonstrated that features of autonomy and connectedness can be demonstrated within given cultures. Thus, the dichotomization of entire cultures as either individualistic or collectivistic has been found to be too simple a characterization.

Similarly, the polarization of genders, where males are depicted as autonomous, whereas females are viewed as connected, has been found wanting. In our own research, we have examined these issues within the framework of features defining the self within a relationship with spouse or partner. We have moved beyond a dichotomous typology that captures the extreme features of orientations defined as either autonomous or connected to consider a trichotomy in which we have added *mutuality* as a style that integrates healthy forms of autonomy and connectedness. Moreover, we have been interested in particular partner combinations, including outcomes, such as the ability to be one's authentic self. Findings supported our hypothesis that certain partner combinations, for example, self-focused, autonomous individuals paired with an other-focused, connected style, would represent liabilities for the other-focused partners. Specifically, we found that other-focused partners in such a relationship felt less validated by their partners, which in turn led to the suppression of their true selves. Mutual individuals who are paired with mutual partners fare the best in terms of feeling validated, as well as being more authentic within the relationship. Moreover, our process model reveals that those who cannot demonstrate true-self behavior with a partner or spouse report lower self-worth and more depressed affect. Thus, there are liabilities associated with the more extreme relationship styles in which self-focused autonomy or other-focused connectedness predominate. Across the various literatures addressing these issues, there would appear to be consensus that a healthy combination of autonomy and connectedness will lead to the most adaptive outcomes across the life span.

CHAPTER TWELVE

Interventions to Promote Adaptive Self-Evaluations

By evolutionary design, the self should perform many positive functions, and for the majority of individuals, such processes do serve organizational, motivational, and protective purposes. However, for others, the genetic and environmental throw of the dice has rendered them less fortunate, making it difficult for a faltering self-system to provide these functions. Moreover, the natural liabilities of self-development can be exacerbated for children who may lack particular abilities and/or experience caregivers who are critical, harshly conditional in their support, neglectful, or rejecting. As a result, we observe numerous children and adolescents who possess unfavorable representations of themselves. In this last chapter, potential interventions to foster more adaptive self-evaluations are addressed. These suggestions build upon the major themes of this volume, namely, that the self is both a cognitive and social construction, and in so doing provide a summary and application of the issues addressed in the preceding chapters.

As a *cognitive* construction, the self-portrait will be profoundly impacted by the particular cognitive-developmental level at which the individual is operating. These normative, age-dependent cognitive processes define, as well as constrain, the particular agentic role that the I-self plays in constructing the Me-self, dictating the various *structural* features that the Me-self assumes at different developmental levels. However, at any given developmental level, there will be individual differences in those cognitive processes that contribute to the *valence* of one's self-representations. These include (1) the ability to discount the importance of domains in which an individual is unsuccessful, (2) the extent to which individuals can make *realistic* self-evaluations, (3) perceptions regarding the stability or malleability of one's self-representations, and (4) personal metatheories about the particular *causes* of personal perceptions of self, as well as directionality of effects. As a *social* construction, self-representations will also be shaped by treatment at the hands of caregivers and other socializing agents. Thus, the particular child-rearing and socialization practices that an individual experiences will be responsible for many of the vast individual differences that can be observed in the content and the valence of self-evaluations. This chapter first describes potential interventions that involve cognitive factors impacting the valence of self-representations, followed by a discussion of intervention strategies that focus on those social factors that influence self-evaluations. Finally, suggestions for effective program evaluation are offered.

GENERAL ISSUES IN PLANNING AN INTERVENTION

Two general issues must be considered before examining potential intervention strategies, namely, the importance of identifying the particular *target* of an intervention, as well as specifying a *model* of the causes and correlates of the self-representations in question. With regard to the first issue, the target of an intervention, should one identify the self-evaluations themselves as the target, for example, by attempting to enhance global self-worth directly, or should one focus primarily on improving actual skills in particular domains? There has been some debate about this issue, particularly within the field of education where various programs have been designed to maintain or enhance academic self-concept and global self-esteem or self-worth. The goals of these different educational programs reflect two competing orientations toward change. As Caslyn and Kenny (1977) have noted, "self-enhancement" theorists believe that efforts should focus on enhancing self-concept and self-esteem directly, for example, by giving students affectively based exercises that encourage them to feel good about themselves. In contrast, "skills" theorists argue that attitudes about the self are consequences of successful achievement and thus pedagogical efforts should be directed toward enhancing specific academic skills. In recent years, the pendulum has clearly shifted toward the skills learning orientation in which interventions target specific domains.

Elsewhere (Harter, 1988a, 1990c), I have suggested the usefulness of distinguishing between the *goal* of a program (e.g., enhanced self-esteem) and the *target* of our interventions, arguing that while self-esteem enhancement may be a goal, intervention strategies should be directed at its *determinants*. For example, attempts to impact global self-worth should first identify the specific *causes* of perceived overall worth as a person, in the design of interventions to ameliorate these causes which should, in turn, enhance global feelings of worth. Attempts to improve competence in domains of importance or to teach social skills that may allow the child to garner more support are examples of such strategies that are derived from our own model. Based on the lack of the success of the more general, affectively based programs in the 1960s and 1970s, it appears that efforts to enhance the child's self-worth *directly* will have little impact, particularly given certain cognitive-developmental limitations during childhood that will preclude the effectiveness of such a strategy (see Harter, 1988a). These limitations are discussed.

Others have offered similar arguments. Greenberg et al. (1995) hypothesize that by encouraging the acquisition of skills and creative achievement, such activities may, as a by-product, produce higher self-esteem that is also more stable. In his meta-analysis of a variety of program interventions, Hattie (1992) concludes that cognitively based programs are consistently and significantly more effective than affectively based programs (see also Strein, 1988). Hattie suggests that the cognitively oriented interventions target smaller, more definable goals that are also more amenable to measurement. Marsh shares this perspective, noting that interventions directed at impacting particular domains, and that are assessed at the domain-specific level, will be the most successful. For example, in his own work, he finds that academic interventions have substantial effects on the academic components of the self-concept but little effect on nonacademic components and vice versa (Craven, Marsh, & Debus, 1991; Hattie & Marsh, 1996; Marsh & Peart, 1988). Bracken (1996) has also argued that the lack of success of certain intervention programs is due to the fact that global self-concept is insufficiently sensitive to specific treatments. Thus, he recommends interventions that directly address the various self-concept components. Given the hierarchical nature of both the Marsh and Bracken models, one would infer that global self-concept at the apex would be enhanced as well, although not to the same degree.

The effectiveness of any intervention effort also hinges on the a priori specification of a *model* that will serve as a guide, since it will clarify the particular causes that represent the targets of the intervention. For example, in our own work (as described in Chapter 8), we have developed a theoretically derived model of the causes and correlates of global self-worth. Thus, we identified two general antecedents, competence or adequacy in domains of importance (from James' formulation on the causes of self-esteem) and approval from significant others (from Cooley's looking-glass-self formulation). Initially we identified five domains: Scholastic Competence, Behavioral Conduct, Physical Appearance, Peer Likability, and Athletic Competence. Sources of support have included peer and parental support.

In addition to specifying potential determinants of global self-worth, we sought to identify certain *correlates* as well. Considerable research, including our own work, has indicated that global self-worth or esteem is highly related to markers for depression, including depressed affect and hopelessness. As noted in Chapter 8, these constructs are so highly intercorrelated that in our own work we have combined them into a depression/adjustment composite. Thus, self-worth, affect or mood (depressed to cheerful), and hopelessness (hopeless to hopeful) are the outcomes we have sought to predict, where domain-specific self-evaluations and perceived approval have been identified as the key predictors. Suicidal ideation, in turn, is predicted by the depression/adjustment composite (see Figure 8.2).

As described in Chapter 8, perceptions of competence/adequacy in the cluster of peer-salient domains (Physical Appearance, Peer Likability, Athletic Competence) yield strong paths to peer approval, which in turn impact the depression/adjustment composite. There is also a direct path from this cluster to the outcome composite of self-worth, affect, and hopelessness. Perceptions of competence/adequacy in the cluster of more parent-salient domains, namely, Scholastic Competence and Behavioral Conduct, manifest strong paths to parental approval which, in turn, impact the depression/adjustment composite. There is also a direct path from this cluster to the composite of outcomes. The cross-paths from peer-salient domains to parent support, and from parent-salient domains to peer support, are smaller in magnitude. This model specifies our *general* expectation for how perceptions of competence or adequacy in different domains, in combination with social support, will impact global self-worth, as well as its correlates. As such, it identifies potential targets for intervention.

However, inspection of individual profiles reveals that not every potential pathway in the model is manifest for a given child or adolescent. Thus, while theoretically driven models, supported by empirical evidence, may document relationships among predictors and outcomes for larger groups of youth, these pathways may not speak to the specific precursors of low self-worth and their correlates for particular individuals. As described in Chapter 8, some children and adolescents with negative evaluations of their overall personal worth may report that they feel inadequate in the peer-salient domains and that they lack peer approval; however, they report relatively high levels of both perceived adequacy in the parent-salient domains and indicate that they have high levels of parental support. Conversely, other profiles reveal the opposite pattern in that low scores are reported for both parent-salient domains and parental support, whereas perceptions of competence/adequacy in the peer-salient domains, as well as perceived peer support, are high. The detection of such profiles led to a more systematic empirical attempt to document the multiple pathways to low self-worth and its correlates (Harter & Whitesell, 1997). As reported in Chapter 8, we identified six different profiles that captured the majority of subjects reporting the combination of low self-worth, depressed affect, and hopelessness.

These findings are important in their implications for intervention. For many at risk for depressive symptomatology, there are very specific pathways to these outcomes that require identification; that is, an intervention strategy for a depressed adolescent who feels inadequate in the domains of Physical Appearance, Peer Likability, and Athletic Competence, and who lacks peer support, would need to be quite different from the strategy with another adolescent whose pathway to depression reflects feelings of inadequacy in the domains of Scholastic Competence and Behavioral Conduct, and who lacks parental support. The same intervention will not be appropriate for both. Thus, interventions need to be tailored to the specific constellation of predictors displayed by a given individual if they are to be maximally effective. One intervention will not fit all.

Not all theorists would support the type of model that we have developed, where self-worth or personal esteem plays a central role. There are those who would question the importance of self-esteem, contending that the focus on perceptions of global worth has been misguided. For example, Damon (1995) and Seligman (1993) have been critical of what they consider to be an overemphasis by educators and clinicians on promoting high self-esteem among our youth or among depressed individuals, particularly when these efforts lead to an inflated sense of esteem. Damon views such efforts as not only misguided but also possibly detrimental, arguing that they divert educators from teaching skills and deprive students of the thrill of actual accomplishment. It is Damon's contention that self-esteem has become an overrated commodity and that the effusive praise that parents or teachers heap on children to make them feel good is often met with suspicion by children; moreover, it interferes with the goal of building specific skills in the service of genuine achievement. In a similar vein, Seligman argues that self-esteem is merely an epiphenomenon, a reflection that one's commerce with the world is going badly, with little explanatory power in and of itself. He contends that if it becomes a focal point in treatment, it will distract clinicians from identifying the more specific causes of psychological problems such as depression.

At one level, global self-esteem or self-worth would appear to have little explanatory power, since as a mediator, it has been causally implicated in so many different child and adolescent problem behaviors, including depression and suicide, eating disorders, antisocial behaviors and delinquency (most recently, gang membership), as well as teen pregnancy (see Mecca, Smelser, & Vasconcellos, 1989, who review evidence on the links between self-esteem and these problem behaviors). Thus, we do not now understand what specific forces lead one individual with low self-worth to terminate his/her *own* life, while another, with an eating disorder, will put his/her life at risk; still another may terminate someone *else's* life (as in gang shootings), and yet another, through pregnancy, will create a *new* life. Knowing that a child or adolescent has low self-esteem or self-worth, therefore, will not allow us to predict which *particular* outcome will ensue.

However, it is very important to emphasize that in our zeal for parsimonious explanatory models, we must not ignore the fact that the *phenomenological* self-theory as experienced by children, adolescents, and adults is not necessarily parsimonious. Self-evaluations, including global self-worth, are very salient constructs in one's working model of self and, as such, can wield powerful influences on affect and behavior. Thus, the challenge is to develop models that identify the specific antecedents of different outcomes, while preserving the critical role of self-representations as phenomenological mediators. This perspective, although not embraced by all theorists in the field, will serve as a framework for the intervention strategies recommended.

The term "strategies" is employed to specify particular *principles* drawn from the material presented in this volume. Specific intervention techniques are not addressed, since there can be different types of interventions that may accomplish similar goals, depending upon the preferences and skills of those designing a program to affect self-perceptions. A wide variety of specific approaches exists in the field today (see the chapter contributions in Brinthaupt & Lipka, 1994). For example, there are more traditional therapeutic approaches based upon behavior-modification interventions (see Kendall, 1991), cognitive therapy (e.g., Beck, 1976; Seligman, 1993), rational therapy (e.g., Ellis, 1958; Zastrow, 1994), and psychoanalytic interventions (e.g., Wexler, 1991) based upon the formulation of Kohut. Other interventions, reviewed by Brinthaupt and Lipka, involve direct attempts to teach particular skills that will eventually alter children's self-concepts. On the educational front, broader strategies are emerging, for example the "ecological approach" (Beane, 1994), in which there is an attempt to alter features of the general school environment such that it provides a more self-enhancing atmosphere (e.g., shifting from an emphasis on external control to self-direction). There are also more circumscribed programs, where the focus may be on art or dance experiences, Ropes courses, Outward Bound experiences, job training, and so forth. The present chapter does not recommend any particular technique. Rather, the focus is on intervention strategies (outlined in Table 12.1) in the form of goals to be achieved by program designers' preferred techniques, which may lead to more adaptive self-functioning. Clearly, there is a need for research to determine which specific techniques lead to the desired goals to be described.

TABLE 12.1. Summary of Intervention Strategies

Intervention strategies directed at cognitive determinants
1. Reduction of discrepancies between aspirations and perceived adequacy
2. Encouragement of relatively accurate self-evaluations
3. The potential for change in the valence of self-representations
4. Attention to individuals' own theories about the causes of their self-representations

Intervention strategies directed at social factors influencing self-evaluations
1. Provisions to increase approval support
2. Internalization of the positive opinions of others

INTERVENTION STRATEGIES DIRECTED AT COGNITIVE DETERMINANTS

Reduction of Discrepancies between Aspirations and Perceived Adequacy

As described in Chapters 6 and 8, James' model of global self-esteem, as well as frameworks that highlight the relationship between real and ideal self-concepts, emphasize the discrepancy between an individual's aspirations and his/her actual accomplishments. The larger the discrepancy, the more negative the perceptions of global worth as a person. Thus, interventions to reduce this discrepancy should serve to enhance feelings of self-worth. There are two potential strategies in this regard. The first is to identify arenas (e.g., academic competence, behavioral conduct) in which there are such discrepancies and implement interventions to improve the skills in those areas. Improved skills should lead to enhanced perceptions of competence or adequacy, thereby reducing the discrepancy. In turn, global self-worth should become more positive. As discussed in Chapter 6, there may be natural limits on the extent to which a given can improve. However, any gains should have a corresponding effect in reducing the discrepancy.

A second strategy focuses on the *importance* component of the discrepancy; that is, interventions that help the individual highlight the importance of arenas in which he/she is skillful and discount those in which he/she is unsuccessful or feels inadequate will serve to reduce discrepancies, which in turn should enhance self-worth. It should be noted that one does not have to be a superstar in the decathlon of life in order maintain high evaluations of one's overall worth as a person. Rather, an individual needs a certain number of domains in which there is a congruence between relatively high levels of success and the value placed upon these activities. It is hoped that the importance of those arenas in which one is less talented can be appropriately discounted. The goal, therefore, is actively opting to spend more psychological time in those life niches where favorable self-appraisals are more common and avoiding arenas in which one feels inadequate.

This same analysis can be applied to the concept of *relational self-worth*, introduced in Chapter 7. The ability to construct different perceptions of one's worth as a person in different relationships may have protective benefits. Our evidence reveals that for the majority of adolescents, there are particular contexts in which individuals report higher self-worth, which is also associated with greater support from the significant others in that context. Thus, an adaptive strategy is to inhabit such domains, either in action or in thought, with greater frequency than contexts in which there is less support and therefore a more negative appraisal of personal worth.

Moreover, one can come to *value* the more supportive contexts, allowing the sense of worth in that interpersonal sphere to generalize to perceptions of *global* self-worth. It is important to appreciate the fact that the concept of global self-worth is not to be laid to rest in the contemporary shift to contextual and multidimensional frameworks. As observed in Chapter 7, such a conceptual burial is unlikely given that global self-worth remains a phenomenological reality in the lives of individuals. There is a voluminous literature on its numerous and meaningful correlates. Of interest in our own data (Harter, Waters, & Whitesell, 1998) is the finding that for the vast majority of individuals, self-worth in one particular relational context is much more highly predictive of global self-worth than is their relational self-worth scores in all other contexts. The specific domain occupying this position varies from adolescent to adolescent. Interestingly, for many adolescents, the relational self-worth score in that particular context is higher than in other domains. Thus, psychological occupancy in that particular context would appear to be very adaptive in that it should promote more positive feelings of global self-worth.

For many individuals, the ability to discount domains in which one feels inadequate or unworthy will represent a potential pathway to enhanced self-worth; that is, the *reduction* of a discrepancy between high aspirations and low competence or adequacy will be the goal of an intervention. However, for other individuals, such a strategy may be undesirable. In fact, *increasing* the discrepancy may be the initial goal. Consider the example of the student described in Chapter 6, whose ratings of both importance and adequacy in the domain of Behavioral Conduct were quite low. It is likely that although this student did not attach great importance to proper conduct, educators, parents, or mental health workers would deem appropriate conduct to be highly desirable. Thus, an initial strategy would involve *creating* a discrepancy by heightening the student's perception of the importance of good conduct, after which interventions to improve his conduct could be attempted. If such efforts were successful, this student should evaluate his conduct more positively which would then reduce the discrepancy between the new level of importance attached to proper conduct and perceptions of improved behavior. The ultimate goal, therefore, is discrepancy reduction in the service of a more adaptive level of self-worth.

Total discrepancy reduction may not be desirable, however. As observed in Chapter 6, some discrepancy, in which an individual's ideals are slightly higher than his/her level of performance, may be motivating. Hattie (1992) concurs, suggesting that providing the child with realistic expectancies that are somewhat higher than the individual's actual level of accomplishment may lead to achievements that in turn will enhance the domain-relevant sense of self-efficacy (Bandura, 1990) as well as self-concept. Thus, both the agentic sense of the I-self and the self-evaluative component of the Me-self can be positively affected.

It should be noted that from a developmental perspective, these strategies will only be appropriate beginning in middle childhood. Younger children not only lack a conscious, verbalizable sense of their worth as a person, but they also have only a rudimentary sense of the importance of particular domains. Moreover, they do not have the cognitive skills to compare aspirations to actual adequacy. Thus, they cannot conceptualize discrepancies and the role they might play in impacting evaluations of self.

Encouragement of Relatively Accurate Self-Evaluations

Another consideration in the design of interventions concerns the *accuracy* of self-evaluations. How critical is it to promote self-evaluations that accurately reflect reality, namely, to encourage positive self-appraisals that are veridical with an individual's actual skills and attributes? That is, should the goal of interventions be *enhancement* of self-evaluations or the fostering of their accuracy? As becomes apparent, there is some controversy on this issue. There are those who tout enhancement as the primarily goal, whereas others point out the dangers of promoting unrealistically high self-evaluations and urge that programs promote more realistic self-perceptions.

As a backdrop, there are normative-developmental as well as individual differences in accuracy. There is a growing body of developmental literature revealing that young children are relatively inaccurate judges of their abilities, but that accuracy increases with age (Harter, 1985a; Harter & Pike, 1984; Leahy & Shirk, 1985; Phillips & Zimmerman, 1990; Stipek, 1981, 1984). The clearest picture emerges when one compares teachers' evaluations with children's self-ratings of competence. Among young children, the correlations are modest to negligible. Findings also indicate that even when young children are exposed to repeated failures, they do not lower their expectations for success; rather, they persist in holding high and unrealistic beliefs about their abilities (Parsons & Ruble, 1977). As argued elsewhere (Harter, 1988a) young children's inaccurate and inflated self-evaluations should be understood as "normative distortions" and the result of their failure to differentiate the *wish* to be competent from reality. Stipek (1984) provides experimental evidence that young children's unrealistically high performance expectations are intruded upon by personal desires.

With increasing development, children's estimates of their ability become more realistic due to several different processes. The emergence of the cognitive ability to engage in social comparison leads to lower and more realistic self-evaluations (e.g., Frey & Ruble, 1985, 1990; Ruble & Frey, 1991). Cognitive-developmental advances also allow one to make the distinction between real and ideal self-concepts (e.g., Glick & Zigler, 1985; Higgins, 1991; Oosterwegel & Oppenheimer, 1993). Moreover, the development of perspective-taking abilities provides the child with a more accurate rendering of others' views of their abilities and attributes (Leahy & Shirk, 1985; Oosterwegel & Oppenheimer, 1993; Selman, 1980) that are incorporated into the looking-glass self. Concomitantly, children manifest an increasing capacity for self-reflection (Leahy & Shirk, 1985). Finally, during childhood, there is an increasing differentiation between concepts of effort and ability, and their relationship to one another (Nicholls, 1990). For example, the realization that extreme effort implies less ability contributes to more realistic appraisals of one's competencies.

There is some evidence that the progression toward more realistic self-evaluations is not completely linear. Findings (Harter, 1982a) have indicated that the correlation between perceived scholastic competence and teachers' ratings of students' competence gradually increased from third through sixth grade. However, the correlation plummeted with the transition to junior high school in seventh grade, after which it recovered substantially in eighth and ninth grades. The new school environment brings different academic expectations and shifting standards of social comparisons in the face of a new social reference group. Initially, these changes may lead to ambiguity that results in unrealistic self-evaluations, requiring that students construct new criteria by which to judge their competence (Harter, Whitesell, & Kowalski, 1992). As a more general consideration, most developmental transitions present new tasks to be mastered, which may cause doubt and anxiety about one's abilities as well as challenge existing self-representations, leading to potential alterations and inaccuracies in self-perceptions (see also Mack, 1983).

There are also *individual differences* in the degree to which self-evaluations are veridical with more objective indices (Harter, 1985a; Leahy & Shirk, 1985; Phillips & Zimmerman, 1990). In our own work, we have identified three groups of middle school children: those who seriously *overrate* their competence relative to the teacher's judgment, those who seriously *underrate* their competence, and those whose ratings are *congruent* with the teacher's. Moreover, there are liabilities associated with both overrating and underrating one's competence. We documented these liabilities in an experimental task in which we brought these three types of students into the laboratory in small groups (8–10), where they were introduced to a mock classroom. They were given workbooks containing anagrams of different difficulty levels and were first told that this was a word game that we were trying to develop for children their age. During this initial phase, we obtained a baseline of each student's actual skill level on the anagram task. We then told them that the next anagrams they were to do would be more like a school test. They would be timed, to see how long it took them to complete each anagram, and would be given a grade (A, B, C, D, or Fail) based on how well they did. Moreover, to create the typical atmosphere of social comparison in regular classrooms, they had to raise their hands when they completed each anagram. During this classroom simulation phase, the students were allowed to choose the difficulty level of the anagrams they preferred to attempt from among three-, four-, five-, and six-letter anagrams. In creating this type of school setting, we anticipated that children's perceptions of academic ability would be made particularly salient.

Given this preference-for-challenge paradigm, we were particularly interested in the difficulty level that each group selected, relative to its own ability level as determined during the first game-like phase of the session. The findings revealed that both underraters and overraters selected much easier anagrams than their ability scores revealed they could perform, unlike more accurate raters, who selected anagrams commensurate with their skill level. Thus, the preferences of the underraters reflected choices based upon self-perceptions of low competence rather than upon their actual ability. The overraters, in contrast, selected anagrams that were more congruent with their moderately low actual ability level than with their inflated sense of competence. The overraters' performance suggests that, at some level, they were aware that they were not nearly as competent as their self-reported evaluations of competence implied. It would appear that to protect what may be a fragile and distorted sense of scholastic ability, they were driven to select the easiest anagrams, in order to avoid failure and its implications for the self. These findings have clear practical implications in that they suggest that both groups of inaccurate raters are avoiding cognitively challenging situations, a pattern that could jeopardize their acquisition of higher-level skills.

Phillips and Zimmerman (1990) have been particularly interested in high-achieving students who seriously underestimate their scholastic competence. They also find that underraters are guided more by their inaccurate self-perceptions than by their actual capabilities. Those who manifested this "illusion of incompetence" reported unrealistically low expectations for success, displayed evaluation anxiety, and were reluctant to perform challenging achievement tasks. Moreover, they believed that significant adults judged their abilities unfavorably, suggesting that they had incorporated these perceived evaluations into their self-concept. Gender differences revealed that, beginning in the ninth grade, girls were overrepresented among underraters and perceived their mothers to expect less of them and to hold them to less stringent achievement standards than those for boys.

With regard to the overestimation of one's abilities, a critical consideration involves the *magnitude* of the discrepancy between perceived and actual competence. Large discrepancies, such as those that defined the overraters and underraters in the studies described here, signal liabilities, for example, they prohibit preference for challenging activities that might promote further learning. However, completely veridical self-evaluations can also be self-limiting. For example, it has been demonstrated that depressed individuals are more likely to report realistic self-appraisals; in contrast, nondepressed persons are likely to view themselves as more capable than they really are (e.g., Alloy & Abramson, 1979; Asarnow & Bates, 1988; Lewinsohn, Mischel, Chaplain, & Barton, 1980).

Some degree of overestimation, if not excessive, represents one of many self-enhancing biases that most (nondepressed) people exhibit (Banaji & Prentice, 1994; Baumeister, Tice, & Hutton, 1989). Thus, high-self-esteem individuals construe events and process information so as to promote positive self-perceptions, which in turn serves to preserve feelings of self-worth (see Blaine & Crocker, 1993; Brown, 1993a, 1993b; Dunning, 1993; Greenwald, 1980; Greenwald & Pratkanis, 1984; Pelham & Swann, 1989; Steele, 1988; Taylor & Brown, 1988). In his "self-affirmation theory," Steele has addressed the strategies through which individuals modify their beliefs about the self in the service of this goal (see also Taylor, 1983; Tesser & Cornell, 1991). While the overestimation strategy represents some distortion, such self-enhancement may improve task performance (Bandura, 1989; Brown, 1993b; Taylor & Brown, 1988). Taylor and Brown conclude that the self-enhancing strategies associated with high self-esteem are functional, as evidenced by the fact that self-esteem is consistently linked to other indices of psychological adjustment. Although most of these efforts have focused on adult subjects, data with children reveal that high-self-esteem students see themselves as slightly more competent than do their teachers in both their most competent and least competent domains (Harter, 1986a). Low-self-esteem children show little tendency to inflate their judgments of competence; in fact, for their lowest competence domain, they view themselves as less capable than do their teachers.

Other self-enhancement strategies displayed by high-self-esteem individuals include downward comparisons in which the self is considered superior to others (Baumeister, 1991a; Brown, 1986, 1993a, 1993b; Markus, Cross, & Wurf, 1990; Wood, 1989). Dunning (1993) reviews those studies that demonstrate this "above average effect" in numerous domains, a strategy that Markus and Kityama (1991) feel is particularly prevalent in Western cultures. In their self-evaluation maintenance theory, Tesser and colleagues (Beach & Tesser, 1995; Tesser, 1988) identify another strategy for self-enhancement, namely, basking in the glory of the accomplishments of a close other (e.g., a spouse) with whom one identifies. Such a process will only serve the intended goal if success in the given domain of comparison is not vitally important to the individual's self-definition. However, these processes have not been examined in children, as a function of age, to determine at what point in their development such mechanisms might emerge.

The functional value of self-enhancement strategies and self-serving biases has been touted by many social psychologists. However, others adopt a less sanguine perspective. Baumeister (1991b; 1993) observes the risks that accompany a preoccupation with self-presentation, high self-monitoring, and the maintenance of a highly positive self-image involving egoistic illusions. He cites the potential for disconfirmation from others, vulnerability to attack, the pressure of living up to the inflated self-image, and overconfidence that may create interpersonal difficulties. Others (Blaine & Crocker, 1993; Brown, 1993a, 1993b; De La Ronde & Swann, 1993) have pointed to similar liabilities. Brown observes that an overemphasis on positive outcomes can undermine the stability of the self-concept. Kernis (1993) finds that those with high but unstable self-esteem are also prone to hostility. De La Ronde and Swann observe that such overestimation can rob individuals of opportunities to gain an understanding of what they are truly like.

Implications for Intervention

What does this pattern of findings imply for intervention? First, from a developmental perspective, it is critical to appreciate the normative developmental changes in the nature of self-representations that can serve as guidelines for what can and cannot expect to be impacted. Instilling realistic images of self in very young children is a dubious goal, given that cognitive-developmental factors conspire with typically positive feedback from benevolent socializing agents to produce normatively inflated evaluations of their attributes. Moreover, as discussed in Chapter 2, the all-or-none thinking of young children will lead most to feel that they are "all smart" or "all nice," and the very nature of these cognitive structures will make them very resistant to attempted alterations.

Among older children and adolescents, there is greater potential for bringing about realistic self-representations. With such individuals, the ultimate goal would appear to be to invoke strategies that would lead children to adopt relatively realistic perceptions of their abilities, namely, to bring their self-evaluations in line with more objective markers that are typically agreed upon by socializing agents (e.g., parents, teachers, coaches) and their peer group. For overraters, bringing perceptions of competence in line with reality requires sensitive strategies to decrease their inflated self-evaluations, without causing excessive anxiety or overwhelming threats to their self-system. Since one liability of overrating, avoidance of challenge, can interfere with actual skills development, these children need to appreciate the fact that they are not as proficient as they claim. Presumably, with a more realistic outlook, they will be in a better position to respond to interventions to improve their actual skills level.

In contrast, strategic interventions for those underrating their competence would appear to be more benevolent in that one needs to convince them that they are really are more competent than they believe. Yet there are challenges in working with this group given that they may be very resistant to attempts to alter their self-perceptions. As becomes apparent in the following section, evidence suggests that many individuals go to great lengths to seek feedback that confirms their self-concepts and typically reject information that threatens the stability of their self-representations. Thus, while instilling relatively realistic images of self may be the purpose of an intervention, there are psychological roadblocks to achieving such a goal in working with those who both overrate and underrate their abilities.

The Potential for Change in the Valence of Self-Representations

Initially, it is important to address the question of whether concepts of self, either at a domain-specific or more global level, are immutable or subject to change. If self-representations are relatively stable, then practitioners should be less sanguine about the possibility of promoting positive self-evaluations in individuals with negative self-images. Alternatively, if self-representations are potentially malleable, then practitioners can be more optimistic, particularly if there is a cogent analysis of the particular *causes* of a given individual's negative self-evaluations.

The initial focus in this section is on literature relevant to the actual stability and/or change in the *valence* of self-representations, namely, how favorably the self is evaluated. Three themes can be identified in this literature:

1. Do self-evaluations change normatively, with *development?*
2. Do they vary as a function of the *situation* (over short time intervals)?
3. Are there individual differences in the stability or change in one's self-evaluations, such that for some, evaluations are quite stable, whereas for others, fluctuation or change is more common?

Attention then turns to the personal metatheories that individuals hold with regard to change, belief systems that are also very relevant to potential changes in their self-representations.

Normative-Developmental Change

With regard to normative developmental change, the evidence reveals that self-evaluative judgments become less positive as children move into middle childhood (Frey & Ruble, 1985, 1990; Harter, 1982a; Harter & Pike, 1984; Stipek, 1981). Investigators attribute such a decline to the greater reliance on social comparison information and external feedback, leading to more realistic judgments about one's capabilities (see also Crain, 1996; Marsh, 1989). A growing number of studies suggest that there is another decline at early adolescence (ages 11–13), after which global evaluations of worth and domain-specific self-evaluations gradually become more positive over the course of adolescence (Dusek & Flaherty, 1981; Engel, 1959; Marsh, Parker, & Barnes, 1985; Marsh, Smith, Marsh, & Owens, 1988; O'Malley & Bachman, 1983; Piers & Harris, 1964; Rosenberg, 1986; Savin-Williams & Demo, 1993; Simmons, Rosenberg, & Rosenberg, 1973).

Many of the changes reported coincide with the educational transition to junior high school. Eccles and colleagues (Eccles & Midgley, 1989; Eccles et al., 1984; Wigfield, Eccles, MacIver, Reuman, & Midgley, 1991), and Simmons and colleagues (Blyth, Simmons, & Carlton-Ford, 1983; Simmons & Blyth, 1987; Simmons, Blyth, Van Cleave, & Bush, 1979; Simmons et al., 1973) have postulated that differences in the school environments of elementary and junior high schools are in part responsible. Junior high school brings more emphasis on social comparison and competition, stricter grading standards, more teacher control, less personal attention from teachers, and disruptions in social networks, all of which lead to a mismatch between the structure of the school environment and the needs of young adolescents. The numerous physical, cognitive, social, and emotional changes further jeopardize the adolescent's sense of continuity, which may in turn threaten self-esteem (Leahy & Shirk, 1985). A number of these studies (e.g., Blyth et al., 1983; Nottelmann, 1987; Rosenberg & Simmons, 1972; Simmons & Rosenberg, 1975; Simmons et al., 1979; Wigfield et al., 1991) also report lower self-esteem for girls than for boys (see also Block & Robins, 1993, who find that the gender gap widens from ages 14 to 23).

The magnitude of the decline in perceptions of overall worth is also related to the timing of school shifts and to pubertal change (Brooks-Gunn, 1988; Brooks-Gunn & Peterson, 1983; Simmons & Blyth, 1987). Those making the shift from sixth to seventh grade show greater losses of self-esteem than those who make the school transition a year later, from seventh to eighth grade. Moreover, students making the earlier change, particularly girls, do not recover these losses during the high school years. Early-maturing girls fare the worst. They are the most dissatisfied with their bodies, in part because they tend to be somewhat heavier and do not fit the cultural stereotype of female attractiveness emphasizing thinness, as described in Chapter 6. This in turn has a negative effect on their self-worth. Furthermore, according to the developmental readiness hypothesis (Simmons & Blyth, 1987), early-maturing girls are not yet emotionally prepared to deal with the social expectations that surround dating, or with the greater independence that early maturity often demands (see Lipka, Hurford, & Litten, 1992, for a general discussion of the effects of being "off-time" in one's level of maturational development).

Several interpretations have been offered for the gradual gains in self-esteem that follow from eighth grade through high school (McCarthy & Hoge, 1982). Gains in personal autonomy may provide more opportunity to select performance domains in which one is competent, consistent with a Jamesian analysis. Increasing freedom may allow more opportunities to select support groups that will provide esteem-enhancing approval, consistent with the looking-glass-self formulation. Increased role-taking ability may also lead teenagers to behave in more socially acceptable ways that garner the acceptance of others. A study by Hart, Fegley, and Brengelman (1993) provides some confirming evidence. In describing their past and present selves, adolescents asserted that with time, they have become more capable, mature, personable, and attractive, describing how they shed undesirable cognitive, emotional, and personality characteristics.

An analysis of changes in *mean* level of self-worth, however, may mask individual differences in response to educational transitions (see also Block & Robins, 1993). Findings from our own laboratory (Harter, 1986a; Johnson & Harter, 1995) on both the transition to junior high school and to college have identified three groups—those whose self-worth increases, decreases, and remains the same. Within our own framework, we contend that self-worth should only be altered if theoretically derived *antecedents* of self-worth change, leading to an examination of instability or stability as a function of those determinants identified by James (competence in domains of importance) and Cooley (approval from significant others). Results indicate that those whose self-worth *increased* across educational transitions displayed greater competence in domains of importance and reported more social approval in the new school environment. Students whose self-worth *decreased* reported both a decline in competence for valued domains and reported less social support after the transition. Students showing no changes in self-worth reported negligible changes in both competence and social support. Demo and Savin-Williams (1992) have also adopted a more idiographic approach, demonstrating that while nearly half of their sample demonstrated stability in their perceptions of overall worth, the remaining subjects manifested varying degrees of instability.

Situational Differences

The extent to which self-representations vary as a function of situation is a second context in which the issue of the stability and malleability of the self-concept has been raised. Within this literature, there is some tension between those who claim that self-representations are relatively enduring and those who contend that self-representations are more malleable. James scooped contemporary theorists and researchers on this issue, arguing that whereas the barometer of our self-esteem rises and falls from one day to another, there is nevertheless a certain average tone of self-feeling, independent of the reasons we may have for momentary self-satisfaction or discontent.

However, there is one camp of investigators that reports evidence that self-concepts are relatively stable. For example, Swann (1985, 1987, 1996) provides evidence demonstrating individuals' elaborate and ingenious strategies for self-verification; people go to great lengths to seek information that confirms their self-concept and are highly resistant to information that threatens their view of self (see also Baumeister, 1993; Epstein, 1991; Greenwald, 1980; Markus, 1977; Rosenberg, 1979). According to Swann, people do not want feedback that may contradict their existing identities; since such identities provide a psychological blueprint for action, they are the guideposts for how we are to behave. Epstein similarly observes that "people have a vested interest in maintaining the stability of their personal theories of reality, for they are the only systems they have for making sense of their world and guiding their behavior" (p. 97). In Swann's (1996) most recent treatment of this topic, he observes that those with negative self-evaluations are actually ambivalent, in that praise puts them in conflict. While on the one hand, favorable evaluations would be welcome, they also require unfavorable evaluative feedback, to the extent that such individuals desire *verification*. He notes that such people are "caught in a crossfire in which the warmth produced by favorable evaluations is chilled by incredulity" (p. 14).

On the other hand, considerable evidence reveals that situational factors can lead to short-term changes in self-evaluation (Baumgardner, Kaufman, & Levy, 1989; Gergen, 1967, 1982; Heatherton & Polivy, 1991; Jones, Rhodewalt, Berglas, & Skelton, 1981; Markus & Kunda, 1986; Rosenberg, 1986; Savin-Williams & Demo, 1983; Tesser, 1988). Gergen's position is perhaps the most extreme, in that he has argued that people are capable of marked shifts in their public presentation that are not necessarily accompanied by self-alienation. In an effort to reconcile these positions, Markus and Kunda have invoked the construct of the "working self-concept." According to their view, the individual possesses a stable universe of core self-conceptions. The working self-concept is a subset of these self-conceptions, a temporary structure elicited by those situational factors that occur at any given point in time. Thus, the self-concept is also malleable to the extent that the content of the working self-concept changes. Their empirical findings strongly support such a position (see also Greenwald & Pratkanis, 1984).

There is a growing consensus that, as James originally suggested, individuals possess both a *baseline* self-concept and a *barometric* self-concept (see reviews by Demo & Savin-Williams, 1992; Rosenberg, 1986). Thus, people have a core sense of self that is relatively consistent over time; however, there are also situational variations around this core self-portrait. Others have come to a similar conclusion, postulating that individuals display both trait and state self-esteem (Heatherton & Polivy, 1991; Leary & Downs, 1995). According to some, an individual's baseline sense of self is difficult to alter. Theorists have argued, within the context of hierarchical models of the self, that higher-order schemas such as global self-worth or esteem are far more resistant to modification than lower-order, situation-specific constructs (Epstein, 1991; Hattie, 1992). Epstein notes that such higher-order schemas have typically been acquired early in development and are often derived from emotionally significant experiences to which the individual may have little conscious access, making the beliefs difficult to alter.

With regard to the barometric self, adolescence is a time when fluctuations appear to be the most flagrant (Blos, 1962; Demo & Savin-Williams, 1992; Harter, 1990b; Leahy & Shirk, 1985; Rosenberg, 1986). Those of a cognitive-developmental persuasion (e.g., Fischer, 1980; Harter, 1990b; Harter & Monsour, 1992; Higgins, 1991) have attributed these fluctuations to limitations in the ability cognitively to control seemingly contradictory self-attributes (shy vs. outgoing), particularly during middle adolescence. Psychoanalytic thinkers (e.g., Blos, 1962; Kohut, 1977) attribute fluctuations to the intense heightened narcissism and self-preoccupation of adolescents whose self-esteem swings from grandiosity to battered self-devaluation. Rosenberg (1986) focuses more on how socialization factors influence the volatility of the self during adolescence. Thus, he observes that the adolescent is preoc-cupied with what others think of the self but has difficulty divining others' impressions, leading to ambiguity about the self. Moreover, different signifi-cant others may have different impressions of the self, creating contradic-tory feedback.

Individual Differences

A focus on individual differences in the extent to which self-evalua-tions are stable or malleable is the third major context in which issues of stability and change in self-evaluations have been examined. Kernis and col-leagues have been the major proponents of such an approach (Greenier, Kernis, & Waschull, 1995; Kernis, 1993; Kernis, Cornell, Sun, Berry, & Harlow, 1993). According to these investigators, those prone to short-term fluctuations in self-esteem demonstrate enhanced sensitivity to evaluative events, ego involvement (vs. task involvement), preoccupation with self-evalu-ation, and overreliance on social sources of self-esteem (see also Deci & Ryan, 1987; Rosenberg, 1986). Our own findings (discussed in Chapter 7) indicating greater fluctuations in self-worth for those who consciously en-dorse a looking-glass-self orientation (approval determines self-worth) are consistent with this individual-difference approach (Harter, Stocker, et al., 1996). Moreover, we speculated that the developmental precursors may have involved parenting characterized by inconsistent and/or conditional approval. Greenier et al. (1995) also conjecture that inconsistent as well as controlling feedback will undermine the development of a stable sense of worth (see also Deci & Ryan, 1987, 1995).

In further support of an individual-difference approach, Kernis and colleagues have distinguished between individuals with stable and unstable self-esteem, at two *levels* of self-esteem, high and low. They have been par-ticularly interested in illuminating the differential reactions to success and failure feedback of those both high and low in self-esteem, those whose self-esteem is *unstable*. For those with high self-esteem, instability is associated with strategies in which individuals continually seek favorable feedback and defensively react to negative feedback (e.g., by questioning its legitimacy) in order to defend their fragile sense of high self-esteem. Another manifesta-tion of defensiveness is a heightened tendency to become angry or hostile. For those with low self-esteem, instability is associated with attempts to avoid continuous, negative feedback that might lead to global conclusions about their inadequacy or worthlessness. Thus, for Kernis and colleagues, it is not sufficient to consider only level of self-esteem, given that different styles are related to the stability of self-esteem as well.

Dweck and colleagues (Dweck, 1991; Dweck & Elliot, 1983; Dweck &

Leggett, 1988) have approached the issue of individual differences from another perspective, examining differences in the actual *theories* that older children actively hold about stability or change in traits over situation or time. Specifically, they have examined the implicit theories that children develop about self-attributes that concern *intelligence,* attributional patterns that have implications for behavior. They identify two types of self-theories, which they label "entity" and "incremental" conceptualizations of intelligence. Children who are entity theorists consider their intellectual ability to be fixed and therefore uncontrollable. Such children focus on performance outcomes and are oriented toward gaining approval and avoiding negative feedback. If they receive negative evaluations, their confidence is eroded and they develop behavior patterns of helplessness in the face of challenge or failure. In contrast, children who are "incremental theorists" believe that their intelligence is malleable. As a result, they are oriented toward learning goals that will allow them to increase their competence. Such children are very mastery oriented in the face of challenge as well as failure. More recently, Dweck and colleagues have extended their analysis to traits in the social realm, with similar implications. This work is particularly important in its demonstration of the *function* of particular self-theories in influencing behavior. Moreover, it suggests that some children's self-evaluations may be more resistant to change than others.

Implications for Intervention

What are the implications of this body of literature for interventions designed to alter the self-evaluations of those with unfavorable views of themselves? First, the literature suggests that there may be particular developmental periods or transitions in which children are more vulnerable to losses in global perceptions of worth. For example, adolescence, in general, and the transition to new school settings during this period in particular, represent potential points of vulnerability. Thus, these may be critical junctures during which practitioners should focus on both prevention against such losses and interventions for those who would appear to have been negatively affected. Implicit in this work is the assumption that self-evaluations are more malleable during these junctures, which also bodes well for potential opportunities to enhance self-worth as well as domain-specific self-evaluations.

However, as argued earlier in this chapter, self-evaluations will be difficult to alter unless one can pinpoint the precise *causes* of unfavorable views of self, antecedents that may well differ across individuals. Our own efforts at examining changes in self-worth during the transitions to junior high school and to college reveal both increases and decreases in perceptions of worth as a person that are directly linked to the antecedent predictors in our model. Even in the face of a careful analysis of particular causes, however, certain self-evaluations may be resistant to change if images of self have become deeply entrenched, particularly from a very early age. Higher-order schemas of self (e.g., global self-worth) may be particularly resistant to alteration if they were derived from emotionally significant experiences that occurred in childhood. Moreover, for victims of severe and chronic child abuse, the conviction that they are fundamentally defective at their core will be quite difficult to alter, as therapists will attest. Such resistance to change will be exacerbated to the extent that representations of self reflect unconscious processes of which one has little awareness, and therefore over which one has minimal control.

Certain theorists identified here would also argue that there are personal motives to preserve the stability of one's self-evaluations that also make change difficult. Thus, while those with low self-worth may, at one level, desire favorable evaluations from others, such feedback violates their own view of self and, as such, is personally threatening. Individual differences in the *metatheories* that children and adolescents hold with regard to the malleability of the self will also impact potential change. As Dweck's work reveals, there are those who consider their intellectual ability to be fixed and therefore uncontrollable, whereas others believe that it is possible to enhance their intelligence through mastery efforts. Thus, reframing strategies, in which there is an attempt to revise perceptions that one's perceived inadequacies are unalterable, may allow such individuals to chart a more adaptive course toward possible change in self-conceptions.

Attention to Individuals' Own Theories about the Causes of Their Self-Representations

The work of Dweck raises the more general issue of the importance of understanding how particular individuals conceptualize the antecedents of the beliefs they hold about themselves. An appreciation for these cognitive constructions may be an important prerequisite to the design of an intervention strategy. Dweck's research converges with the efforts of investigators examining those *attributional* variables that influence one's sense of self and accompanying depressive symptomatology. For example, external attributions in which others are viewed as responsible for one's successes will impede self-concept change (Gold, 1994; Tice, 1994), as will internal attributions for negative events that are global and stable because they are associated with low self-esteem and accompanying depressed affect (Seligman & Peterson, 1986). Thus, strategies in which there is a cognitive/verbal reframing of one's attributions, shifting to global, stable, internal attributions for one's successes, rather than failures, have been suggested as another form of intervention (see Pope, McHale, & Craighead, 1988; Seligman, 1993). These suggestions are consistent with the findings of Grusec and colleagues (e.g., Grusec & Redler, 1980), who observed that children who attribute their prosocial behavior to a trait were found to engage in more prosocial behavior than those who attributed the same behavior to external factors (see also Eisenberg, Cialdini, McCreath, & Shell, 1987, who link children's views on the value of consistency to prosocial behaviors).

Pope et al. (1988) offer an attributional analysis of individuals' perceptions of their attractiveness which, as discussed in an earlier chapter, is highly related to global self-worth. They contend that it is important to shift the individual's attribution away from stable and global attributions about unattractiveness (e.g., "I'm ugly, and will always be ugly"; "I'm ugly and therefore worthless"). Although they suggest that some counseling around dress and hygiene may be appropriate, they do not recommend cosmetic overhauls that pander to the ideals of attractiveness touted in the media. Rather, they suggest that interventionists communicate the fact that such ideals are virtually unattainable; therefore, individuals should alter the standards for what they should look like. As noted earlier in this chapter, reducing the discrepancy between one's ideal body image and perceptions of one's looks should serve to bolster self-worth from a Jamesian perspective, for example, by discounting the importance of appearance as defined by media standards. Consistent with our own analysis, Pope et al. also recommend cognitive restructuring such that individuals shift their focus from concerns about appearance to other domains (academic, athletic, interpersonal, or moral) where they are, or can be, more successful.

In addition to identifying the types of attributions that individuals bring to bear on their self-representations, it is important to determine the broader theory that they have adopted with regard to the antecedents of their own self-representations. It is all well and good for theorists to specify a model of the causes and correlates of global self-worth, for example, as we have done. However, if a given individual holds a *different* theory, intervention efforts that require the conscious cooperation of the child or adolescent may well falter if his/her theory is not taken into account. For example, what are the constructs in a given individual's own cognitive interpretation of the causes and correlates of his/her self-worth, to what extent does the individual perceive the links, and what are the directions of influence as he/she understands them?

For example, in our own work (see Chapter 6), we have asked adolescents to reflect upon the directionality of the link between appearance and global self-worth, and have identified two subgroups, those who feel that their appearance determines their worth as a person, and those who feel that their self-worth impacts their perceptions of their attractiveness. Those adopting the first perspective, especially if they are females, are particularly at risk for low self-worth and depressed affect. These findings suggest that a reframing intervention may be appropriate; that is, efforts should attempt to shift perceptions to the conviction that an emphasis on other desirable qualities (e.g., kindness, fairness, empathy, intelligence) will lead to the approval of their *inner* self as a worthwhile person, which in turn will provoke an acceptance of their *outer* self, namely, how they think they look.

These suggestions imply that healthy self-development should be promoted by the conscious appreciation for the *origins* of self-perceptions, such that the individual can be an active agent of change in altering negative self-evaluations. With the I-self at the helm, one may alter Me-self development, steering it along a more favorable course. Insight-oriented interventions and therapies may prove beneficial in this regard. They may aid individuals to uncover causes initially beyond their control, for example, negative treatment by socializing agents that instilled negative self-perceptions. With such insight can come the realization that as a child, one was not totally to blame for the events that provoked unfavorable self-perceptions. Although the early induction of negative evaluations may render them more resistant to change, the very *knowledge* of their external origins should offer some sense of current, *cognitive* control. An understanding of the impact of one's early history can also allow for corrective experiences to redress the psychological damage caused by neglectful, rejecting, or abusive child-rearing agents.

Insight-oriented interventions that require an awareness of the nature of self-processes themselves are unlikely to be very effective before adolescence, however. From both neo-Freudian and cognitive-developmental perspectives, there is evidence that children have little interest in, or capacity for, an analysis of the origins of their self-attributes (see Harter, 1988a). As observed in Chapter 2, Anna Freud (1965) has written cogently on this topic, pointing out that children naturally direct their interest toward the outer world of events rather than to the inner world of intrapsychic experiences. She notes that children do not naturally take themselves as the object of their own observation; they do not normally engage in introspection. As a result, psychological issues and/or conflicts are externalized, and environmental solutions are preferred to internal or intrapsychic analysis and change.

Cognitive-developmental theory and evidence provide a complementary perspective in alerting us to factors that mitigate against the child's ability to engage in self-observation. Among young children, their confounding of wishes and reality, their inability to engage in logical thinking, and their egocentrism each preclude thoughtful reflection on the self. With the emergence of concrete operational thought, there are newly developed capacities; however, these make it unlikely that the child will engage in self-observation; that is, the newfound logical abilities to emerge during this period are directed toward an analysis of concrete events in the external world, as the title of this stage implies. Thus, children show little interest in analyzing internal events such as self-attributes, their causes, and their potential impact on affective and motivational processes. The ability to treat one's own thoughts as objects of reflection, to introspect about one's attributes, and to create metatheories about their origins, does not begin to develop until early adolescence (see Harter, 1990b).

For adolescents and adults, fostering insights about the origins of self-perceptions may help to offset the fact that constructs at or near the apex of a hierarchy of self-representations are often more resistant to change. Such a conclusion is most likely for those who can become cognizant of the lower-order postulates that formed the basis for the construction of the more abstract, global self-representations at the top of the hierarchy; that is, an awareness of the process through which such higher-order generalizations were constructed, including an appreciation for the origins of the *content* of lower-order attributes, may allow one to dismantle the hierarchy, particularly if it is no longer realistic. For example, in the third grade, I constructed the trait label "dumb" that I applied to myself, due to the fact that I was relatively unsuccessful at cursive writing and at certain math concepts. Between second and third grades, I had switched from a very progressive private school that had focused on reading and a variety of creative arts opportunities, to a more traditional public school that emphasized the three R's, two of which I had not yet educationally encountered. Some years later, I could appreciate the basis on which this trait label was constructed, allowing me to "deconstruct" it in an examination of the particular external events and experiences upon which it was founded. Thus, I no longer concluded that I was "dumb." A cardinal tenet of cognitive-developmental theorizing is that more mature cognitive structures demonstrate "reversibility"; that is, one can move facilely up and down within a given hierarchy, cognitively appreciating the links. Scaffolding these skills with regard to the hierarchies that come to define the self and to recontrust hierarchies would appear to represent an important avenue to healthy self-development.

Scaffolding to help adolescents develop more adaptive links between seemingly contradictory attributes that define their multiple selves, as described in Chapter 3, is also recommended as a strategy for those experiencing conflict over such opposing characteristics. For example, at a specific level, aiding adolescents to see that their tendencies to be both cheerful and depressed across different relational contexts can be subsumed under the higher-order construct of "moody" may reduce the perceived conflict. At the more general level, seemingly contradictory attributes in different contexts can be integrated under the larger conceptual umbrella of a self-system that is guiding one to behave "appropriately" or "flexibly" in different situations.

Another solution for resolving potential contradictions within one's self-portrait is offered by those theorists who have emphasized the role of autobiograpical *narratives* in the construct of the adult self (Freeman, 1992; Gergen & Gergen, 1988; McAdams, 1997; Oyserman & Markus, 1993). In developing a self-narrative, the individual creates a sense of continuity over time as well as coherent connections among self-relevant life events. In constructing such a life story, the I-self is assigned an important agentic role as author, temporally sequencing the Me-selves into a coherent self-narrative that provides meaning and a sense of future direction. Moreover, narrative construction is a continuous process, as we not only craft but also revise the story of our lives, creating new blueprints that facilitate further architectural development of the self. Interventions that help adolescents or adults to create such a meaningful narrative may help to resolve apparent conflicts between different attributes, allowing individuals to preserve some sense of a unified self. As with many of the other strategies suggested, cognitive reframing can serve to promote healthier self-development.

INTERVENTION STRATEGIES DIRECTED AT SOCIAL FACTORS INFLUENCING SELF-EVALUATIONS

Provisions to Increase Approval Support

As described in Chapter 7 on social sources of self-evaluation, a looking-glass-self perspective alerts us to the impact of approval or disapproval from significant others on global self-worth. Thus, those most at risk for low self-worth are children and adolescents who lack support and may actively experience disapproval or, in the extreme, rejection. An initial goal should be the determination of whether the child's perceptions are *realistic*. Just as the accuracy of self-perceptions about one's competence or adequacy is critical to successful adaptation, as described earlier, so is the ability to accurately appraise the level of support that one is actually receiving. For those children or adolescents who underestimate the level of parental approval, efforts should focus on helping such individuals to develop a more realistic appreciation for the support that parents are providing. For those low-self-worth individuals whose perceptions are relatively accurate, strategies designed to reduce disapproval as well as increase levels of approval should help to redress this psychological situation.

For those experiencing lack of support at the hands of parents, interventions may follow more traditional therapeutic procedures, including family therapy designed to assess the interpersonal dynamics between parents and child and to recommend corrective solutions. For those parents who primarily offer harsh *conditional* approval, communicating that they will only approve of their child as a person if he/she meets highly demanding and often unrealistic parental standards, therapeutic efforts should focus on techniques that encourage the parents to accept the child for who he/she is as a person. Our model reveals that success in the domains of academic competence and behavioral conduct are likely to garner parental support; thus, strategies to promote greater success in these domains should lead to higher levels of support. However, parents, particularly those whose support is conditional, need to be encouraged to display more respect for the child's personal agenda, including strengths in domains that may be less highly valued by the parents. For example, there may be mismatches between the expectations of parents and the potential talents of the child. Thus, parents of a child who finds it hard to achieve academically for good reason (level of intelligence, presence of learning disabilities) but who is athletically capable, should be encouraged to reward the child's athletic accomplishments rather than critically hound the child for his/her lack of academic success.

For those experiencing lack of *peer* support, the initial efforts should also be directed at determining whether the child's perceptions are realistic. For example, certain children, those who are rejected and/or aggressive, not only inflate their sense of competence or adequacy but also appear to overestimate the extent to which they are valued by peers, whereas neglected children are more realistic (see Boivin, Thomassin, & Alain, 1989; Crick & Dodge, 1994; Patterson, Kupersmidt, & Griesler, 1990; Rubin, Chen, & Hymel, 1993). Other children, in contrast, who are reasonably well liked, may underestimate peer support. Thus, for those who are misreading the more objective level of peer support, interventions should focus on encouraging children to be more realistic. However, just as we saw that inaccurate self-perceptions of one's abilities may be resistant to alteration, so may unrealistic perceptions of support be difficult to change.

For children who are accurately aware of negative peer reactions, attempts should focus on understanding the particular causes of their lack of acceptance. Do the children lack attributes that are valued by peers, for example, attractiveness, athletic ability, and interpersonal qualities that make them likable? If the deficiencies reside in the child, efforts may be directed toward improving the child's skills in these areas, realizing that there will be natural limits on the extent to which the child may be able to improve. For certain children who are neglected or rejected, social skills training programs may be appropriate in the service of improving their likability (see Asher, 1985; Asher & Renshaw, 1981). For other children, removing them from an unsupportive peer-group situation and placing them with individuals who are likely to provide more support may represent a strategy for improving their global self-worth.

To the degree to which it is realistic, children should be encouraged to inhabit those interpersonal contexts in which support is forthcoming, compared to those in which they do not garner support and which, therefore, contribute to more negative appraisals of self. Such a strategy follows from our previous analysis of relational self-worth; that is, for most individuals, self-worth will be higher in some interpersonal contexts than others. Thus, one should be encouraged to value those contexts, allowing the sense of worth in that social domain to generalize to perceptions of *global* self-worth. This strategy may not be realistic, however, given that children with disapproving parents do not have the option to avoid the family context, nor can those who experience neglect or rejection from peers in the classroom opt out of attending school.

In cases where the strategies suggested appear unworkable, providing some type of *compensatory* support may represent an alternative. For example, among children and adolescents experiencing disapproval, rejection, or neglect at the hands of parents, providing nonparental adult support may serve to offset the negative effects of lack of parent support. Within both the resiliency and social support literature, there has been increasing emphasis on the positive roles that can be played by such special adults (Cauce, Reid, Landesman, & Gonzales, 1990; Masten, in press; Masten, Best, & Garmezy, 1994; Rutter, 1987). Programs such as Big Sisters and Big Brothers build upon this strategy more formally, as do a variety of mentoring programs.

There is relatively little empirical work on this issue, however. As described in Chapter 7, we have begun to address the role of special adults within our own research program. Our initial findings reveal that about 60% of middle school students report that they have such a special adult in their lives. Moreover, these young adolescents indicate that their special adults provide a number of types of support including approval, emotional support, instrumental help, as well as positive challenges to achievement and mastery goals (Talmi & Harter, 1998). The most common special adults reported include relatives (e.g., grandparents, aunts or uncles), adult friends of parents, and parents of their friends. Others include coaches, teachers, counselors, and ministers. With regard to the compensatory effect of special adult support, we hypothesized that those with low levels of parental support who had a special adult would report higher levels of global self-worth than those who did not have such a person in their lives.

The findings only partially confirmed this hypothesis, in that compensatory effects were demonstrated for only a subset of adolescents. Further inspection of the data revealed that those who appeared to profit from special adult support reported higher competence/adequacy scores, particularly in what we labeled earlier as the more parent-salient domains of Scholastic Competence and Behavioral Conduct, compared to those who showed no effect of special adult support. Two interpretations suggest themselves. The first is that special adult support cannot overcome the negative contribution of low competence/adequacy to global self-worth among those who appeared not to profit from such support. The second is that for the group that did seem to profit, special adult support served to bolster perceptions of scholastic competence and behavioral conduct, which, in turn, positively impacted global self-worth. Although this particular data set does not allow us to determine directly which interpretation is more appropriate, it is of interest that special adult support will not necessarily benefit all recipients given that other factors in our model, namely, competence or adequacy, also contribute to global self-worth.

Internalization of the Positive Opinions of Others

Although the approval and opinions of significant others are critical to the child's self-definition, there is considerable consensus that the healthiest developmental course is one in which realistic standards and positive opinions are *internalized,* such that they become truly *self*-evaluations that the child comes to personally own (see Connell & Wellborn, 1991; Damon & Hart, 1988; Higgins, 1991; Stipek et al., 1992). As discussed in Chapters 2 and 3, cognitive-developmental advances during childhood and adolescence facilitate this process in that the I-self gradually becomes able to directly evaluate the Me-self. Although the origins of self-representations are decidedly social in nature, it becomes critical, through such an internalization process, that the I-self assume responsibility for the construction and content of the Me-self, as well as experience self-affects in the form of *pride* over personal accomplishments.

The importance of *internalizing* the positive messages of socializing agents during childhood can be observed in our own findings revealing the liabilities of continuing to operate according to a looking-glass-self perspective in adolescence. Those who indicated that their self-worth depended directly upon the opinions of others were far more preoccupied with others' evaluations and reported fluctuations in perceived approval, as well as an unstable sense of self-worth. To the extent that one continues to base perceptions of worth as a person upon what are perceived to be the fluctuating evaluations of others, one's self-image will necessarily be chimerical. The greater preoccupation with the opinions of others also leads these looking-glass-self adolescents to become socially distracted from their schoolwork, as judged by teachers. Finally, these individuals reported lower *levels* of support, as well as self-worth compared to those who felt that their self-worth was causally prior to the opinions of others. This latter group, therefore, gave evidence of the type of internalization process that constitutes a healthier pattern of development, as indicated by more positive correlates.

In addition, the individual who continues to base his/her self-worth on the external standards of others is at risk for false-self behavior, as our own work has demonstrated. Deci and Ryan (1995) concur, citing the dangers of developing a false self if self-esteem is based primarily on impression management and is contingent upon living up to the externally imposed evaluation criteria of others. Such "contingent self-esteem" is contrasted to "true self-esteem," derived from more autonomous actions that involve self-determination based upon internal standards, leading to a genuine sense of efficacy. Deci and Ryan argue that the latter orientation leads to a more stable and integrated sense of self that can be shared with others in a more mutual, authentic relationship.

Thus, the continuing preoccupation with either external standards or evaluations of others poses liabilities, particularly with increasing levels of development. Our findings on autonomy and connectedness as dimensions of adult relationship styles have also revealed that those other-focused individuals who appear to be overly connected to their partners are detrimentally preoccupied with relationship issues (see Chapter 9). Individuals endorsing this style reported the lowest levels of validation from their partners, as well as difficulty in being their authentic self within the relationship. Although the internalization of a relatively autonomous set of standards and self-appraisals would appear to be an important goal of development, there are also liabilities for those self-focused, autonomous individuals who appear to have eschewed meaningful connectedness with a partner. The highest levels of validation, authentic-self behavior and self-worth, were reported by those who strove for mutuality, balancing healthy forms of autonomy and connectedness that did not threaten the relationship or compromise their self-system.

How one actually fosters the healthy internalization of the opinions and approval of others has received far less attention. Maccoby and Martin (1983), in reviewing techniques to enhance the internalization of moral standards, report that strategies in which the child is made to feel actively responsible for his/her actions, what they label as "induction" techniques, represent one such avenue. With regard to performance-oriented goals, therefore, emphasizing *children's* role in producing positive outcomes, as well highlighting the fact that they must feel very proud of *themselves*, should also foster internalization. Helping children to establish personal ideals toward which they strive (as opposed to merely meeting the ideals of others) is another strategy for promoting the internalization of standards. In contrast, conditional support, in which the child must meet the high and unrealistic standards of others in order to obtain approval, as well as inconsistent support, should undermine the internalization process. Encouraging children not to place such heavy reliance on social comparison with others, but rather evaluate their present performance in relation to their own past performance, constitutes a related strategy for fostering personal goals and standards that they can realistically achieve. The more positive self-evaluations that such a focus should produce will, in turn, impact overall evaluations of worth. Thus, there are a variety of potential strategies that can be derived from those social factors that influence perceptions of worth.

THE NEED FOR EFFECTIVE PROGRAM EVALUATION

A major problem with many intervention efforts is their failure to employ an adequate program evaluation strategy in their assessments of potential change over time; that is, the particular program may have many positive features. However, weaknesses in the evaluation strategy do not allow potential effects to be detected. Toward the goal of maximizing the demonstration of intervention effects, a number of suggestions are offered (see also Harter, 1990c).

1. *Do not put the methodological cart before the theoretical horse.* It is imperative that the evaluator first identify the particular issue, question, or problem that is at the heart of one's inquiry. Then, formulate a set of hypotheses that are based upon a particular model or conceptual framework from which these issues can be thoughtfully considered. The specific identification of both a research problem and a conceptual framework will, in turn, dictate the choice of measures. The selection of an instrument will seem distressingly arbitrary if an investigator is not clear about his/her specific purpose, the appropriate conceptual framework, as well as the precise meaning assigned to the self given its many different definitions. Too often, investigators attempt to design a study around a measure (often, one of ours), rather than around an interesting or compelling research question and set of thoughtful hypotheses. The former strategy will do little to illuminate our understanding of self-processes and their function. Moreover, in the absence of a clear set of questions, the wrong measure (often, one of ours) may well be inappropriately selected.

2. *Select an instrument that specifically taps the dimensions of interest.* Often, investigators do not select measures that are sensitive to the dimensions that have peaked their interest. For example, investigators often express their desire to assess self-concept in children. However, upon further reflection, it becomes evident that they are actually interested in such constructs as

creativity, ego strength, fine-motor competence, social skills, resiliency, nurturance, discipline, and so on, that may bear a *relationship* to self-concept but are not its defining features. If self-concept *is* to be examined, which of the many measures now available should one choose? The dizzying array of domains that have proliferated (as described in Chapter 5) will undoubtedly lead to perplexity, if not paralysis, for the psychometrically challenged. It is critical, therefore, that evaluators be as precise as possible about the particular construct under scrutiny, in order to be able to select an instrument that specifically operationalizes that construct. Failure to be clear about one's formulation will inevitably lead to the choice of instruments that will be insensitive to potential hypotheses that may well have considerable merit.

In choosing an instrument, researchers are also faced with decisions about the *level* of measurement, namely, should they select more molar or molecular measures of the self? Given the shift to multidimensional measures that differentiate between an increasing number of domains, there is currently the implicit assumption by many that the more domains, the better the instrument. However, the value of those more molecular approaches requires justification, both theoretically and empirically; that is, the choice of a more global versus differentiated measure will depend entirely upon the particular research questions and hypotheses one has chosen to address. Investigators need to consider thoughtfully what level of specificity their research question requires. For example, if an educator is interested in evaluating the effect of a new math curriculum on perceptions of arithmetic competence, he/she may well opt for a more molecular measure such as the Math Self-Concept subscale on Marsh's Self-Description Questionnaire (1993) or on our own Self-Perception Profile for Learning-Disabled Students (Renick & Harter, 1988), which can also be used successfully with normally achieving students.

However, if an investigator were more interested in documenting the relationship between a child's intrinsic motivation for schoolwork in general and his/her overall feelings of scholastic competence (e.g., Harter, Whitesell, & Kowalski, 1992), assessment would more reasonably proceed at the level of a scholastic competence subscale, such as on our Life-Span Battery of Self-Perception Profiles (see Chapter 5). Toward other research goals, a more global index may be desirable. For example, if one were intrigued by the hypothesis that positive regard from significant others may influence the overall positive regard that one has for the self, then the Rosenberg Self-Esteem Scale (1979), the Global Self-Worth subscale from our measures, or the General Self-Concept subscales on the measures by Marsh and Bracken, would be the appropriate choice.

3. *Clearly distinguish between a concern with the actual stability of the construct and test–retest reliability.* The substantive issue of stability versus change

in self-representations also interacts with a particular psychometric consideration, namely, the appropriateness of employing test–retest reliability as
an index of the adequacy of one's measure; that is, one must first give thoughtful consideration to whether a given self-construct is realistically expected to
change over time. If we have reason to believe that particular self-representations in question are subject to legitimate and meaningful *change*, then test–
retest reliability is inappropriate as an index of the merit of an instrument.
Under these circumstances, one may well wish to examine change; however,
the focus will be on the stability of the construct itself and not a cause for
psychometric concern should scores change over time. If, on the other hand,
one has good reason to consider a given self-construct to be *stable*, then test–
retest reliability assessments can be justified. Thus, investigators need to be
clear about their framework before examining potential change or stability
over time. In our own work, we have been impressed with the potential for
self-concept scores and/or self-worth to change, meaningfully, if their causes
are altered. Thus, a comparison of scores over time represents an index of
actual change rather than an assessment of test–retest reliability (unless one
opts for a very short time interval, e.g., 3–4 weeks).

4. *Clearly distinguish between the accuracy of self-evaluations and the issue of
validity.* There is another potential source of psychometric confusion in considering the topic of accuracy, in that often it is confounded with the issue
of *validity*. Consider the following types of comparisons: (a) perceived scholastic competence is correlated with teachers' judgments of the students'
scholastic competence, with GPA, or with achievement test scores; (b) perceived social acceptance is correlated with sociometric ratings of popularity;
(c) perceived physical appearance is correlated with independent judges' ratings of attractiveness, based on concurrent photographs. On the surface,
these all seem like legitimate comparisons, however, comparisons for what
purpose? Are such relationships to be taken as evidence for the validity of
the self-report instrument itself? Or, alternatively, do they say more about
how the *self*-perceptions of children and adolescents may legitimately differ
from the supposedly more "objective" judgments of outside raters such as
parents, teachers, and peers? That is, there may be the potentially different
bases on which children and adolescents evaluate their attributes in such
domains leading to discrepancies that do not necessarily cast doubt on the
validity of the self-report measure. Self-perceptions are just that, self-perceptions. Thus, validity can only be assessed through other self-report instruments.

In our own work, we have found that such comparisons between self-
perceptions and the judgments of others speak more to the nature of the
evaluation process than to the validity of the instrument. Moreover, the
very term "accuracy" may be a misnomer; that is, subjective self-judgments

that do not correspond to an external criterion considered to be "objective" become interesting in their own right. Such discrepancies suggest, for example, that subjective and objective judgments may depend upon different sources of information. Lack of congruence does not, therefore, necessarily lead to the conclusion that a given self-report instrument is invalid. For example, in one study, we identified middle school students whose judgments of their scholastic competence were either much higher than, much lower than, or corresponded to the evaluations of their teachers. In addition to teachers' evaluations, we also obtained parents' ratings of their children's scholastic competence. We found that the children's judgments of their competence were much more congruent with their *parents'* evaluations than with those of their teachers. We interpreted these findings to mean that students were more likely to incorporate their parents' evaluations than their teachers' perceptions in coming to conclusions about their scholastic abilities. While students' judgments may have appeared "inaccurate" in relation to teachers' observations, the more interesting outcome was the illumination of the particular *process* through which children were making their judgments. From a looking-glass-self perspective, the opinions of certain significant others may have a more powerful impact on self-evaluations than feedback from others.

5. *Attempt to specify a pattern of predictions.* The investigator interested in potential self-concept change will gain increasing predictive power to the extent that he/she can anticipate what facets of the self-concept should not only change, but also be *unaffected* by a particular manipulation or treatment. Consider the earlier example in which an investigator wishes to evaluate the effectiveness of a given math program on children's math self-concept. As noted, one would initially select a measure specific to math self-concept. However, program evaluators may well want to include other subscales, predicting that *math* self-concept *should* change as a result of the intervention, whereas other dimensions, for example, perceptions of social acceptance or perceived physical appearance, would *not* be expected to change. To the extent that a researcher can predict a differentiated pattern of scores, and these hypotheses are supported, he/she is in a much better position to draw meaningful conclusions about the impact of a particular intervention.

In other situations, one may predict that an intervention in a given domain *would* have an impact upon another dimension of the self-concept. For example, in a school setting where athletic prowess is highly valued and therefore a route to social acceptance, skills interventions designed to enhance athletic performance may well augment children's perceived popularity. However, within such an environment, enhanced academic performance in math, to pursue the earlier example, would *not* be expected to influence a child's perceptions of peer acceptance.

6. *Include measures of the processes thought to be responsible for self-concept*

change. Too often, pre–post designs focus exclusively on the potential product of a given intervention and do not directly assess those processes thought to be responsible for self-concept change. Thus, there is no way of knowing whether the postulated reasons for such change are in fact the actual factors that produced the differences observed. Investigators cannot simply *infer* that their hypotheses have been supported. Positive self-image changes as a result of a remedial educational program, for example, may have as much to do with the individualized attention given to the student as with the particular academic content that has been selected. In therapy, to take another example, the regard that the therapist communicates by thoughtfully listening to the client may be just as critical to self-concept change as the more direct suggestions that the therapist may make about altering certain behaviors or attitudes. Thus, it becomes critical at the outset to attempt to identify the mechanisms thought to responsible for self-concept change, in order to include measures that will tap these processes, in addition to outcomes.

We have recently had good success with the design of self-report items that tap adolescents' own perceptions of the *link* between the features of an intervention and outcomes. Such questions address the issue of whether adolescents are aware that program features have had their intended effect. For example, in our study of special adults (Talmi & Harter, 1998), we wrote questions such as "The approval that I get from my special adult makes me like myself better as a person" in evaluating perceptions of the link between approval and self-worth. In another study of the effects of adolescent girls' sports participation upon a number of outcomes, we crafted items such as "Playing on the team has led me to be more competitive." Other outcomes included enhancing one's athletic ability, developing friendships, becoming more disciplined academically, improving relationships with parents, and enhancing self-worth. We found that those who perceived the links reported better outcomes, suggesting the importance of making the purpose of an intervention clear to its recipients.

7. *Clarify expectations about the directionality of change.* Often, the investigator interested in self-concept change begins with an implicit, benevolent hope that all subjects will manifest gains, defined as enhanced self-concept. In fact, much of the self-concept intervention research of the 1960s was based on such a vision, reflecting the general Camelot-like optimism that pervaded this period of history. The notion that a very positive self-image might be unrealistic was far from the forefront of our thinking. As described earlier in this chapter, from a mental health perspective, a more worthy goal may be the establishment of a relatively realistic self-concept. Investigators' expectations in this regard have implications for their measurement strategy and anticipated outcome. For example, an orientation designed to instill realistic self-judgments would lead to the expectation that subjects with an inflated sense of self might report less positive judgments at the end of a

given intervention. If a program evaluator adopted such a framework, he/she would not employ a single group design with the expectation that all scores would show gains. Rather, he/she would want to identify subgroups of subjects at the outset, where the goal would be increases in self-concept for some and lowered scores for others as a function of the intervention.

Another implication here is that one may be less interested in the actual level of the self-concept score, in favor of a score that tapped the *discrepancy* between perceived competence, for example, and actual competence assessed independently. A focus on the establishment of a realistic self-concept, therefore, would lead to the expectation that, in a pre–post design, such a discrepancy score would be reduced as a result of the particular treatment. Thus, clarity about the anticipated directionality of change scores will allow one to interpret more meaningfully the pattern of findings.

8. *Single group versus subgroup designs.* The preceding discussion has implied that in certain cases, an investigator may wish to examine self-concept change within particular subgroups of interest. Three different strategies may be suggested in this regard. One possibility is to identify subgroups of subjects on an a priori basis given their particular psychological characteristics, for example, children who tend to overestimate versus underestimate their self-concept, to pursue the previous discussion. There may well be other psychological dimensions of interest on which subjects are selected, dimensions independent of self-concept itself. One may, for example, be interested in academic self-concept change among children who are identified as intrinsically versus extrinsically motivated. Alternatively, subjects may be identified based on group membership (e.g., mainstreamed vs. nonmainstreamed learning-disabled children). One is then in a position to advance hypotheses about how an intervention may differentially affect the groups selected.

Often, an investigator may not have a clear pattern of a priori predictions, although there may be the general expectation that not all subjects will show equal gains. For example, self-concept change may partly be a product of where one started initially. Thus, a second strategy would be to identify subgroups based upon initial self-concept scores (e.g., high, medium, and low). One possible pattern is that subjects at the pretest with relatively high scores cannot realistically be expected to show gains, since ceiling effects leave little room for improvement. Subjects with extremely low scores may not be expected to show gains, since, often, psychological factors contributing to such a pattern initially may mitigate against their responsiveness to intervention. For example, it may be very difficult to increase the very negative academic self-concept of a child's whose educational history has repeatedly conveyed the message that he/she is intellectually inadequate. An intervention designed to improve the perceived behavioral conduct of delinquent adolescents may have little impact on those who have a stake in maintaining their image as troublemakers if it provides them with peer acceptance or other forms of secondary gain. It may well be, therefore, that the investigator would anticipate that subjects whose scores fall within some midrange, initially upon pretest, will have the greatest potential for self-concept gain.

A third strategy for examining subgroups may involve the identification, upon *posttest*, of those participants who actually did manifest increases, decreases, or no change in self-concept. One may then be in a position to determine what might have been different about these subjects initially, factors causing them to be more or less receptive to change in a particular direction. Such a strategy would be more appropriate in the exploratory phases of a project, when one is not yet in a position to make explicit hypotheses about conditions under which self-concept change might be expected to occur. Thus, findings based upon such a strategy could be employed to design more prospective studies in which factors expected to influence self-concept change could then be selected or manipulated.

9. *Carefully consider statistical issues such as regression to the mean.* The strategies suggested above represent various logical alternatives to understanding differential patterns of self-concept change. However, there are statistical considerations of which one must also be aware, for example, regression to the mean, or the use of difference scores, to name but two common concerns. Detailed discussions of these issues can be found in most textbooks on statistical issues in assessment and should be consulted accordingly. Regression to the mean is particularly problematic given the earlier suggestion that self-concept change be examined as a function of whether one's pretest scores were high, medium, or low, as one possible subgroup strategy. Statistically, it would be anticipated that those with high scores at the pretest should manifest decreases upon a second testing, whereas those with low scores initially should show gains. To the extent that a different pattern was evidenced, based on an alternative set of a priori hypotheses, one would be in a much stronger position to interpret data supporting that pattern.

In our own work, where we have been concerned about regression to the mean effects in examining scholastic self-concept change as a function of the transition from elementary to junior high school, we have employed one statistical procedure that attempts to control for such effects. Our design is one in which we have sought to identify three subgroups of students, those who perceptions of scholastic competence (a) increase, (b) decrease, or (c) remain the same across this transition. We first determine the correlation between perceived scholastic scores at the two time periods, sixth-grade elementary school and seventh-grade junior high school. We then calculate what level of perceived competence would be predicted for each individual student in the seventh grade, based on the regression line established for the group as a whole. Increasers are defined as those students whose scores increased (more than the standard error of measurement) above the predicted value; by the same logic, decreasers are those whose scores decreased in relation to the predicted value. No change was defined as seventh-grade scores that were consistent with the prediction equation. This procedure controls for regression to the mean, since increases or decreases in the seventh grade are rendered independent of the student's level of perceived scholastic competence in the sixth grade. This is but one possible procedure that deals with certain, though by no means all, of the statistical concerns in dealing with score-change data. In implementing any of the strategies suggested earlier, careful consideration should be given to such issues in the analysis and interpretation of one's results.

CONCLUSION

Despite the protective functions performed by the self-system, there are also potential liabilities associated with self-development. Some of these liabilities represent normative-developmental phenomena and thus are experienced by the majority of individuals, for example, conflict over the multiple selves that proliferate in adolescence. Other liabilities reflect individual differences that are linked to the particular socialization histories that children and adolescents experience. Thus, some individuals develop favorable representations of self, whereas others come to adopt very negative perceptions of their competence, personal adequacy, and overall sense of self-worth. For the latter group, intervention strategies may aid in fostering more positive self-evaluations.

The intervention strategies suggested in this chapter build upon the major themes of this volume, beginning with the observation that the self is both a cognitive and a social construction. Thus, a range of both cognitive and social intervention strategies may be effective. Any such strategies will only be effective to the extent that one first specifies a model of the causes of negative self-representations that will serve to pinpoint the particular target of an intervention. This perspective does not imply that one should attempt to impact directly the original cause of negative self-perceptions. For example, if a child has experienced lack of approval, neglect, or active rejection at the hands of caregivers, one may not be able to redress these antecedents. However, provisions for compensatory support as well as the fostering of insight about these initial causes, particularly for older children or adolescents, may have corrective influences.

General models of the causes, correlates, and consequences of self-representations provide an initial framework for identifying potential intervention strategies. The suggested strategies in this chapter build upon our own model, which has specified determinants derived from James (competence in domains of importance) and Cooley (approval from significant others). However, it has become apparent in our own work that there are multiple pathways to low self-worth and associated features of depression. Not all of the pathways in the general model are observed in all individuals. To date, we have documented six different patterns of antecedents leading to low self-worth and associated depression. A similar theme has been addressed within the clinical literature, where theorists (see Kendall, Lerner, & Craighead, 1984; Shirk & Russell, 1996) have challenged the "uniformity myth," namely, that the precursors of a given disorder (e.g., depression, conduct diagnoses) are necessarily similar across individuals so diagnosed. Thus, it is unlikely that one therapy or one intervention strategy will fit all, leading to challenges in the design of effective strategies that will be appropriate for particular individuals or subgroups that may share a common pattern of antecedents. Moreover, features of the self-system itself, for example, the need to verify self-representations, may well lead individuals to resist change, despite the benevolent intentions of intervenors.

The cognitive and social strategies suggested in this chapter have potential merit not only as interventions in the lives of those with unfavorable self-evaluations but also represent principles that may *prevent* the development of negative self-representations. Cognitive strategies include the following:

1. Reduction of the discrepancy between domain-specific perceived incompetence or inadequacy and the importance of success in those arenas. Fostering a focus on domains in which one does display competencies, while discounting those domains in which one is less adequate (to the extent that this is possible), should enhance global self-worth.

2. Encouragement of relatively realistic self-perceptions given the documented liabilities of inaccurate conceptions of self.

3. Assessment of the individual's belief system with regard to the potential for self-concept change, where efforts are directed toward encouraging the belief that most positive self-evaluations can and should be achieved.

4. Appreciation for the particular folk theory that an individual holds with regard to the causes of his/her negative self-evaluations, including the perceived directionality of effects that may be at variance with a more general model of causes, correlates, and consequences of self-worth.

5. For older children and adolescents, scaffolding an understanding of the actual *origins* of their negative self-perceptions, which should aid individuals to gain insights into antecedents, and in turn promote more positive self-evaluations.

For adolescents in particular, support for higher-level conceptualizations of those self-attributes perceived as contradictory or conflictual may be achieved by providing more integrative personal constructs (e.g., their cheerful and depressed attributes can be subsumed under the higher-order construct of moody). Further encouragement of attributions of appropriateness or flexibility for characteristics viewed as contradictory, as well as the construction of personal narratives that can give meaning to multiplicity, should also serve to enhance feelings of self-understanding and self-worth.

Strategies directed toward the more social determinants of negative self-representations can also be derived from the themes addressed in this volume. These include the following:

1. Provide for more support from parents, peers, or compensatory sources (e.g., special adults) for those children whose negative self-evaluations stem from neglect, disapproval, unconditional support, rejection, or abuse.
2. Encourage individuals to place more psychological emphasis on those interpersonal contexts in which they are experiencing support, to the extent that this is possible.
3. Use techniques that foster the internalization of the positive opinions of others, in order that the individual comes to personally adopt such representations as defining features of the self.

Finally, our understanding of the effectiveness of any given intervention strategy depends heavily upon appropriate program evaluation methodologies. Potentially effective intervention programs may not be demonstrated to be successful because there was no clear conceptual framework dictating the choice of measures. Moreover, other limitations include failing to assess features of the program itself, the confounding of substantive and psychometric issues such as reliability and validity, and/or the use of data-analytic strategies that are not sufficiently sensitive to patterns of individual or subgroup change.

The strategies suggested seem to call attention to self-constructs. However, the ultimate paradox is that those most preoccupied with perceptions of self are likely to experience the most unfavorable evaluations of their capabilities and their worth as a person. Moreover, those who *consciously adopt* a Jamesian perspective with regard to the impact of perceived appearance on self-worth and/or a looking-glass-self perspective, in which they remain preoccupied with the opinions of others, are most at risk for negative self-evaluations. While these processes set the stage for the development of attitudes about the self, the healthiest self-development will result from socialization experiences that (1) foster the belief that one's inner qualities (competence, kindness, morality) are more important than one's outer appearance, and (2) provide positive feedback about these qualities that can be internalized in the form of representations that one comes naturally to own as personal constructions of the Me-self by the I-self. Toward these goals let us all strive, in our own lives, and in the lives of others.

References

Abramson, L. Y., Metalsky, G. I., & Alloy, L. B. (1989). Hopelessness and depression: A theory-based subtype of depression. *Psychological Review, 96,* 358-372.

Abramson, L. Y., Seligman, M. E. P., & Teasdale, J. D. (1978). Learned helplessness in humans: Critique and reformulation. *Journal of Abnormal Psychology, 87,* 49-74.

Achenbach, T. M., Conners, C. K., & Quay, H. C. (1985). *The ACQ Behavior Checklist.* Unpublished manual, University of Vermont, Burlington.

Achenbach, T. M., & Edelbrock, C. S. (1983). *Manual for the Child Behavior Checklist and Revised Child Behavior Profile.* Burlington: University of Vermont.

Adams, G. R. (1982). Physical attractiveness. In A. G. Miller (Ed.), *In the eye of the beholder: Contemporary issues in stereotyping* (pp. 130-159). New York: Praeger.

Ahmed, K., & Harter, S. (1996). *Variations in self-esteem across different relational contexts among ethnic minority youth.* Unpublished manuscript, University of Denver, Denver, CO.

Ainsworth, M. (1973). The development of infant-mother attachment. In B. Caldwell & H. Ricciuto (Eds.), *Review of child development research* (Vol. 3, pp. 1-94). Chicago: University of Chicago Press.

Ainsworth, M. (1974). Infant-mother attachment and social development: Socialization as a product of reciprocal responsiveness to signals. In M. Richards (Ed.), *The integration of the child into the social world* (pp. 99-135). Cambridge, UK: Cambridge University Press.

Ainsworth, M. (1979). Infant-mother attachment. *American Psychologist, 34,* 932-937.

Alcohol, Drug Abuse, and Mental Health Administration. (1989). *Report of the Secretary's Task Force on Youth Suicide* (DHHS Publication No. ADM 89-1621). Washington, DC: U.S. Government Printing Office.

Alessandri, S. M., & Lewis, M. (1993). Parental evaluation and its relation to shame and pride in young children. *Sex Roles, 29,* 335-343.

Allen, J. P., Hauser, S. T., Bell, K. L., & O'Connor, T. G. (1994). Longitudinal assessment of autonomy and relatedness in adolescent-family interactions as predictors of adolescent ego development and self-esteem. *Child Development, 64,* 179-194.

Allgood-Merten, B., Lewinsohn, P. M., & Hops, R. (1990). Sex differences and adolescent depression. *Journal of Abnormal Psychology, 99,* 55–63.

Alloy, L., & Abramson, L. (1979). Judgment of contingency in depressed and nondepressed students: Sadder but wiser? *Journal of Experimental Psychology, 108,* 441–485.

Allport, G. W. (1961). *Pattern and growth in personality.* New York: Holt, Rinehart & Winston.

American Association of University Women. (1992). *How schools shortchange girls.* Washington, DC: American Association of University Women Educational Foundation.

Andersen, A. E. (1992). Diet vs. shape content of popular male and female magazines: A dose–response relationship to the incidence of eating disorders? *International Journal of Eating Disorders, 11,* 283–287.

Archer, S. L. (1989). Gender differences in identity development: Issues of process, domain, and timing. *Journal of Adolescence, 12,* 117–138.

Asarnow, J. R., & Bates, S. (1988). Depression in child psychiatric inpatients: Cognitive and attributional patterns. *Journal of Abnormal Child Psychology, 16,* 601–615.

Asch, S. S. (1966). Depression: Three clinical variations. *Psychological Study of the Child, 21,* 150–171.

Asendorpf, J. B., & van Aken, M. A. G. (1993). Deutsche versionen der Selbstkonzeptskalen von Harter. *Zeitscrift für Entwicklungspsychologie und Padagogische Psychologie, 25,* 64–86.

Asher, S. R. (1985). An evolving paradigm in social skill training research with children. In B. H. Schneider, E. H. Rubin, & J. E. Ledingham (Eds.), *Children's peer relations: Issues in assessment and intervention* (pp. 157–171). New York: Springer-Verlag.

Asher, S. R., & Renshaw, P. D. (1981). Children without friends: Social knowledge and social skill training. In S. R. Asher & J. M. Gottman (Eds.), *The development of children's friendships* (pp. 273–296). Cambridge, UK: Cambridge University Press.

Ashmore, R. D., & Ogilvie, D. M. (1992). He's such a nice boy . . . when he's with Grandma: Gender and evaluation in self-with-other representations. In T. M. Brinthaupt & R. P. Lipka (Eds.), *The self: Definitional and methodological issues* (pp. 236–290). Albany: State University of New York Press.

Bagley, C., & McDonald, M. (1984). Adult mental health sequelae of child sexual abuse, physical abuse, and neglect in maternally separated children. *Canadian Journal of Community Mental Health, 3,* 15–26.

Baker, D. (1986). Sex differences in classroom interactions in secondary science. *Journal of Classroom Interaction, 22,* 212–218.

Baldwin, J. M. (1895). *Mental development of the child and the race: Methods and processes.* New York: Macmillan.

Baldwin, J. M. (1897). *Social and ethical interpretations in mental development: A study in social psychology.* New York: Macmillan.

Banaji, M. R., & Prentice, D. A. (1994). The self in social contexts. In L. W. Porter & M. R. Rosenzweig (Eds.), *Annual review of psychology* (Vol. 45, pp. 297–325). New Haven, CT: Yale University Press.

Bandura, A. (1977). Self-efficacy: Toward a unifying theory of behavioral change. *Psychological Review, 84,* 191–215.

Bandura, A. (1978). The self system in reciprocal determinism. *American Psychologist, 33,* 344–358.

Bandura, A. (1989). Self-regulation of motivation and action through internal standards and goal systems. In L. Pervin (Ed.), *Goal concepts in personality and social psychology* (pp. 19–86). Hillsdale, NJ: Erlbaum.

Bandura, A. (1990). Conclusion: Reflections on nonability determinants of competence. In R. J. Sternberg & J. Kolligian, Jr. (Eds.), *Competence considered* (pp. 316–352). New Haven, CT: Yale University Press.

Bandura, A. (1991). Self-regulation of motivation through anticipatory and self-regulatory mechanisms. In R. A. Dienstbier (Ed.), *Perspectives on motivation: Nebraska Symposium on Motivation* (Vol. 38, pp. 79–94). Lincoln: University of Nebraska Press.

Bannister, D., & Agnew, J. (1977). The child's construing of self. In J. Cole (Ed.), *Nebraska Symposium on Motivation* (Vol. 26, pp. 99–125). Lincoln: University of Nebraska Press.

Barbar, R., & Cardinale, L. (1991). Are females invisible students? An investigation of teacher–student questioning interactions, *School Science and Mathematics, 91,* 306–310.

Barnes, E. J. (1980). The black community as a source of positive self-concept for Black children: A theoretical perspective. In R. Jones (Ed.), *Black psychology* (pp. 231–250). New York: Harper & Row.

Barnett, M. A., McMinimy, V., Flouer, G., & Masbad, I. (1987). Adolescents' evaluations of peers' motives for helping. *Journal of Youth and Adolescence, 16,* 579–586.

Barrett, K. C. (1995). A functionalist approach to shame and guilt. In J. P. Tangney & K. W. Fischer (Eds.), *Self-conscious emotions: The psychology of shame, guilt, embarrassment, and pride* (pp. 25–63). New York: Guilford Press.

Barrett, K. C., & Campos, J. (1987). Perspectives on emotional development: II. A functionalist approach to emotions. In J. Osofsky (Ed.), *Handbook of infant development* (2nd ed., pp. 555–578). New York: Wiley.

Bartholomew, K. (1990). Avoidance of intimacy: An attachment perspective. *Journal of Social and Personal Relationships, 7,* 147–178.

Bartolome, L. I. (1994). Beyond the methods fetish: Toward a humanizing pedagogy. *Harvard Educational Review, 64,* 173–194.

Basow, S. A. (1992). *Gender stereotypes and roles* (3rd ed.). Pacific Grove, CA: Brooks/Cole.

Bates, E. (1990). Language about me and you: Pronominal reference and the emerging concept of self. In D. Cicchetti & M. Beeghly (Eds.), *The self in transition: Infancy to childhood* (pp. 1–15). Chicago: University of Chicago Press.

Battle, J. (1987). Relationship between self-esteem and depression among children. *Psychological Reports, 60,* 1187–1190.

Baumeister, R. F. (1987). How the self became a problem: A psychological review of historical research. *Journal of Personality and Social Psychology, 52,* 163–176.

Baumeister, R. F. (1990). Suicide as escape from self. *Psychological Review, 97,* 90–113.

Baumeister, R. F. (1991a). *Escaping the self.* New York: Basic Books.

Baumeister, R. F. (1991b). *Meanings of life.* New York: Guilford Press.

Baumeister, R. F. (1993). Understanding the inner nature of low self-esteem: Uncertain, fragile, protective, and conflicted. In R. F. Baumeister (Ed.), *Self-esteem: The puzzle of low self-regard* (pp. 201–218). New York: Plenum.

Baumeister, R. F., Stillwell, A. M., & Heatherton, T. F. (1995). Interpersonal aspects of guilt: Evidence from narrative studies. In J. P. Tangney & K. W. Fischer (Eds.), *Self-conscious emotions: The psychology of shame, guilt, embarrassment, and pride* (pp. 255–273). New York: Guilford Press.

Baumeister, R. F., Tice, D. M., & Hutton, D. G. (1989). Self-presentational motivations and personality differences in self-esteem. *Journal of Personality, 57,* 547–579.

Baumgardner, A. H., Kaufman, C. M., & Levy, P. E. (1989). Regulating affect interpersonally: When low self-esteem leads to greater enhancement. *Journal of Personality and Social Psychology, 56,* 907–921.

Baumrind, D. (1966). The effects of authoritative parental control on child behavior. *Child Development, 37,* 887–907.

Baumrind, D. (1971). Current patterns of parental authority. *Developmental Psychology Monographs, 4,* 1–102.

Baumrind, D. (1989). Rearing competent children. In W. Damon (Ed.), *Child development today and tomorrow* (pp. 349–378). San Francisco: Jossey-Bass.

Beach, S. R. H., & Tesser, A. (1995). Self-esteem and the extended self-evaluation maintenance model: The self in social contest. In M. H. Kernis (Ed.), *Efficacy, agency, and self-esteem* (pp. 145–168). New York: Plenum.

Beale, C. R. (1994). *Boys and girls: The development of gender roles.* New York: McGraw-Hill.

Beane, J. A. (1994). Cluttered terrain: The schools' interest in the self. In T. M. Brinthaupt & R. P. Lipka (Eds.), *Changing the self* (pp. 69–88). Albany: State University of New York Press.

Beck, A. T. (1967). *Depression: Clinical, experimental and theoretical aspects.* New York: Harper & Row.

Beck, A. T. (1975). *Depression: Causes and treatments.* Philadelphia: University of Pennsylvania Press.

Beck, A. T. (1976). *Cognitive therapy and the emotional disorders.* New York: New American Library.

Beck, A. T. (1987, May). *Hopelessness as a prediction of ultimate suicide.* Paper presented at the joint meetings of the American Association of Suicidology and the International Association for Suicide Prevention, San Francisco, CA.

Beeghly, M., Carlson, V., & Cicchetti, D. (1986, April). *Child maltreatment and the self: The emergence of internal state language in low SES 30-month olds.* Paper presented at the International Conference on Infant Studies, Beverly Hills, CA.

Belenky, M. F., Clinchy, B. M., Goldberger, N. R., & Tarule, J. M. (1986). *Women's ways of knowing: The development of self, voice, and mind.* New York: Basic Books.

Bell, L. A. (1989). Something's wrong here and it's not me: Challenging the dilemmas that block girls' success. *Journal for the Education of the Gifted, 12*, 118–130.

Bem, S. (1985). Androgyny and gender schema theory. In T. B Sonderegger (Ed.), *Nebraska Symposium on Motivation* (Vol. 32, pp. 180–226). Lincoln: University of Nebraska Press.

Berndt, T. J., & Burgy, L. (1996). The social self-concept. In B. A. Bracken (Ed.), *Handbook of self-concept* (pp. 171–209). New York: Wiley.

Berscheid, E., Walster, E., & Bohrnstedt, G. (1973, November). Body image: The happy American body: A survey report. *Psychology Today*, pp. 119–131.

Bertenthal, B. I., & Fischer, K. W. (1978). Development of self-recognition in the infant. *Developmental Psychology, 14*, 44–50.

Biaggio, M. K., & Goodwin, W. H. (1987). Relation of depression to anger and hostility constructs. *Psychological Reports, 61*, 87–90.

Bibring, E. (1953). The mechanism of depression. In P. Greenacre (Ed.), *Affective disorders: Psychoanalytic contribution to their study* (pp. 13–48). New York: International Universities Press.

Birtchnell, S. A., Dolan, B. M., & Lacey, J. H. (1987). Body image distortion in non-eating disordered women. *International Journal of Eating Disorders, 6*, 385–391.

Blaine, B., & Crocker, J. (1993). Self-esteem and self-serving biases in reactions to positive and negative events: An integrative review. In R. F. Baumeister (Ed.), *Self-esteem: The puzzle of low self-regard* (pp. 55–81). New York: Plenum.

Blatt, S. J. (1974). Levels of object representation in anaclitic and introjective depression. *Psychoanalytic Study of the Child, 29*, 107–157.

Blatt, S. J. (1990). Interpersonal relatedness and self-definition: Two personality configurations and their implications for psychopathology and psychotherapy. In J. L. Singer (Ed.), *Repression and dissociation: Implications for personality theory, psychopathology and health* (pp. 299–335). Chicago: University of Chicago Press.

Blatt, S. J. (1995). Representational structures in psychopathology. In D. Cicchetti & S. Toth (Eds.), *Rochester Symposium on Developmental Psychopathology: Emotion, cognition, and representation* (Vol. 6, pp. 1–34). Rochester, NY: University of Rochester Press.

Bleiberg, E. (1984). Narcissistic disorders in children. *Bulletin of the Menninger Clinic, 48*, 501–517.

Block, J. H. (1983). Differential premises arising from differential socialization of the sexes: Some conjectures. *Child Development, 54*, 1335–1354.

Block, J. H., & Block, J. (1980). The role of ego-control and ego-resiliency in the organization of behavior. In W. A. Collins (Ed.), *Development of cognition, affect, and social relations: The Minnesota Symposia on Child Psychology* (Vol. 13, pp. 39–101). Hillsdale, NJ: Erlbaum.

Block, J. H., & Robins, R. W. (1993). A longitudinal study of consistency and change in self-esteem from early adolescence to early adulthood. *Child Development, 64,* 909-923.

Blos, P. (1962). *On adolescence.* New York: Free Press.

Blyth, D. A., Simmons, R. G., & Carlton-Ford, S. (1983). The adjustment of early adolescents to school transitions. *Journal of Early Adolescence, 3,* 105-120.

Boivin, M., Thomassin, L., & Alain, M. (1989). Peer rejection and self-perception among early elementary school children: Aggressive rejectees vs. withdrawn rejectees. In B. Schneider, J. Nadel, G. Attili, & R. Weissberg (Eds.), *Social competence in developmental perspective* (pp. 392-394). Norwell, MA: Kluwer.

Boivin, M., Vitaro, F., & Gagnon, C. (1992). A reassessment of the Self-Perception Profile for Children: Factor structure, reliability, and convergence validity of a French version among second through sixth grade children. *International Journal of Behavioral Development, 15,* 275-290.

Boldizar, J. P. (1991). Assessing sex-typing and androgyny in children: The children's sex-role inventory. *Developmental Psychology, 27,* 505-515.

Bolognini, M., Plancheral, B., Bettschart, W., & Halfon, O. (1996). Self-esteem and mental health in early adolescence: Development and gender differences. *Journal of Adolescence, 19,* 233-245.

Bonner, R. L., & Rich, A. R. (1987). Toward a predictive model of suicidal ideation and behavior: Some preliminary data in college students. *Suicide and Life-Threatening Behavior, 17,* 50-63.

Bowlby, J. (1969). *Attachment and loss: Vol. 1. Attachment.* New York: Basic Books.

Bowlby, J. (1973). *Attachment and loss: Vol. 2. Separation.* New York: Basic Books.

Bowlby, J. (1979). *The making and breaking of affectional bonds.* London: Tavistock.

Bowlby, J. (1980). *Attachment and loss: Vol. 3. Loss, sadness, and depression.* New York: Basic Books.

Bracken, B. (1992). *Multidimensional Self Concept Scale.* Austin, TX: PRO-ED.

Bracken, B. (1996). Clinical applications of a context-dependent multi-dimensional model of self-concept. In B. Bracken (Ed.), *Handbook of self-concept* (pp. 463-505). New York: Wiley.

Breckler, S. J., & Greenwald, A. G. (1982, August). *Charting coordinates for the self-concept in multidimensional trait space.* Paper presented at a symposium, "Functioning and Measurement of Self-Esteem," conducted at the annual meeting of the American Psychological Association, Washington, DC.

Bretherton, I. (1987). New perspectives on attachment relations: Security, communication, and internal working models. In J. D. Osofsky (Ed.), *Handbook of infant development* (2nd ed., pp. 1061-1101). New York: Wiley.

Bretherton, I. (1991). Pouring new wine into old bottles: The social self as internal working model. In M. R. Gunnar & L. A. Sroufe (Eds.), *Self processes and development: The Minnesota Symposia on Child Development* (Vol. 23, pp. 1-41). Hillsdale, NJ: Erlbaum.

Bretherton, I. (1992). The origins of attachment theory: John Bowlby and Mary Ainsworth. *Developmental Psychology, 28,* 759-775.

Bretherton, I. (1993). From dialogue to internal working models: The co-construction of self in relationships. In C. A. Nelson (Ed.), *Memory and affect: Minnesota Symposia on Child Psychology* (Vol. 26, pp. 237–263). Hillsdale, NJ: Erlbaum.

Bretherton, I., & Beeghly, M. (1982). Talking about internal states: The acquisition of an explicit theory of mind. *Developmental Psychology, 18,* 906–921.

Bretherton, I., Fritz, J., Zahn-Waxler, C., & Ridgeway, D. (1986). Learning to talk about emotions: A functionalist perspective. *Child Development, 57,* 529–548.

Briere, J. (1989). *Therapy for adults molested as children.* New York: Springer.

Briere, J. (1992). *Child abuse trauma: Theory and treatment of the lasting effects.* Newbury Park, CA: Sage.

Briere, J., & Runtz, M. (1988). Symptomatology associated with childhood sexual victimization in a non-clinical sample. *Child Abuse and Neglect, 12,* 51–59.

Briere, J., & Woo, R. (1991, August). *Child abuse sequelae in adult psychiatric emergency room patients.* Paper presented at the annual meeting of the American Psychological Association, San Francisco, CA.

Brim, O. B. (1976). Life span development of the theory of oneself: Implications for child development. In H. W. Reese (Ed.), *Advances in child development and behavior* (Vol. 11, pp. 82–103). New York: Academic Press.

Brinthaupt, T. M., & Lipka, R. P. (Eds.). (1994). *Changing the self: Philosophies, techniques, and experiences.* Albany: State University of New York Press.

Brody, L. R. (1985). Gender differences in emotional development: A review of theories and research. *Journal of Personality, 53,* 102–149.

Brooks-Gunn, J. (1988). Antecedents and consequences of variations in girls' maturational timing. *Journal of Adolescent Health Care, 9,* 365–373.

Brooks-Gunn, J., & Peterson, A. (1983). *Girls at puberty: Biological and psychological perspectives.* New York: Plenum.

Brophy, J. (1981). Teacher praises: A functional analysis. *Review of Educational Research, 51,* 5–32.

Brophy, J. (1985). Interactions of male and female students with male and female teachers. In L. C. Wilkenson & C. B. Marrett (Eds.), *Gender influences in classroom interaction* (pp. 107–130). Orlando, FL: Academic Press.

Broughton, J. (1978). The development of the concepts of self, mind, reality, and knowledge. In W. Damon (Ed.), *Social cognition* (pp. 75–100). San Francisco: Jossey-Bass.

Broughton, J. (1981). The divided self in adolescence. *Human Development, 24,* 13–32.

Broughton, J. M. (1987). The psychology, history, and ideology of the self. In K. S. Larsen (Ed.), *Dialectics and ideology in psychology* (pp. 128–164). Norwood, NJ: Ablex.

Brown, B. B. (1990). Peer groups and peer cultures. In S. S. Feldman & G. Elliot (Eds.), *At the threshold: The developing adolescent* (pp. 171–196). Cambridge, MA: Harvard University Press.

Brown, J. D. (1986). Evaluations of self and others: Self-enhancement biases in social judgments. *Social Cognition, 4,* 353–376.

Brown, J. D. (1993a). Motivational conflict and the self: The double-bind of low self-esteem. In R. F. Baumeister (Ed.), *Self-esteem: The puzzle of low self-regard* (pp. 117–127). New York: Plenum.

Brown, J. D. (1993b). Self-esteem and self-evaluation: Feeling is believing. In J. Suls (Ed.), *Psychological perspectives on the self* (Vol. 4, pp. 27–58). Hillsdale, NJ: Erlbaum.

Brown, L., & Gilligan, C. (1992). *Meeting at the crossroads: Women's psychology and girls' development.* Cambridge, MA: Harvard University Press.

Browne, A., & Finkelhor, D. (1986). Impact of child sexual abuse: A review of the research. *Psychological Bulletin, 99,* 66–77.

Bruner, J. (1990). *Acts of meaning.* Cambridge, MA: Harvard University Press.

Buddin, B. (1998). *The effects of parental role modeling and support for voice on level of voice among high school students.* Unpublished doctoral dissertation, University of Denver, Denver, CO.

Buhrmester, D., & Furman, W. (1987). The development of companionship and intimacy. *Child Development, 58,* 1101–1113.

Bukowsky, W. M. (1992). Sexual abuse and maladjustment considered from the perspective of normal developmental processes. In W. O'Donohue & J. H. Geer (Eds.), *The sexual abuse of children: Theory and research* (Vol. 1, pp. 261–282). Hillsdale, NJ: Erlbaum.

Burgess, E. W., & Locke, H. J. (1948). *The family: From institution to companionship.* New York: Amsterdam.

Buss, A. H. (1980). *Self-consciousness and social anxiety.* San Francisco: Freeman.

Butler, J. M., & Haigh, G. V. (1954). Changes in the relation between self-concepts and ideal concepts consequent upon client-centered counseling. In C. R. Rogers & R. F. Dymond, (Eds.), *Psychotherapy and personality change* (pp. 55–75). Chicago: University of Chicago Press.

Bynner, J. M., O'Malley, P. M., & Bachman, J. C. (1981). Self-esteem and delinquency revisited. *Journal of Youth and Adolescence, 10,* 407–441.

Byrne, D. E. (1996). Academic self-concept: Its structure, measurement, and relation with academic achievement. In B. A. Bracken (Ed.), *Handbook of self-concept* (pp. 287–316). New York: Wiley.

Calverley, R. M., Fischer, K. W., & Ayoub, C. (1994). Complex splitting of self-representations in sexually abused adolescent girls. *Development and Psychopathology, 6,* 195–213.

Campos, J., & Stenberg, C. (1980). Perception, appraisal, and emotion: The onset of social referencing. In M. Lamb & L. Sherrod (Eds.), *Infant social cognition* (pp. 273–314). Hillsdale, NJ: Erlbaum.

Cantor, N., & Mischel, W. (1979). Prototypes in person perception. In L. Berkowitz (Ed.), *Advances in experimental social psychology* (Vol. 12, pp. 3–52). New York: Academic Press.

Cantor, P. (1987). *Young people in crisis; How you can help.* A film presentation of the National Committee on Youth Suicide Prevention and American Association of Suicidology, in consultation with Harvard Medical School, Department of Psychiatry, Cambridge Hospital, Cambridge, MA.

Carlson, G. A., & Cantwell, D. P. (1980). Unmasking masked depression in children and adolescents. *American Journal of Psychiatry, 137,* 443–449.

Carlson, G. A., & Garber, J. (1986). Developmental issues in the classification of depression in children. In M. Rutter, C. E. Izard, & P. B. Read (Eds.), *Depression in young people: Developmental and clinical perspectives* (pp. 399–434). New York: Guilford Press.

Carroll, J. J., & Steward, M. S. (1984). The role of cognitive development in children's understandings of their own feelings. *Child Development, 55,* 1486–1492.

Carver, C. S., & Scheier, M. F. (1990). Origins and functions of positive and negative affect: A control-process. *Psychological Review, 97,* 19–35.

Carver, C. S., & Scheier, M. F. (1991). Self-regulation and the self. In J. Strauss & G. R. Goethals (Eds.), *The self: Interdisciplinary approaches* (pp. 168–207). New York: Springer-Verlag.

Case, R. (1985). *Intellectual development: Birth to adulthood.* New York: Academic Press.

Case, R. (1991). Stages in the development of the young child's first sense of self. *Developmental Review, 11,* 210–230.

Case, R. (1992). *The mind's staircase.* Hillsdale, NJ: Erlbaum.

Case, R., & Griffin, S. (1990). Child cognitive development: The role of central conceptual structures in the development of scientific and social thought. In C. A. Hauert (Ed.), *Developmental psychology: Cognitive, perceptuo-motor and psychological perspectives* (pp. 211–239). Amsterdam: Elsevier/North Holland.

Caslyn, R. J., & Kenny, D. A. (1977). Self-concept of ability and perceived evaluation of others: Cause or effect of academic achievement. *Journal of Educational Psychology, 69,* 136–145.

Cassidy, J. (1988). Child–mother attachment and the self at age six. *Child Development, 57,* 331–337.

Cassidy, J. (1990). Theoretical and methodological considerations in the study of attachment and the self in young children. In M. T. Greenberg, D. Cicchetti, & E. M. Cummings (Eds.), *Attachment in the preschool years: Theory, research, and intervention* (pp. 87–120). Chicago: University of Chicago Press.

Cassidy, J., & Kobak, R. R. (1988). Avoidance and its relationship to other defensive processes. In J. Belsky & T. Nezworski (Eds.), *Clinical implications of attachment* (pp. 300–326). Hillsdale, NJ: Erlbaum.

Cauce, A. M., Reid, M., Landesman, S., & Gonzales, N. (1990). Social support in young children: Measurement, structure, and behavioral impact. In B. R. Sarason, I. G. Sarason, & G. R. Pierce (Eds.), *Social support: An interactional view* (pp. 64–94). New York: Wiley.

Cavior, N., & Lombardi, D. A. (1973). Developmental aspects of judgment of physical attractiveness in children. *Developmental Psychology, 8,* 67–71.

Chandler, M. (1997). Stumping for progress in a post-modern world. In E. Amsel & K. A. Renninger (Eds.), *Change and development: Issues of theory, method, and application* (pp. 1–26). Hillsdale, NJ: Erlbaum.

Chodorow, N. (1989). *Feminism and psychoanalytic theory.* New Haven, CT: Yale University Press.

Christensen, A. (1988). Dysfunctional interaction patterns in couples. In P. Noller & M. A. Fitzpatrick (Eds.), *Perspectives on marital interaction* (pp. 31–52). Clevedon, Avon, UK: Multilingual Matters.

Christensen, A., & Heavey, C. L. (1990). Gender and social structure in the demand/withdraw pattern of marital conflict. *Journal of Personality and Social Psychology, 59,* 73–81.

Cicchetti, D. (1989). How research on child maltreatment has informed the study of child development: Perspectives from developmental psychology. In D. Cicchetti & V. Carlson (Eds.), *Child maltreatment: Theory and research on the causes and consequences of child abuse and neglect* (pp. 309–350). New York: Cambridge University Press.

Cicchetti, D. (1990). The organization and coherence of socioemotional, cognitive, and representational development: Illustrations through a developmental psychopathology perspective on Down syndrome and child maltreatment. In R. Thompson (Ed.), *Nebraska Symposium on Motivation: Socioemotional development* (Vol. 36, pp. 266–375). Lincoln: University of Nebraska Press.

Cicchetti, D. (1991). Fractures in the crystal: Developmental psychopathology and the emergence of self. *Developmental Review, 11,* 271–287.

Cicchetti, D., & Beeghly, M. (1990). Perspectives on the study of the self in transition. In D. Cicchetti & M. Beeghly (Eds.), *The self in transition: Infancy to childhood* (pp. 1–15). Chicago: University of Chicago Press.

Cicchetti, D., Beeghly, M., Carlson, V., & Toth, S. (1990). The emergence of the self in atypical populations. In D. Cicchetti & M. Beeghly (Eds.), *The self in transition: Infancy to childhood* (pp. 309–344). Chicago: University of Chicago Press.

Cicchetti, D., & Carlson, V. (Eds.). (1989). *Child maltreatment: Theory and research on the causes and consequences of child abuse and neglect.* New York: Cambridge University Press.

Cicchetti, D., & Schneider-Rosen, K. (1986). An organizational approach to childhood depression. In M. Rutter, C. E. Izard, & P. B. Read (Eds.), *Depression in young people: Developmental and clinical perspectives.* (pp. 71–134). New York: Guilford Press.

Cohn, L. D., Adler, N. E., Irwin, C. E., Jr., Millstein, S. G., Kegeles, S. M., & Stone, G. (1987). Body-figure preferences in male and female adolescents. *Journal of Abnormal Psychology, 96,* 276–279.

Collins, W. A. (1990). Parent–child relationships in the transition to adolescence: Continuity and change in interaction, affect, and cognition. In R. Montemayor, G. R. Adams, & T. P. Gullota (Eds.), *From childhood to adolescence: A transitional period?* (Vol. 2, pp. 85–106). Newbury Park, CA: Sage.

Condry, J. C., & Ross, D. F. (1985). Sex and aggression: The influence of gender label on the perception of aggression in children. *Child Development, 51,* 943–967.

Connell, J. P. (1985). A new multidimensional measure of children's perceptions of control. *Child Development, 56,* 1018–1041.

Connell, J. P., Spencer, M. B., & Aber, J. L. (1994). Educational risk and resilience in African-American youth: Context, self, action, and outcomes in school. *Child Development, 65,* 493–506.

Connell, J. P., & Wellborn, J. G. (1991). Competence, autonomy, and relatedness: A motivational analysis of self-system processes. In M. R. Gunnar & L. A. Sroufe (Eds.), *Self processes and development: The Minnesota Symposia on Child Development* (Vol. 23, pp. 43–78). Hillsdale, NJ: Erlbaum.

Cooley, C. H. (1902). *Human nature and the social order.* New York: Charles Scribner's Sons.

Coons, P. M. (1984). The differential diagnosis of multiple personality: A comprehensive review. *Psychiatric Clinics of North America, 7,* 51–65.

Cooper, C. R., Grotevant, H. D., & Condon, S. M. (1983). Individuality and connectedness both foster adolescent identity formation and role taking skills. In H. D. Grotevant & C. R. Cooper (Eds.), *Adolescent development in the family: New directions for child development* (pp. 43–59). San Francisco: Jossey-Bass.

Cooper, C. R., Jackson, J. F., Azmitia, M., Lopez, E., & Dunbar, N. (1995). Bridging students' multiple worlds: African American and Latino youth in academic outreach programs. In R. F. Macias & R. G. Garcia-Ramos (Eds.), *Changing schools for changing students: An anthology of research on language minorities* (pp. 211–234). Santa Barbara: University of California Linguistic Minority Research Institute.

Coopersmith, S. (1967). *The antecedents of self-esteem.* San Francisco: Freeman.

Costanzo, P. R. (1991). Morals, mothers, and memories: The social context of developing social cognition. In R. Cohen & R. Siegel (Eds.), *Context and development* (pp. 91–132). Hillsdale, NJ: Erlbaum.

Coster, W. J., Gersten, M. S., Beeghly, M., & Cicchetti, D. (1989). Communicative functioning in maltreated toddlers. *Developmental Psychology, 25,* 1020–1029.

Cousins, S. D. (1989). Culture and self-perception in Japan and the United States. *Journal of Personality and Social Psychology, 56,* 124–131.

Crain, R. M. (1996). The influences of age, race, and gender on child and adolescent multidimensional self-concept. In B. A. Bracken (Ed.), *Handbook of self-concept* (pp. 395–420). New York: Wiley.

Craven, R. G., Marsh, H. W., & Debus, R. (1991). Effects of internally focused feedback and attributional feedback on the enhancement of academic self-concept. *Journal of Educational Psychology, 83,* 17–26.

Crawford, M. (1989). Agreeing to differ: Feminist epistemologies and women's ways of knowing. In M. Crawford, & M. Gentry (Eds.), *Gender and thought: Psychological perspectives* (pp. 128–145). New York: Springer.

Crick, N. R., & Dodge, K. A. (1994). A review and reformulation of social information processing mechanisms in children's social adjustment. *Psychological Bulletin, 115,* 74–101.

Crittenden, P. M. (1981). Abusing, neglecting, problematic, and adequate dyads: Differentiating by patterns of interaction. *Merrill–Palmer Quarterly, 27,* 201–208.

Crittenden, P. M. (1985). Maltreated infants: Vulnerability and resilience. *Journal of Child Psychology and Psychiatry, 26,* 85–96.

Crittenden, P. M. (1988). Relationships at risk. In J. Belsky & T. Nezworski (Eds.), *Clinical implications of attachment* (pp. 136–174). Hillsdale, NJ: Erlbaum.

Crittenden, P. M. (1990). Internal representational models of attachment relationships. *Infant Mental Health Journal, 11,* 259–277.

Crittenden, P. M. (1994). Peering into the black box: An exploratory treatise on the development of self in young children. In D. Cicchetti & S. L. Toth (Eds.), *Rochester Symposium on Developmental Psychopathology: Disorders and dysfunctions of the self* (Vol. 5, pp. 79–148). Rochester, NY: University of Rochester Press.

Crittenden, P. M., & Ainsworth, M. D. S. (1989). Child maltreatment and attachment theory. In D. Cicchetti & V. Carlson (Eds.), *Child maltreatment: Theory and research on the causes and consequences of child abuse and neglect* (pp. 432–463). New York: Cambridge University Press.

Crocker, P. R. E., & Ellsworth, J. P. (1990). Perceptions of competence in physical education students, *Canadian Journal of Sports Science,15,* 262–266.

Cross, W. E. (1985). Black identity: Rediscovering the distinction between personal identity and reference group orientation. In M. B. Spencer, G. C. Brookings, & W. R. Allen (Eds.), *Beginnings: The social and affective development of black children* (pp. 155–171). Hillsdale, NJ: Erlbaum.

Crowther, J. H., & Chernyk, B. (1986). Bulimia and binge eating in adolescent females: A comparison. *Addictive Behaviors, 11,* 415–424.

Culbertson, J. L., & Willis, D. J. (1998). Interventions with young children who have been multiply abused. In B. B. R. Rossman & M. S. Rosenberg (Eds.), *Multiple victimization of children: Conceptual, developmental, research, and treatment issues* (pp. 207–232). New York: Haworth Press.

Curran, D. K. (1987). *Adolescent suicidal behavior.* Washington, DC: Hemisphere.

Damon, W. (1995). *Greater expectations: Overcoming the culture of indulgence in America's homes and schools.* New York: Free Press.

Damon, W., & Hart, D. (1988). *Self-understanding in childhood and adolescence.* New York: Cambridge University Press.

Danis, B., & Harter, S. (1996). *Self-perceptions of anorectic and bulimic female college students.* Unpublished manuscript, University of Denver, Denver, CO.

Darling, N. (1991). The influence of challenging and supportive relationships on the academic achievement of adolescents. In S. F. Hamilton (Ed.), *Unrelated adults in adolescents' lives* (pp. 12–30). Ithaca, NY: Western Societies Program.

Darling, N., Hamilton, S. F., & Niego, S. (1996). Adolescents' relations with adults outside the family. In G. R. Adams, R. Montemayor, & T. P. Gullotta (Eds.), *Psychosocial development during adolescence* (pp. 216–235). Thousand Oaks, CA: Sage.

Davies, E., & Furnham, A. (1986). Body satisfaction in adolescent girls. *British Journal of Medical Psychology, 59,* 279–287.

de Beauvoir, S. (1952). *The second sex.* New York: Knopf.

Deci, E. L., & Ryan, R. M. (1987). The support of autonomy and the control of behavior. *Journal of Personality and Social Psychology, 53,* 1024–1037.

Deci, E. L., & Ryan, R. M. (1995). Human autonomy: The basis for true self-esteem. In M. H. Kernis (Ed.), *Efficacy, agency, and self-esteem* (pp. 31-46). New York: Plenum.

De La Ronde, C., & Swann, W. B., Jr. (1993). Caught in the crossfire: Positivity and self-verification strivings among people with low self-esteem. In R. F. Baumeister (Ed.), *Self-esteem: The puzzle of low self-regard* (pp. 147-161). New York: Plenum.

Delpit, L. D. (1993). The silenced dialogue: Power and pedagogy in educating other people's children. In L. Weis & M. Fine (Eds.), *Beyond silenced voices* (pp. 119-139). Albany: State University of New York Press.

Demo, D. H., & Savin-Williams R. C. (1992). Self-concept stability and change during adolescence. In R. P. Lipka & T. M. Brinthaupt (Eds.), *Self-perspectives across the life span* (pp. 116-150). Albany: State University of New York Press.

Deutsch, H. (1955). The imposter: Contribution to ego psychology of a type of psychopath. *Psychoanalytic Quarterly, 24,* 483-505.

Dickstein, E. (1977). Self and self-esteem: Theoretical foundations and their implications for research. *Human Development, 20,* 129-140.

Dodge, K. A. (1991). The structure and function of reactive and proactive aggression. In D. Pepler & K. H. Rubin (Eds.), *The development and treatment of childhood aggression* (pp. 201-218). Hillsdale, NJ: Erlbaum.

Doi, T. (1973). *Anatomy of dependence* (J. Bester, Trans.). Tokyo: Kodansha.

Doi, T. (1986). *The anatomy of conformity: The individual versus society.* Tokyo: Kodansha.

Donaldson, S. K., & Westerman, M. A. (1986). Development of children's understanding of ambivalence and causal theories of emotion. *Developmental Psychology, 22,* 655-662.

Dunn, J. (1987). The beginnings of moral understanding: Development in the second year. In J. Kagan & S. Lamb (Eds.), *The emergence of morality in young children* (pp. 91-111). Chicago: University of Chicago Press.

Dunn, J. (1988). *The beginnings of social understanding.* Cambridge, MA: Harvard University Press.

Dunn, J., Brown, J., & Beardsall, L. (1991). Family talk about feeling states and children's later understanding of others' emotions. *Developmental Psychology, 27,* 445-448.

Dunning, D. (1993). Words to live by: The self and definitions of social concepts and categories. In J. Suls (Ed.), *Psychological perspectives on the self* (Vol. 4, pp. 99-126). Hillsdale, NJ: Erlbaum.

Dusek, J. B., & Flaherty, J. (1981). The development of the self during the adolescent years. *Monograph of the Society for Research in Child Development, 46*(Whole No. 191), 1-61.

Duvall, S., & Wicklund, R. A. (1972). *A theory of self-awareness.* New York: Academic Press.

Dweck, C. S. (1991). Self-theories and goals: Their role in motivation, personality and development. In R. Dienstbier (Ed.), *Nebraska Symposium on Motivation* (Vol. 38, pp. 199-235). Lincoln: University of Nebraska Press.

Dweck, C. S., & Elliott, E. S. (1983). Achievement motivation. In P. Mussen & E. M. Hetherington (Eds.), *Handbook of child psychology: Vol 4. Socialization, personality, and social development* (pp. 643–691). New York: Wiley.

Dweck, C. S., & Leggett, E. L. (1988). A social-cognitive approach to motivation and personality. *Psychological Review, 95,* 256–273.

Eagly, A. (1987). *Sex differences in social behavior: A social role interpretation.* Hillsdale, NJ: Erlbaum.

Eagly, A. H. (1995). The science and politics of comparing women and men. *American Psychologist, 50,* 145–158.

Eccles, J. S., & Blumenfeld, P. (1985). Classroom experiences and student gender: Are there differences and do they matter? In L. C. Wilkinson & C. B. Marrett (Eds.), *Gender influences in classroom interaction* (pp. 79–114). Orlando, FL: Academic Press.

Eccles, J. S., & Midgley, C. (1989). Stage/environment fit: Developmentally appropriate classrooms for early adolescents. In R. Ames & C. Ames (Eds.), *Research on motivation in education* (Vol. 3, pp. 139–181). San Diego: Academic Press.

Eccles, J. S., Midgley, C., & Adler, T. (1984). Grade-related changes in the school environment: Effects on achievement motivation. In J. G. Nicholls (Ed.), *The development of achievement motivation* (pp. 283–331). Greenwich, CT: JAI Press.

Eccles, J. S., Wigfield, A., & Schiefele, U. (1998). Motivation to succeed. In W. Damon (Series Ed.) & N. Eisenberg (Vol. Ed.), *Handbook of child psychology: Vol. 3. Social, emotional, and personality development* (5th ed., pp. 1017–1096). New York: Wiley.

Eder, R. A., Gerlach, S. G., & Perlmutter, M. (1987). In search of children's selves: Development of the specific and general components of the self-concept. *Child Development, 58,* 1044–1050.

Eichenbaum, L., & Orbach, S. (1983). *Understanding women: A feminist psychoanalytic approach.* New York: Basic Books.

Eisenberg, A. (1985). Learning to describe past experiences in conversation. *Discourse Processes, 8,* 177–204.

Eisenberg, N., Cialdini, R. B., McCreath, J., & Shell, R. (1987). Consistency based compliance: When and why do consistency procedures have immediate effects? *Journal of Behavioral Development, 12,* 351–368.

Eisenberg, N., & Lennon, R. (1983). Sex differences in empathy and related capacities. *Psychological Bulletin, 94,* 100–131.

Eisenberg, N., Martin, C. L., & Fabes, R. A. (1996). Gender development and gender effects. In D. C. Berliner, & R. C. Calfee (Eds.), *Handbook of educational psychology* (pp. 358–396). New York: Simon & Schuster/Macmillan.

Elkind, D. (1967). Egocentrism in adolescence. *Child Development, 38,* 1025–1034.

Elkind, D. (1979). Growing up faster. *Psychology Today, 12,* 38–45.

Elkind, D. (1984). *All grown up and no place to go: Teenagers in crisis.* Reading, MA: Addison-Wesley.

Elliot, D. M., & Briere, J. (1992). Sexual abuse trauma among professional women:

Validating the Trauma Symptom Checklist (TSC-40). *Child Abuse and Neglect,* 16, 391–398.

Ellis, A. (1958). Rational psychotherapy. *Journal of General Psychology,* 58, 35–49.

Emde, R. N. (1988). Development terminable and interminable: Innate and motivational factors from infancy. *International Journal of Psychoanalysis,* 69, 23–25.

Emde, R. N. (1994). Individuality, context, and the search for meaning. *Child Development,* 65, 719–737.

Emde, R. N., Biringen, A., Clyman, R. B., & Oppenheim, D. (1991). The moral self of infancy: Affective core and procedural knowledge. *Developmental Review,* 11, 251–270.

Emde, R. N., & Oppenheim, D. (1995). Shame, guilt, and the oedipal drama: Developmental considerations concerning morality and the referencing of critical others. In J. P. Tangney & K. W. Fischer (Eds.), *Self-conscious emotions: The psychology of shame, guilt, embarrassment, and pride* (pp. 413–436). New York: Guilford Press.

Emery, P. E. (1983). Adolescent depression and suicide. *Adolescence,* 18, 245–258.

Engel, M. (1959). The stability of the self-concept in adolescence. *Journal of Abnormal and Social Psychology,* 58, 211–217.

Epstein, S. (1973). The self-concept revisited or a theory of a theory. *American Psychologist,* 28, 405–416.

Epstein, S. (1981). The unity principle versus the reality and pleasure principles, or the tale of the scorpion and the frog. In M. D. Lynch, A. A. Norem-Hebeisen, & K. Gergen (Eds.), *Self-concept: Advances in theory and research* (pp. 82–110). Cambridge, MA: Ballinger.

Epstein, S. (1990). The self-concept, the traumatic neuroses, and the structure of personality. In D. Ozer, J. M. Healy, Jr., & A. J. Stewart (Eds.), *Perspectives on personality* (Vol. 3, pp. 31–59). Greenwich, CT: JAI Press.

Epstein, S. (1991). Cognitive-experiential self theory: Implications for developmental psychology. In M. R. Gunnar & L. A. Sroufe (Eds.), *Self processes and development: The Minnesota Symposia on Child Development* (Vol. 23, pp. 111–137). Hillsdale, NJ: Erlbaum.

Epstein, S., & Morling, B. (1995). Is the self motivated to do more than enhance and/or verify itself? In M. H. Kernis (Ed.), *Efficacy, agency, and self-esteem* (pp. 9–26). New York: Plenum.

Erickson, M. F., Egeland, B., & Pianta, R. (1989). The effects of maltreatment on the development of young children. In D. Cicchetti & V. Carlson (Eds.), *Child maltreatment: Theory and research on the causes and consequences of child abuse and neglect* (pp. 647–684). New York: Cambridge University Press.

Erikson, E. H. (1950). *Childhood and society* (2nd ed.). New York: Norton.

Erikson, E. H. (1959). Identity and the life cycle. *Psychological Issues,* 1, 18–164.

Erikson, E. H. (1968). *Identity, youth, and crisis.* New York: Norton.

Fallon, A. E., & Rozin, P. (1985). Sex differences in perceptions of desirable body shape. *Journal of Abnormal Psychology,* 94, 102–105.

Faludi, S. (1991). *Backlash: The undeclared war against women.* New York: Crown.

Feingold, A. (1992). Good-looking people are not what we think. *Psychological Bulletin, 111,* 304–341.

Feiring, C., & Taska, L.S. (1996). Family self-concept: Ideas on its meaning. In B. Bracken (Ed.), *Handbook of self-concept* (pp. 317–373). New York: Wiley.

Feldman, D. H. (1994). *Beyond universals in cognitive development* (2nd ed.). Norwood, NJ: Ablex.

Felson, R. B. (1993). The (somewhat) social self: How others affect self-appraisals. In J. Suls (Ed.), *Psychological perspectives on the self* (Vol. 4, pp. 1–26). Hillsdale, NJ: Erlbaum.

Felson, R., & Zielinski, M. (1989). Children's self-esteem and parental support. *Journal of Marriage and the Family, 51,* 727–735.

Fenichel, O. (1945). *The psychoanalytic theory of neurosis.* New York: Norton.

Ferguson, T. J., & Stegge, H. (1995). Emotional states and traits in children: The case of guilt and shame. In J. P. Tangney & K. W. Fischer (Eds.), *Self-conscious emotions: The psychology of shame, guilt, embarrassment, and pride* (pp. 174–197). New York: Guilford Press.

Fine, M. (1991). *Framing dropouts: Notes on the politics of an urban public high school.* Albany: State University Press of New York.

Finkelhor, D. (1979). *Sexually victimized children.* New York: Free Press.

Finkelhor, D. (1984). *Child sexual abuse: New theory and research.* New York: Free Press.

Fischer, K. W. (1980). A theory of cognitive development: The control and construction of hierarchies of skills. *Psychological Review, 87,* 477–531.

Fischer, K. W., & Ayoub, C. (1994). Affective splitting and dissociation in normal and maltreated children: Developmental pathways for self in relationships. In D. Cicchetti & S. Toth (Eds.), *Rochester Symposium on Developmental Psychopathology: Disorders and dysfunctions of the self* (Vol. 5, pp. 149–222). Rochester, NY: University of Rochester Press.

Fischer, K. W., & Canfield, R. (1986). The ambiguity of stage and structure in behavior: Person and environment in the development of psychological structure. In I. Levin (Ed.), *Stage and structure: Reopening the debate* (pp. 246–267). New York: Plenum.

Fischer, K. W., Hand, H. H., Watson, M. W., Van Parys, M., & Tucker, J. (1984). Putting the child into socialization: The development of social categories in preschool children. In L. Katz (Ed.), *Current topics in early childhood education* (Vol. 5, pp. 27–72). Norwood, NJ: Ablex.

Fischer, K. W., & Pipp, S. L. (1984). Development of the structures of unconscious thought. In K. Bowers & D. Meichenbaum (Eds.), *The unconscious reconsidered* (pp. 88–148). New York: Wiley.

Fischer, K. W., Shaver, P., & Carnochan, P. (1990). How emotions develop and how they organize development. *Cognition and Emotion, 4,* 81–127.

Fischer, K. W., Wang, L., Kennedy, B., & Cheng, C. (in press). Culture and biology in emotional development. In D. Sharma & K. W. Fischer (Eds.), *Socioemotional development across cultures: New directions for child development.* San Francisco: Jossey-Bass.

Fitzpatrick, M. A. (1988). *Between husbands and wives: Communication in marriage.* Newbury Park, CA: Sage.

Fivush, R. (1987). Scripts and categories: Interrelationships in development. In U. Neisser (Ed.), *Concepts and conceptual development: Ecological and intellectual factors in categorization.* Cambridge, UK: Cambridge University Press.

Fivush, R., Gray, J. T., & Fromhoff, F. A. (1987). Two-year-olds talk about the past. *Cognitive Development, 2,* 393–409.

Fivush, R., & Hamond, N. R. (1990). Autobiographical memory across the preschool years: Toward reconceptualizing childhood amnesia. In R. Fivush & J. A. Hudson (Eds.), *Knowing and remembering in young children* (pp. 223–248). New York: Cambridge University Press.

Fivush, R., & Hudson, J. A. (Eds.). (1990). *Knowing and remembering in young children.* New York: Cambridge University Press.

Flavell, J. H. (1985). *Cognitive development* (2nd ed.). Englewood Cliffs, NJ: Prentice-Hall.

Flavell, J. H., Miller, P. H., & Miller, S. A. (1993). *Cognitive development* (3rd ed.). Englewood Cliffs, NJ: Prentice Hall.

Floyd, F., & Markman, H. J. (1983). Observational biases in spouse observation: Toward a cognitive/behavioral model of marriage. *Journal of Consulting and Clinical Psychology, 51,* 450–457.

Fox, K., Page, A., Armstrong, N., & Kirby, B. (1994). Dietary restraint and self-perceptions in early adolescence. *Personality and Individual Differences, 17,* 87–96.

Frank, E., Carpenter, L. L., & Kupfer, D. J. (1988). Sex differences in recurrent depression: Are there any that are significant? *American Journal of Psychiatry, 145,* 41–45.

Franzoi, S. L., & Shields, S. A. (1984). The body esteem scale: Multidimensional structure and sex differences in a college population. *Journal of Personality Assessment, 48,* 173–178.

Freeman, M. (1992). Self as narrative: The place of life history in studying the life span. In T. M. Brinthaupt & R. P. Lipka (Eds.), *The self: Definitional and methodological issues* (pp. 15–43). Albany: State University of New York Press.

Freud, A. (1965). *Normality and pathology in childhood.* New York: International Universities Press.

Freud, S. (1952). *A general introduction to psychoanalysis.* New York: Washington Square Press.

Freud, S. (1968). Mourning and melancholia. In J. Strachey (Ed. and Trans.), *The standard edition of the complete psychological works of Sigmund Freud* (Vol. 14, 237–260). London: Hogarth Press. (Original work published 1917)

Frey, K. S., & Ruble, D. N. (1985). What children say when the teacher is not around: Conflicting goals in social comparison and performance assessment in the classroom. *Journal of Personality and Social Psychology, 48,* 550–562.

Frey, K. S., & Ruble, D. N. (1990). Strategies for comparative evaluation: Maintaining a sense of competence across the life span. In R. J. Sternberg & J. Kolligian,

Jr. (Eds.), *Competence considered* (pp. 167–189). New Haven, CT: Yale University Press.

Frijda, N. H. (1986). *The emotions.* Cambridge, UK: Cambridge University Press.

Furman, W., & Bierman, K. (1984). Children's conceptions of friendships: A multimethod study of developmental changes. *Developmental Psychology, 20,* 925–931.

Galbo, J. J., & Mayer-Demetrulias, D. (1996). Recollections of nonparental significant adults during childhood and adolescence. *Youth and Society, 27,* 403–420.

Garbarino, J., Guttman, E., & Seeley, J. (1986). *The psychologically battered child: Strategies for identification, assessment, and intervention.* San Francisco: Jossey-Bass.

Garner, D. M., Garfinkel, P. E., Schwartz, D., & Thompson, M. (1980). Cultural expectations of thinness in women. *Psychological Reports, 47,* 483–491.

Garrison, C. Z. (1989). The study of suicidal behavior in the schools. *Suicide and Life-Threatening Behavior, 19,* 120–130.

Gavin, D. A. W., & Herry, Y. (1996). The French Self-Perception Profile for Children: Score validity and reliability. *Educational and Psychological Measurement, 56,* 678–700.

Gecas, V. (1972). Parental behavior and contextual variations in adolescent self-esteem. *Sociometry, 36,* 332–345.

Gergen, K. J. (1967). To be or not to be the single self. In S. M. Journal (Ed.), *To be or not to be: Existential perspectives on the self* (pp. 104–132). Gainesville: University of Florida Press.

Gergen, K. J. (1968). Personal consistency and the presentation of self. In C. Gordon & J. Gergen (Eds.), *The self in social interaction* (pp. 299–308). New York: Wiley.

Gergen, K. J. (1977). The social construction of self-knowledge. In T. Mischel (Ed.), *The self: Psychological and philosophical issues* (pp. 139–169). Totowa, NJ: Rowman & Littlefield.

Gergen, K. J. (1982). From self to science: What is there to know? In J. Suls (Ed.), *Psychological perspectives on the self* (Vol. 1, pp. 129–149). Hillsdale, NJ: Erlbaum.

Gergen, K. J. (1991). *The saturated self.* New York: Basic Books.

Gergen, K. J., & Gergen, M. M. (1988). Narrative and the self as relationship. In L. Berkowitz (Ed.), *Advances in experimental social psychology* (Vol. 21, pp. 17–56). New York: Academic Press.

Gesell, A., & Ilg, F. (1946). *The child from five to ten.* New York: Harper & Row.

Gilligan, C. (1982). *In a different voice: Psychological theory and women's development.* Cambridge, MA: Harvard University Press.

Gilligan, C. (1993). Joining the resistance: Psychology, politics, girls, and women. In L. Weis & M. Fine (Eds.), *Beyond silenced voices* (pp. 143–168). Albany: Suny University of New York Press.

Gilligan, C., Lyons, N., & Hanmer, T. J. (1989). *Making connections.* Cambridge, MA: Harvard University Press.

Gilligan, C., Rogers, A. G., & Tolman, D. L. (Eds.). (1991). *Women, girls, and psychotherapy: Reframing resistance.* New York: Haworth Press.

Gispert, M., Davis, M. C., Marsh, L., & Wheeler, K. (1987). Predictive factors in repeated suicide attempts by adolescents. *Hospital and Community Psychology*, *38*, 390–393.

Glick, M., & Zigler, E. (1985). Self-image: A cognitive-developmental approach. In R. Leahy (Ed.), *The development of the self* (pp. 1–54). New York: Academic Press.

Gnepp, J., McKee, E., & Domanic, J. A. (1987). Children's use of situational information to infer emotion: Understanding emotionally equivocal situations. *Developmental Psychology*, *23*, 114–123.

Goffman, E. (1959). *The presentation of self in everyday life*. Garden City, NY: Doubleday.

Gold, M. (1994). Changing the delinquent self. In T. M. Brinthaupt & R. P. Lipka (Eds.), *Changing the self* (pp. 89–108). Albany: State University of New York Press.

Gordon, C. (1968). Self-conceptions: Configurations of content. In C. Gordon & K. J. Gergen (Eds.), *The self is social interaction* (pp. 115–136). New York: Wiley.

Gottman, J. M., & Krokoff, L. J. (1989). Marital interaction and satisfaction: A longitudinal view. *Journal of Consulting and Clinical Psychology*, *57*, 47–52.

Gralinsky, J., Fesbach, N. D., Powell, C., & Derrington, T. (1993, April). *Self-understanding: Meaning and measurement of maltreated children's sense of self*. Paper presented at the meeting of the Society for Research in Child Development, New Orleans, LA.

Granlese, J., & Joseph, S. (1993). Factor analysis of the Self-Perception Profile for Children. *Personality and Individual Differences*, *15*, 343–345.

Graziano, W. G., & Waschull, S. B. (1995). Social development and self-monitoring. In N. Eisenberg (Ed.), *Social development: Review of personality and social psychology* (Vol. 15, pp. 233–260). London: Sage.

Green, A. H. (1982). Child abuse. In J. Lachenmeyer & M. Gibbs (Eds.), *Psychopathology in childhood* (pp. 91–123). New York: Gardner Press.

Greenberg, J., Pyszczynski, T., & Solomon, S. (1995). Toward a dual-motive depth psychology of self and social behavior. In M. H. Kernis (Ed.), *Efficacy, agency, and self-esteem* (pp. 73–101). New York: Plenum.

Greenfeld, D., Quinlan, D. M., Harding, P., Glass, E., & Bliss, A. (1987). Eating behavior in an adolescent population. *International Journal of Eating Disorders*, *6*, 99–111.

Greenier, K. D., Kernis, M. H., & Waschull, S. B. (1995). Not all high or low self-esteem people are the same: Theory and research on stability of self-esteem. In M. H. Kernis (Ed.), *Efficacy, agency, and self-esteem* (pp. 51–68). New York: Plenum.

Greenwald, A. G. (1980). The totalitarian ego: Fabrication and revision of personal history. *American Psychologist*, *7*, 603–618.

Greenwald, A. G., & Pratkanis, A. R. (1984). The self. In R. S. Wyer & T. K. Srull (Eds.), *Handbook of social cognition* (Vol. 3, pp. 129–178). Hillsdale, NJ: Erlbaum.

Griffin, N., Chassin, L., & Young, R. D. (1981). Measurement of global self-concept versus multiple role-specific self-concepts in adolescents. *Adolescence*, *16*, 49–56.

Griffin, S. (1992). Structural analysis of the development of their inner world: A neo-structural analysis of the development of intrapersonal intelligence. In R. Case (Ed.), *The mind's staircase* (pp. 189–206). Hillsdale, NJ: Erlbaum.

Griffin, S. (1995). A cognitive-developmental analysis of pride, shame, and embarrassment in middle childhood. In J. P. Tangney & K. W. Fischer (Eds.), *Self-conscious emotions: The psychology of shame, guilt, embarrassment, and pride* (pp. 219–236). New York: Guilford Press.

Gross, J., & Rosen, J. C. (1988). Bulimia in adolescents: Prevalence and psychosocial correlates. *International Journal of Eating Disorders, 7,* 51–61.

Grotevant, H. D., & Cooper, C. R. (Eds.). (1983). *Adolescent development in the family: New directions for child development.* San Francisco: Jossey-Bass.

Grotevant, H. D., & Cooper, C. R. (1986). Individuation in family relationships. *Human Development, 29,* 83–100.

Grusec, J. E. (1983). The internalization of altruistic dispositions: A cognitive analysis. In E. T. Higgins, D. N. Ruble, & W. W. Hartup (Eds.), *Social cognition and social development: A sociocultural perspective* (pp. 275–293). New York: Cambridge University Press.

Grusec, J. E., & Redler, E. (1980). Attribution, reinforcement, and altruism: A developmental analysis. *Developmental Psychology, 16,* 525–535.

Guardo, C. J., & Bohan, J. B. (1971). Development of a sense of self-identity in children. *Child Development, 42,* 1909–1921.

Guisinger, S., & Blatt, S. J. (1993). Individuality and relatedness: Evolution of a fundamental dialectic. *American Psychologist, 49,* 104–111.

Hagborg, W. J. (1994). The Rosenberg Self-Esteem Scale and Harter's Self-Perception Profile for Adolescents: A concurrent validity study. *Psychology in the Schools, 30,* 132–136.

Hagen, J. W., Barclay, C. R., Anderson, B. J., Feeman, D. J., Segal, S. S., Bacon, G., & Goldstein, G. W. (1990). Intellective functioning and strategy use in children with insulin-dependent diabetes. *Child Development, 61,* 1714–1727.

Haltiwanger, J. (1989, April). *Behavioral referents of presented self-esteem in young children.* Paper presented at the meeting of the Society for Research in Child Development, Kansas City, MO.

Haltiwanger, J., & Harter, S. (1994). *Presented self-esteem in young children.* Unpublished manuscript, University of Denver, Denver, CO.

Hamilton, S. F., & Darling, N. (1989). Mentors in adolescents' lives. In K. Hurrelmann & U. Engel (Eds.), *The social world of adolescents: International perspectives* (pp. 121–139). Hawthorne, NY: DeGruyter.

Hammen, C., & Goodman-Brown, T. (1990). Self-schemas and vulnerability to specific life stress in children at risk for depression. *Cognitive Therapy and Research, 14,* 215–227.

Hansen, S., Walker, J., & Flom, B. (1995). *Growing smart: What's working for girls in school.* Washington, DC: American Association of University Women Educational Foundation.

Harris, P. L. (1983a). What children know about the situations that provoke emotion. In M. Lewis & C. Saarni (Eds.), *The socialization of affect* (pp. 162–185). New York: Plenum.

Harris, P. L. (1983b). Children's understanding of the link between situation and emotion. *Journal of Experimental Child Psychology, 36,* 490–509.

Harris, P. L., Olthof, T., & Meerum-Terwogt, M. (1981). Children's knowledge of emotion. *Journal of Child Psychology and Psychiatry, 45,* 247–261.

Hart, D. (1988). The adolescent self-concept in social context. In D. K. Lapsley & F. C. Power (Eds.), *Self, ego, and identity* (pp. 71–90). New York: Springer-Verlag.

Hart, D., & Edelstein, W. (1992). Self-understanding and development in cross-cultural perspective. In T. M. Brinthaupt & R. P. Lipka (Eds.), *The self: Definitional and methodological issues* (pp. 291–322). Albany: State University of New York Press.

Hart, D., Fegley, S., & Brengelman, D. (1993). Perceptions of past, present and future selves among children and adolescents. *British Journal of Developmental Psychology, 11,* 265–282.

Hart, S. N., Germain, R., & Brassard, M. R. (1987). The challenge: To better understand and combat the psychological maltreatment of children and youth. In M. R. Brassard, R. Germain, & S. N. Hart (Eds.), *Psychological maltreatment of children and youth* (pp. 3–24). New York: Pergamon.

Hart, D., & Karmel, M. P. (in press). Self-awareness and self-knowledge in humans, apes, and monkeys. In A. Russon, K. Bard, & S. Parker (Eds.), *Reaching into thought.* New York: Cambridge University Press.

Harter, S. (1977). A cognitive-developmental approach to children's expression of conflicting feelings and a technique to facilitate such expression in play therapy. *Journal of Consulting and Clinical Psychology, 45,* 417–432.

Harter, S. (1982a). The perceived competence scale for children. *Child Development, 53,* 87–97.

Harter, S. (1982b). Cognitive-developmental considerations in the conduct of play therapy. In C. E. Schafer & K. J. O'Connor (Eds.), *Handbook of play therapy* (pp. 119–160). New York: Wiley.

Harter, S. (1983). Developmental perspectives on the self-system. In P. Mussen & E. M. Hetherington (Eds.), *Handbook of child psychology: Vol. 4. Socialization, personality, and social development* (4th ed., pp. 275–385). New York: Wiley.

Harter, S. (1985a). Competence as a dimension of self-evaluation: Toward a comprehensive model of self-worth. In R. Leahy (Ed.), *The development of the self* (pp. 55–122). New York: Academic Press.

Harter, S. (1985b). *The Self-Perception Profile for Children.* Unpublished manual, University of Denver, Denver, CO.

Harter, S. (1985c). *The Social Support Scale for Children.* Unpublished manual, University of Denver, Denver, CO.

Harter, S. (1986a). Processes underlying the construction, maintenance, and enhancement of the self-concept in children. In J. Suls, & A. G. Greenwald (Eds.), *Psychological perspectives on the self* (Vol. 3, pp. 137–181). Hillsdale, NJ: Erlbaum.

Harter, S. (1986b). Cognitive-developmental processes in the integration of concepts about emotions and the self. *Social Cognition, 4,* 119–151.

Harter, S. (1987). The determinants and mediational role of global self-worth in children. In N. Eisenberg (Ed.), *Contemporary issues in developmental psychology* (pp. 219–242). New York: Wiley.

Harter, S. (1988a). Developmental and dynamic changes in the nature of the self-concept: Implications for child psychotherapy. In S. Shirk (Ed.), *Cognitive development and child psychotherapy* (pp. 119–160). New York: Plenum.

Harter, S. (1988b). *The Self-Perception Profile for Adolescents.* Unpublished manual, University of Denver, Denver, CO.

Harter, S. (1990a). Causes, correlates and the functional role of global self-worth: A life-span perspective. In R. Sternberg & J. Kolligian, Jr., (Eds.), *Competence considered* (pp. 67–98). New Haven, CT: Yale University Press.

Harter, S. (1990b). Adolescent self and identity development. In S. S. Feldman & G. R. Elliot (Eds.), *At the threshold: The developing adolescent* (pp. 352–387). Cambridge, MA: Harvard University Press.

Harter, S. (1990c). Issues in the assessment of the self-concept of children and adolescents. In A. La Greca (Ed.), *Childhood assessment: Through the eyes of a child* (pp. 292–235). New York: Allyn & Bacon.

Harter, S. (1990d). Developmental differences in the nature of self-representations: Implications for the understanding and treatment of maladaptive behaviors. *Cognitive Therapy and Research, 14,* 113–142.

Harter, S. (1993). Causes and consequences of low self-esteem in children and adolescents. In R. F. Baumeister (Ed.), *Self-esteem: The puzzle of low self-regard* (pp. 87–116). New York: Plenum.

Harter, S. (1996a). Developmental changes in self-understanding across the 5 to 7 year shift. In A. Sameroff & M. Haith (Eds.), *Reason and responsibility: The passage through childhood* (pp. 204–236). Chicago: University of Chicago Press.

Harter, S. (1996b). Teacher and classmate influences on scholastic motivation, self-esteem, and choice. In K. Wentzel & J. Juvonen (Eds.), *Social motivation: Understanding children's school adjustment* (pp. 11–42). Cambridge, UK: Cambridge University Press.

Harter, S. (1997). The personal self in social context: Barriers to authenticity. In R. D. Ashmore & L. Jussim (Eds.), *Self and identity: Fundamental issues* (pp. 81–105). New York: Oxford University Press.

Harter, S. (1998a). The development of self-representations. In W. Damon (Series Ed.) & N. Eisenberg (Vol. Ed.), *Handbook of child psychology: Vol. 3. Social, emotional, and personality development* (5th ed., pp. 553–617). New York: Wiley.

Harter, S. (1998b). The effects of child abuse on the self-system. In B. B. Rossman & M. S. Rosenberg (Eds.), *Multiple victimization of children: Conceptual, developmental, research, and treatment issues* (pp. 147–170). New York: Haworth Press.

Harter, S. (in press). Symbolic interactionism revisited: Potential liabilities for the self constructed in the crucible of interpersonal relationships. *Merrill–Palmer Quarterly.*

Harter, S., Bresnick, S., Bouchey, H. A., & Whitesell, N. R. (1997). The development of multiple role-related selves during adolescence. *Development and Psychopathology, 9,* 835–854.

Harter, S., & Buddin, B. J. (1987). Children's understanding of the simultaneity of two emotions: A five-stage developmental acquisition sequence. *Developmental Psychology, 23,* 388–399.

Harter, S., & Jackson, B. K. (1992). Trait versus non-trait conceptualizations of intrinsic/extrinsic motivational orientation. *Motivation and Emotion, 16,* 209–230.

Harter, S., & Jackson, B. K. (1993). Young adolescents' perceptions of the link between low self-worth and depressed affect. *Journal of Early Adolescence, 33,* 383–407.

Harter, S., & Johnson, C. (1993). *Changes in self-esteem during the transition to college.* Unpublished manuscript, University of Denver, Denver, CO.

Harter, S., & Kreinik, P. (1998). *The Self-Perception Profile for Late Adulthood.* Unpublished manual, University of Denver, Denver, CO.

Harter, S., & Marold, D. B. (1993). The directionality of the link between self-esteem and affect: Beyond causal modeling. In D. Cicchetti & S. L. Toth (Eds.), *Rochester Symposium on Developmental Psychopathology: Disorders and dysfunctions of the self* (Vol. 5, pp. 333–370). Rochester, NY: University of Rochester Press.

Harter, S., Marold, D. B., & Whitesell, N. R. (1992). A model of psychosocial risk factors leading to suicidal ideation in young adolescents. *Development and Psychopathology, 4,* 167–188.

Harter, S., Marold, D. B., Whitesell, N. R., & Cobbs, G. (1996). A model of the effects of parent and peer support on adolescent false self behavior, *Child Development, 67,* 360–374.

Harter, S., & Monsour, A. (1992). Developmental analysis of conflict caused by opposing attributes in the adolescent self-portrait. *Developmental Psychology, 28,* 251–260.

Harter, S., Nowakowski, M., & Marold, D. B. (1988). *The Dimensions of Depression Profile.* Unpublished manual, University of Denver, Denver, CO.

Harter, S., & Pike, R. (1984). The pictorial scale of perceived competence and social acceptance for young children. *Child Development, 55,* 1969–1982.

Harter, S., & Silon, E. L. (1985). The assessment of perceived competence, motivational orientation, and anxiety in segregated and mainstreamed educable mentally retarded children. *Journal of Educational Psychology, 77,* 217–230.

Harter, S., Stocker, C., & Robinson, N. S. (1996). The perceived directionality of the link between approval and self-worth: The liabilities of a looking glass self orientation among young adolescents. *Journal of Research on Adolescence, 6,* 285–308.

Harter, S., Waters, P. L., Pettitt, L., Whitesell, N., Kofkin, J., & Jordan, J. (1997). Autonomy and connectedness as dimensions of relationship styles in adult men and women. *Journal of Social and Personal Relationships, 14,* 147–164.

Harter, S., Waters, P., & Whitesell, N. R. (1997). False self behavior and lack of voice among adolescent males and females. *Educational Psychologist, 32,* 153–173.

Harter, S., Waters, P., & Whitesell, N. R. (1998). Relational self-worth: Differences in perceived worth as a person across interpersonal contexts. *Child Development, 69,* 756–766.

Harter, S., Waters, P. L., Whitesell, N. R., & Kastelic, D. (1998). Predictors of level of voice among high school females and males: Relational context, support, and gender orientation. *Developmental Psychology, 34,* 1–10.

Harter, S., & Whitesell, N. R. (1989). Developmental changes in children's understanding of single, multiple and blended emotion concepts. In C. Saarni & P. L. Harris (Eds.), *Children's understanding of emotion* (pp. 81–116). Cambridge, UK: Cambridge University Press.

Harter, S., & Whitesell, N. R. (1996). Multiple pathways to self-reported depression and adjustment among adolescents. *Development and Psychopathology, 9,* 835–854.

Harter, S., Whitesell, N. R., & Junkin, L. J. (in press). Similarities and differences in domain-specific and global self-evaluations of learning-disabled, behaviorally-disordered, and normally-achieving adolescents. *American Educational Research Journal.*

Harter, S., Whitesell, N., & Kowalski, P. (1992). Individual differences in the effects of educational transitions on young adolescents' perceptions of competence and motivational orientation. *American Educational Research Journal, 29,* 777–808.

Hatfield, E., & Sprecher, S. (1986). *Mirror, mirror . . . The importance of appearance in everyday life.* New York: State University of New York Press.

Hattie, J. (1992). *Self-concept.* Hillsdale, NJ: Erlbaum.

Hattie, J., & Marsh, H. W. (1996). Theoretical perspectives on the structure of self-concept. In B. A. Bracken (Ed.), *Handbook of self-concept* (pp. 38–90). New York: Wiley.

Hawton, K. (1986). *Suicide and attempted suicide among children and adolescents.* Beverly Hills, CA: Sage.

Hazan, C., & Shaver, P. (1987). Romantic love conceptualized as an attachment process. *Journal of Personality and Social Psychology, 52,* 511–524.

Heatherton, T. F., & Baumeister, R. F. (1991). Binge eating as escape from self-awareness. *Psychological Bulletin, 110,* 86–108.

Heatherton, T. F., & Polivy, J. (1991). Development and validation of a scale for measuring state self-esteem. *Journal of Personality and Social Psychology, 60,* 895–910.

Heavey, C. L., Layne, C., & Christensen, A. (1993). Gender and conflict structure in marital interaction: A replication and extension. *Journal of Consulting and Clinical Psychology, 61,* 16–27.

Hendrick, S. S., & Hendrick, C. (1993). Lovers as friends. *Journal of Social and Personal Relationships, 10,* 459–466.

Herman, J. (1992). *Trauma and recovery.* New York: Basic Books.

Herman, J. L., Russell, D., & Trocki, K. (1986). Long-term effects of incestuous abuse in childhood. *American Journal of Psychiatry, 143,* 1293–1296.

Higgins, E. T. (1987). Self-discrepancy: A theory relating self and affect. *Psychological Review, 94,* 319–340.

Higgins, E. T. (1989). Self-discrepancy theory: What patterns of self-beliefs cause people to suffer? In L. Berkowitz (Ed.), *Advances in experimental social psychology* (Vol. 22, pp. 23–63). New York: Academic Press.

Higgins, E. T. (1991). Development of self-regulatory and self-evaluative processes: Costs, benefits, and tradeoffs. In M. R. Gunnar & L. A. Sroufe (Eds.), *Self processes and development: The Minnesota Symposia on Child Development* (Vol. 23, pp. 125–166). Hillsdale, NJ: Erlbaum.

Higgins, E. T., & Bargh, J. A. (1987). Social cognition and social perception. *Annual Review of Psychology, 38,* 369–425.

Hill, J. P., & Lynch, M. E. (1983). The intensification of gender-related role expectations during early adolescence. In J. Brooks-Gunn & A. C. Petersen (Eds.), *Girls at puberty* (pp. 201–228). New York: Plenum.

Hill, J. P., & Holmbeck, G. N. (1986). Attachment and autonomy during adolescence. In G. J. Whitehurst (Ed.), *Annals of child development* (Vol. 3, pp. 145–189). Greenwich, CT: JAI Press.

Hoffman, M. L. (1975). Developmental synthesis of affect and cognition and its implications for altruistic motivation. *Developmental Psychology, 11,* 605–622.

Hoffman, M. L. (1977). Sex differences in empathy and related behaviors. *Psychological Bulletin, 84,* 712–722.

Hoffman, M. L. (1982). Development of prosocial motivation: Empathy and guilt. In N. Eisenberg (Ed.), *Development of prosocial behavior* (pp. 281–313). New York: Academic Press.

Hoffman, M. L. (1983). Empathy, guilt, and social cognition. In W. F. Overton (Eds.), *The relationship between social and cognitive development* (pp. 1–51). Hillsdale, NJ: Erlbaum.

Hopper, C. (1988). Self-concept and motor performance of hearing impaired boys and girls. *Adapted Physical Activity Quarterly, 5,* 293–304.

Horney, K. (1945). *Our inner conflicts.* New York: Norton.

Horney, K. (1950). *Neurosis and human growth.* New York: Norton.

Howe, M. L., & Courage, M. L. (1993). On resolving the enigma of infantile amnesia. *Psychological Bulletin, 113,* 305–326.

Hsu, F. L. K. (1983). *Rugged individualism reconsidered.* Knoxville: University of Tennessee Press.

Hudson, J. A. (1990a). Constructive processes in children's autobiographical memory. *Developmental Psychology, 26,* 180–187.

Hudson, J. A. (1990b). The emergence of autobiographical memory in mother–child conversation. In R. Fivush & J. A. Hudson (Eds.), *Knowing and remembering in young children* (pp. 166–196). New York: Cambridge University Press.

Humberstone, B. (1990). Gender, change, and adventure education. *Gender and Education, 2,* 199–215.

Huston, A. C. (1983). Sex-typing. In P. H. Mussen & E. M. Hetherington (Eds.), *Handbook of child psychology* (Vol. 4, pp. 387–467). New York: Wiley.

Iheanacho, S. O. (1988). Minority self-concept: A research review. *Journal of Instructional Psychology, 15,* 3–11.

Izard, C. E. (1984). Emotion-cognition relationships and human development. In C. E. Izard, J. Kagan, & R. B. Zajonc (Eds.), *Emotions, cognition, and behavior* (pp. 389–413). Cambridge, UK: Cambridge University Press.

Jackson, L. A. (1992). *Physical appearance and gender: Sociobiological and sociocultural perspectives.* New York: State University of New York Press.

Jacobs, D. H. (1983). Learning problems, self-esteem, and delinquency. In J. E. Mack & S. L. Ablon (Eds.), *The development and sustenance of self-esteem in childhood* (pp. 209–222). New York: International Universities Press.

Jacobs, J. E. (1992). The influence of gender stereotypes on parent and child math attitudes. *Journal of Educational Psychology, 83,* 518–527.

Jacobs, J. E., & Eccles, J. S. (1992). The influence of parent stereotypes on parent and child ability beliefs in three domains. *Journal of Personality and Social Psychology, 63,* 932–944.

Jacobson, N. S. (1989). The politics of intimacy. *Behavior Therapist, 12,* 29–32.

James, W. (1890). *Principles of psychology.* Chicago: Encyclopedia Britannica.

James, W. (1892). *Psychology: The briefer course.* New York: Henry Holt.

Janoff-Bulman, R. (1992). *Shared assumptions: Towards a new psychology of trauma.* New York: Free Press.

Jehu, D. (1988). *Beyond sexual abuse: Therapy with women who were childhood victims.* Chichester, UK: Wiley.

John, O. P., & Robbins, R. W. (1994). Accuracy and bias in self-perception: Individual differences in self-enhancement and the role of narcissism. *Journal of Personality and Social Psychology, 66,* 206–219.

Johnson, C., & Harter, S. (1995). *The effect of the transition to college on students' self-esteem.* Unpublished manuscript, University of Denver, Denver, CO.

Johnson, E. (1993). *The impact of self-blame versus a sense of responsibility on self-perceptions of competence and worth as a person.* Unpublished master's thesis, University of Denver, Denver, CO.

Johnson, E. (1995). *The role of social support and gender orientation in adolescent female development.* Unpublished doctoral dissertation, University of Denver, Denver, CO.

Jones, E. E., Rhodewalt, E., Berglas, S., & Skelton, J. A. (1981). Effect of strategic self-presentation in subsequent self-esteem. *Journal of Personality and Social Psychology, 41,* 407–421.

Jones, G. M., & Wheatley, J. (1990). Gender differences in teacher–student interactions in science classrooms. *Journal of Research in Science Teaching, 27,* 861–864.

Jordan, J. V. (1991). The relational self: A new perspective for understanding women's development. In J. Strauss & G. Goethals (Eds.), *The self: Interdisciplinary approaches* (pp. 136–149). New York: Springer-Verlag.

Jordan, J. V., Kaplan, A. G., Miller, J. B., Stiver, I. P., & Surrey, J. L. (1991). *Women's growth in connection: Writings from the Stone Center.* New York: Guilford Press.

Josephs, R. A., Markus, H., & Tafarodi, R. W. (1992). Gender differences in the source of self-esteem. *Journal of Personality and Social Psychology, 63,* 391–402.

Juhasz, A. M. (1992). Significant others in self-esteem development: Methods and problems in measurement. In T. M. Brinthaupt & R. P. Lipka (Eds.), *The self: Definitional and methodological issues* (pp. 204–235). Albany: State University of New York Press.

Jung, C. G. (1928). *Two essays on analytical psychology.* New York: Dodd, Mead.

Kagan, J. (1981). *The second year: The emergence of self-awareness.* Cambridge, MA: Harvard University Press.

Kagan, J. (1984). *The nature of the child.* New York: Basic Books.

Kagan, J., & Lamb, S. (Eds.). (1987). *The emergence of morality in young children.* Chicago: University of Chicago Press.

Kanfer, F. H. (1980). Self-management methods. In F. H. Kanfer & A. P. Goldstein (Eds.), *Helping people change: A textbook of methods* (2nd ed., pp. 232–258). New York: Pergamon Press.

Kanfer, F. H., & Phillips, J. S. (1970). *Learning foundations of behavior therapy.* New York: Wiley.

Kaplan, H. (1980). *Deviant behavior in defense of self.* New York: Academic Press.

Kaslow, N. J., Rehm, L. P., & Siegel, A. W. (1984). Social-cognitive and cognitive correlates of depression in children. *Journal of Abnormal Child Psychology, 12,* 605–620.

Katz, E. R., Rubinstein, C. L., Hubert, N. C., & Blew, A. (1988). School and social reintegration of children with cancer. *Journal of Psychosocial Oncology, 6,* 123–139.

Kaufman, J. (1985). *Shame: The power of caring.* Cambridge, MA: Schenkman.

Kaufman, J., & Cicchetti, D. (1989). Effects of maltreatment on school age children's socio-emotional development: Assessment in a day camp setting. *Developmental Psychology, 25,* 516–524.

Kaye, W. H., Gwirtsman, H. E., George, D. T., Weiss, S. R., & Jimerson, D. C. (1986). Relationship of mood alterations to bingeing behaviour in bulimia. *British Journal of Psychiatry, 149,* 479–485.

Kazdin, A. E., Moser, J., Colbus, D., & Bell, R. (1985). Depressive symptoms among physically abused and psychiatrically disturbed children. *Journal of Abnormal Psychology, 94,* 298–307.

Keating, D. P. (1990). Adolescent thinking. In S. S. Feldman, & G. Elliot (Eds.), *At the threshold: The developing adolescent* (pp. 54–90). Cambridge, MA: Harvard University Press.

Keith, L. K., & Bracken, B. A. (1996). Self-concept instrumentation: An historical and evaluative review. In B. A. Bracken (Ed.), *Handbook of self-concept* (pp. 91–170). New York: Wiley.

Kelly, G. A. (1955). *The psychology of personal constructs.* New York: Norton.

Kendall, P. C. (Ed.). (1991). *Child and adolescent therapy: Cognitive-behavioral procedures.* New York: Guilford Press.

Kendall, P. C., Cantwell, D. P., & Kazdin, A. E. (1989). Depression in children and adolescents: Assessment issues and recommendations. *Cognitive Therapy and Research, 13,* 109–146.

Kendall, P. C., Lerner, R., & Craighead, W. (1984). Human development and intervention in child psychopathology. *Child Development, 55,* 71–82.

Kendall-Tackett, K. A., Williams, L. M., & Finkelhor, D. (1993). Impact of sexual abuse on children: A review and synthesis of recent empirical studies. *Psychological Bulletin, 113,* 164–180.

Kennedy, B. (1994). *The development of self-understanding in adolescence.* Unpublished doctoral dissertation, Harvard University, Cambridge, MA.

Kenny, D. (1988). Interpersonal perception: A social relations analysis. *Journal of Social and Personal Relationships, 5,* 247–261.

Kernberg, O. F. (1975). Borderline conditions and pathological narcissism. New York: Aronson.

Kernis, M. H. (1993). The roles of stability and level of self-esteem in psychological functioning. In R. F. Baumeister (Ed.), *Self-esteem: The puzzle of low self-regard* (pp. 167–180). New York: Plenum.

Kernis, M. H., Cornell, D. P., Sun, C., Berry, A., & Harlow, T. (1993). There's more to self-esteem than whether it is high or low: The importance of stability of self-esteem. *Journal of Personality and Social Psychology, 65,* 1190–1204.

Khan, A. U. (1987). Heterogeneity of suicidal adolescents. *Journal of the American Academy of Child and Adolescent Psychiatry, 26,* 92–96.

Kihlstrom, J. F. (1993). What does the self look like? In T. K. Srull & R. S. Wyer, Jr. (Eds.), *The mental representation of trait and autobiographical knowledge about the self: Advances in social cognition* (Vol. 5, pp. 79–90). Hillsdale, NJ: Erlbaum.

Kihlstrom, J. F., & Cantor, N. (1984). Mental representations of the self. In L. Berkowitz (Ed.), *Advances in experimental social psychology* (Vol 17, pp. 2–40). New York: Academic Press.

Kilbourne, J. (1994). Still killing us softly: Advertising and the obsession with thinness. In P. Fallon, M. Katzman, & S. Wooley (Eds.), *Feminist perspectives on eating disorders* (pp. 395–418). New York: Guilford Press.

Kim, U., & Berry, J. W. (1993). *Indigenous psychologies: Research and experience in cultural context.* Newbury Park, CA: Sage.

King, C. A., Naylor, M. W., Segal, H. G., Evans, T., & Shain, B. N. (1993). Global self-worth, specific self-perceptions of competence, and depression in adolescents. *Journal of the American Academy of Child and Adolescent Psychiatry, 32,* 745–752.

Kitayama, S., Markus, H. R., & Matsumoto, H. (1995). Culture, self, and emotion: A cultural perspective on "self-conscious" emotions. In J. P. Tangney & K. W. Fischer (Eds.), *Self-conscious emotions: The psychology of shame, guilt, embarrassment, and pride* (pp. 439–464). New York: Guilford Press.

Kitchner, K. S. (1986). The reflective judgment model: Characteristics, evidence, and measurement. In R. A. Mines & K. S. Kitchener (Eds.), *Adult cognitive development: Methods and models* (pp. 76–91). New York: Praeger.

Klein, H. A., O'Bryant, K., & Hopkins, H. R. (1996). Recalled parental authority style and self-perception in college men and women. *Journal of Genetic Psychology, 157,* 5–17.

Klein, S. B., & Kihlstrom, J. F. (1986). Elaboration, organization, and the self-reference effect in memory. *Journal of Experimental Psychology: General, 115,* 26–38.

Kobak, R. R., & Sceery, A. (1988). Attachment in late adolescence: Working models, affect regulation, and perceptions of self and others. *Child Development, 59,* 135–146.

Kohlberg, L. (1976). Moral stages and moralization. In T. Lickona (Ed.), *Moral development and behavior* (pp. 72–98). New York: Holt, Rinehart & Winston.

Kohut, H. (1977). *The restoration of the self.* New York: International Universities Press.

Kolligian, J., Jr. (1990). Perceived fraudulence as a dimension of perceived incompetence. In R. J. Sternberg & J. Kolligian, Jr. (Eds.), *Competence considered* (pp. 261–285). New Haven, CT: Yale University Press.

Korabik, K., & Pitt, E. J. (1980). Self concept, objective appearance and profile self perception. *Journal of Applied Social Psychology, 10,* 482–489.

Kovacs, M., & Beck, A. T. (1977). An empirical–clinical approach towards a definition of childhood depression. In J. G. Schulterbrandt & A. Raskin (Eds.), *Depression in childhood: Diagnosis, treatment, and conceptual models* (pp. 1–25). New York: Raven Press.

Kovacs, M., & Beck, A. T. (1978). Maladaptive cognitive structures in depression. *American Journal of Psychiatry, 135,* 525–533.

Kovacs, M., & Beck, A. T. (1986). Maladaptive cognitive structures in depression. In J. C. Coyne (Ed.), *Essential papers on depression* (pp. 212–239). New York: New York University Press.

Kuiper, N. A. (1981). Convergent evidence for the self as a prototype: The "inverted-U RT effect" for self and other judgments. *Personality and Social Psychology Bulletin, 7,* 438–443.

Lamborn, S. D., Mounts, N. S., Steinberg, L., & Dornbusch, S. M. (1991). Patterns of competence and adjustment among adolescents from authoritative, authoritarian, indulgent and neglectful families. *Child Development, 62,* 1049–1065.

Lamborn, S. D., & Steinberg, L. (1993). Emotional autonomy redux: Revisiting Ryan and Lynch. *Child Development, 64,* 483–499.

Langlois, J. H. (1981). Beauty and the beast: The role of physical attractiveness in the development of peer relations and social behavior. In S. S. Brehm, S. M. Kassin, & F. X. Gibbons (Eds.), *Developmental social psychology: Theory and research* (pp. 47–63). New York: Oxford University Press.

Lapsley, D. K., & Rice, K. (1988). The "new look" at the imaginary audience and personal fable: Toward a general model of adolescent ego development. In D. K. Lapsley & F. C. Power (Eds.), *Self, ego, and identity: Integrative approaches* (pp. 109–129). New York: Springer-Verlag.

Lazarus, R. S. (1982). Thoughts on the relations between emotion and cognition. *American Psychologist, 37,* 1019–1024.

Lazarus, R. S. (1984). On the primacy of cognition: A functional approach to a semantic controversy. *Cognition and Emotion, 1,* 124–129.

Leahy, R. L. (1985). The costs of development: Clinical implications. In R. L. Leahy (Ed.), *The development of the self* (pp. 267–294). New York: Academic Press.

Leahy, R. L., & Shirk, S. R. (1985). Social cognition and the development of the self. In R. L. Leahy (Ed.), *The development of the self* (pp. 123–150). New York: Academic Press.

Leary, M. R., & Downs, D. L. (1995). Interpersonal functions of the self-esteem motive: The self-esteem system as a sociometer. In M. H. Kernis (Ed.), *Efficacy, agency, and self-esteem* (pp. 123–140). New York: Plenum.

Lecky, P. (1945). *Self-consistency: A theory of personality.* New York: Island Press.

L'Ecuyer, R. (1992). An experiential–developmental framework and methodology to study the transformations of the self-concept from infancy to old age. In T. M. Brinthaupt & R. P. Lipka (Eds.), *The self: Definitional and methodological issues* (pp. 96–136). Albany: State University of New York Press.

Lee, J. (1993). Perceptions of competence among Special Olympics partipants. Unpublished doctoral thesis, University of Denver, Denver, CO.

Lee, V. E., Bryk, A. S., & Smith, J. B. (1993). The organization of effective secondary schools. *Review of Research in Education, 19,* 230–231.

Lerner, H. G. (1989). *The dance of intimacy.* New York: Harper & Row.

Lerner, H. G. (1993). *The dance of deception.* New York: HarperCollins.

Lerner, R. M., & Brackney, B. E. (1978). The importance of inner and outer body parts attitudes in the self-concept of late adolescents. *Sex Roles, 4,* 225–238.

Lerner, R. M., & Karabenick, S. A. (1974). Physical attractiveness, body attitudes, and self-concept in late adolescents. *Journal of Youth and Adolescence, 3,* 307–316.

Lerner, R. M., Karabenick, S. A., & Stuart, J. L. (1973). Relations among physical attractiveness, body attitudes, and self-concept in male and female college students. *Journal of Psychology, 85,* 119–129.

Lerner, R. M., Orlos, J. B., & Knapp, J. R. (1976). Physical attractiveness, physical effectiveness, and self-concept on late adolescents. *Adolescence, 11,* 313–326.

Leventhal, H. L., & Scherer, K. (1987). The relationship of emotion to cognition: A functional approach to a semantic controversy. *Cognition and Emotion, 1,* 3–28.

Lewinsohn, P. M., Mischel, W., Chaplain, W., & Barton, R. (1980). Social competence and depression: The role of illusory self-perceptions. *Journal of Abnormal Psychology, 89,* 203–212.

Lewis, D. O., Mallouh, C., & Webb, V. (1989). Child abuse, delinquency, and violent criminality. In D. Cicchetti & V. Carson (Eds.), *Child maltreatment: Theory and research on the causes and consequences of child abuse and neglect* (pp. 702–721). New York: Cambridge University Press.

Lewis, H. B. (1971). *Shame and guilt in neurosis.* New York: International Universities Press.

Lewis, H. B. (1987). *The role of shame in symptom formation.* Hillsdale, NJ: Erlbaum.

Lewis, M. (1991). Ways of knowing: Objective self-awareness or consciousness. *Developmental Review, 11,* 231–243.

Lewis, M. (1994). Myself and me. In S. T. Parker, R. W. Mitchell, & M. L. Boccia (Eds.), *Self-awareness in animals and humans: Developmental perspectives* (pp. 20–34). New York: Cambridge University Press.

Lewis, M., Allesandri, S. M., & Sullivan, M. W. (1992). Differences in shame and pride as a function of children's gender and task difficulty. *Child Development, 63,* 630–638.

Lewis, M., & Brooks-Gunn, J. (1979). *Social cognition and the acquisition of self.* New York: Plenum.

Liakopoulou, M., Korvessi, M., & Dacou-Voutetakis, C. (1992). Personality characteristics, environmental factors and glycemic control in adolescents with diabetes. *European Child and Adolescent Psychiatry, 1,* 62–88.

Lifton, R. J. (1993). *The protean self.* New York: Basic Books.

Lindsay-Hartz, J., De Rivera, J., & Mascolo, M. F. (1995). Differentiating guilt and shame and their effects on motivation. In J. P. Tangney & K. W. Fischer (Eds.), *Self-conscious emotions: The psychology of shame, guilt, embarrassment, and pride* (pp. 274–300). New York: Guilford Press.

Linville, P. W. (1987). Self-complexity as a cognitive buffer against stress-related illness and depression. *Journal of Personality and Social Psychology, 52,* 663–676.

Lipka, R. P., Hurford, D. P., & Litten, M. J. (1992). Self in school: Age and school experience effects. In R. P. Lipka & T. M. Brinthaupt (Eds.), *Self-perspectives across the life span* (Vol. 3, pp. 93–115). Albany: State University of New York Press.

Lipovsky, J. A., Saunders, B. E., & Murphy, S. M. (1989). Depression, anxiety, and behavior problems among victims of father–child sexual assault and nonabused siblings. *Journal of Interpersonal Violence, 4,* 452–468.

Lockheed, M. E. (1986). Classroom organization and climate. In S. Klein (Ed.), *Achieving sex equity through education* (pp. 113–142). Baltimore: Johns Hopkins University Press.

Logan, R. D. (1987). Historical change in prevailing sense of self. In K. Yardley & T. Honess (Eds.), *Self and identity: Psychological perspectives* (pp. 13–26). Chicester, UK: Wiley.

Longo, L. C., & Ashmore, R. D. (1995). The looks–personality relationship: Self-orientations as shared precursors of subject physical attractiveness and self-ascribed traits. *Journal of Applied Social Psychology, 25,* 371–398.

Lord, C. G., Gilbert, D. T., & Stanley, M. A. (1983). *Idiographic self-schema and cognitive efficiency: Associations or affect?* Unpublished manuscript, Princeton University, Princeton, NJ.

Maccoby, E. (1980). *Social development.* New York: Wiley.

Maccoby, E. E. (1990). Gender and relationships: A developmental account. *American Psychologist, 45,* 513–520.

Maccoby, E. E. (1994). Commentary: Gender segregation in childhood. In C. Leaper

(Ed.), *Childhood gender segregation: Causes and consequences* (pp. 87–98). San Francisco: Jossey-Bass.

Maccoby, E., & Martin, J. (1983). Socialization in the context of the family: Parent–child interaction. In P. Mussen & E. M. Hetherington (Eds.), *Handbook of child psychology: Vol. 4. Socialization, personality and social development* (pp. 1–102). New York: Wiley.

Mack, J. E. (1983). Self-esteem and its development: An overview. In J. E. Mack & S. L. Ablong (Eds.), *The development and sustaining of self-esteem* (pp. 1–44). New York: International Universities Press.

Maeda, K. (1997). *The Self-Perception Profile for Children administered to a Japanese sample.* Unpublished data, Ibaraki Prefectural University of Health Sciences, Ibaraki, Japan.

Maher, F. A., & Tetreault, M. K. T. (1994). *The feminist classroom.* New York: Basic Books.

Mahler, M. S. (1967). On human symbiosis and the vicissitudes of individuation. *Journal of the American Psychoanalytic Association, 15,* 740–763.

Mahler, M. S. (1968). *On human symbiosis and the vicissitudes of individuation: Vol. 1. Infantile psychosis.* New York: International Universities Press.

Main, M., & Solomon, J. (1990). Procedures for identifying infants as disorganized/disoriented during the Ainsworth Strange Situation. In M. Greenberg, D. Cicchetti, & M. Cummings (Eds.), *Attachment during the preschool years: Theory, research, and intervention* (pp. 121–160). Chicago: University of Chicago Press.

Makris-Botsaris, E., & Robinson, W. P. (1991). Harter's Self-Perception Profile for Children: A cross-cultural validation in Greece. *Evaluation and Research in Education, 5,* 135–143.

Maloney, M. J., McGuire, J. B., & Daniels, S. R. (1988). Reliability testing of a children's version of the Eating Attitude Test. *Journal of the American Academy of Child and Adolescent Psychiatry, 27,* 541–543.

Markman, H. J., & Kraft, S. A. (1989). Men and women in marriage: Dealing with gender differences in marital therapy. *Behavior Therapist, 12,* 51–56.

Markus, H. (1977). Self-schemata and processing information about the self. *Journal of Personality and Social Psychology, 35,* 63–78.

Markus, H. (1980). The self in thought and memory. In D. M. Wegner & R. R. Vallacher (Eds.), *The self in social psychology* (pp. 42–69). New York: Oxford University Press.

Markus, H., & Cross, S. (1990). The interpersonal self. In L. A. Pervin (Ed.), *Handbook of personality: Theory and research* (pp. 576–608). New York: Guilford Press.

Markus, H., Cross, S., & Wurf, E. (1990). The role of the self-system in competence. In R. J. Sternberg & J. Kolligian, Jr. (Eds.), *Competence considered* (pp. 205–226). New Haven, CT: Yale University Press.

Markus, H. R., & Kityama, S. (1991). Culture and the self: Implications for cognition, emotion, and motivation. *Psychological Review, 98,* 224–253.

Markus, H., & Kunda, Z. (1986). Stability and malleability of the self-concept. *Journal of Personality and Social Psychology, 51,* 858–866.

Markus, H., & Nurius, P. (1986). Possible selves. *American Psychologist, 41,* 954–969.

Markus, H., & Sentis, K. (1982). The self in social information processing. In J. Suls (Ed.), *Social psychological perspectives on the self* (Vol. 1, pp. 41–70). Hillsdale, NJ: Erlbaum.

Markus, H., & Wurf, E. (1987). The dynamic self-concept: A social psychological perspective. In M. R. Rosenweig & L. W. Porter (Eds.), *Annual Review of Psychology, 38,* 299–337.

Marold, D. B. (1998). Into the haunted house mirrors: The treatment of multiply-traumatized adolescents. In B. R. Rossman & M. S. Rosenberg (Eds.), *Multiple victimization of children: Conceptual, developmental, research, and treatment issues* (pp. 253–272). New York: Haworth Press.

Marsh, H. W. (1986). Global self-esteem: Its relation to specific facets of self-concept and their importance. *Journal of Personality and Social Psychology, 51,* 1224–1236.

Marsh, H. W. (1987). The hierarchical structure of self-concept and the application of hierarchical confirmatory factor analysis. *Journal of Educational Measurement, 24,* 17–19.

Marsh, H. W. (1988). *Self-Description Questionnaire–I.* San Antonio, TX: Psychological Corporation.

Marsh, H. W. (1989). Age and sex effects in multiple dimensions of self-concept: Preadolescence to early adulthood. *Journal of Educational Psychology, 81,* 417–430.

Marsh, H. W. (1990). The structure of academic self-concept: The Marsh/Shavelson model. *Journal of Educational Psychology, 82,* 623–636.

Marsh, H. W. (1991). *Self-Description Questionnaire–III.* San Antonio, TX: Psychological Corporation.

Marsh, H. W. (1993). Academic self-concept: Theory, measurement, and research. In J. Suls (Ed.), *Psychological perspectives on the self* (Vol. 4, pp. 59–98). Hillsdale, NJ: Erlbaum.

Marsh, H. W., Byrne, B. M., & Shavelson, R. J. (1992). A multidimensional, hierarchical self-concept. In T. M. Brinthaupt & R. P. Lipka (Eds.), *The self: Definitional and methodological issues* (pp. 44–95). Albany: State University of New York Press.

Marsh, H. W., & Hattie, J. (1996). Theoretical perspectives on the structure of self-concept. In B. A. Bracken (Ed.), *Handbook of self-concept* (pp. 38–90). New York: Wiley.

Marsh, H. W., & Jackson, S. A. (1986). Multidimensional self-concepts, masculinity, and femininity as a function of women's involvement in athletics. *Sex Roles, 15,* 391–415.

Marsh, H. W., Parker, J., & Barnes, J. (1985). Multidimensional adolescent self-concepts: Their relationship to age, sex, and academic measures. *American Educational Research Journal, 22,* 422–444.

Marsh, H. W., & Peart, N. (1988). Competitive and cooperative physical fitness training programs for girls: Effects on physical fitness and on multidimensional self-concepts. *Journal of Sport and Exercise Psychology, 10,* 390–407.

Marsh, H. W., Smith, I. D., Marsh, M. R., & Owens, L. (1988). The transition from single-sex to coeducational high schools: Effects on multiple dimensions of self-concept and on academic achievement. *American Educational Research Journal, 25,* 237–269.

Mascolo, M. F., & Fischer, K. W. (1995). Developmental transformations in appraisals for pride, shame, and guilt. In J. P. Tangney & K. W. Fischer (Eds.), *Self-conscious emotions: The psychology of shame, guilt, embarrassment, and pride* (pp. 64–113). New York: Guilford Press.

Maslow, A. H. (1954). *Motivation and personality.* New York: Harper & Row.

Masten, A. S. (in press). Resilience in the 90s: Moving beyond risk and protective factors. In R. J. Haggerty, N. Garmezy, M. Rutter, & L. Sherrod (Eds.), *Risk and resilience in children: Developmental approaches.* New York: Cambridge University Press.

Masten, A. S., Best, K. M., & Garmezy, N. (1990). Resilience and development: Contributions from the study of children who overcome adversity. *Development and Psychopathology, 2,* 425–444.

Mathes, E. W., & Kahn, A. (1975). Physical attractiveness, happiness, neuroticism, and self-esteem. *Journal of Psychology, 90,* 27–30.

McAdams, D. (1997). The unity of identity. In R. D. Ashmore & L. Jussim (Eds.), *Self and identity: Fundamental issues* (pp. 46–80). New York: Oxford University Press.

McCann, I. L., & Pearlman, L. A. (1992). *Psychological trauma and the adult survivor* (pp. 211–259). New York: Brunner/Mazel.

McCarthy, J., & Hoge, D. (1982). Analysis of age effects in longitudinal studies of adolescent self-esteem. *Developmental Psychology, 18,* 372–379.

McCaulay, M., Mintz, L., & Glenn, A. A. (1988). Body image, self-esteem, and depression proneness: Closing the gender gap. *Sex Roles, 18,* 381–391.

McCauley, E., Mitchell, J. R., Burke, P., & Moss, S. (1988). Cognitive attributes of depression in children and adolescents. *Journal of Consulting and Clinical Psychology, 56,* 903–908.

McGregor K. N., Mayleben, M. A., Buzzanga, V. L., Davis, S. F., & Becker, A. H. (1992). Selected personality characteristics of first-generation college students. *College Student Journal, 18,* 231–234.

McGregor, L., Eveleigh, M., Syler, J. C., & Davis, S. F. (1991). Self-perception of personality characteristics and the Tyle A behavior pattern. *Bulletin of the Psychonomic Society, 29,* 320–322.

McGuire, W. (1981). The spontaneous self-concept as affected by personal distinctiveness. In A. A. Norem-Hebeisen & M. Lynch (Eds.), *Self-concept* (pp. 211–239). Cambridge, MA: Ballinger.

McGuire, W., & McGuire, C. V. (1980). Significant others in self-space: Sex differences and developmental trends in the social self. In J. Suls (Ed.), *Social psychological perspectives on the self* (Vol. 1, pp. 97–144). Hillsdale, NJ: Erlbaum.

Mead, G. H. (1925). The genesis of the self and social control. *International Journal of Ethics, 35,* 251–273.

Mead, G. H. (1934). *Mind, self, and society from the standpoint of a social behaviorist.* Chicago: University of Chicago Press.

Mecca, A. M., Smelser, N. J., & Vasconcellos, J. (Eds.). (1989). *The social importance of self-esteem.* Berkeley: University of California Press.

Meece, J. L. (1987). The influence of school experiences on the development of gender schemata. In L. S. Liben & M. L. Signorella (Eds.), *Children's gender schemata* (pp. 57–73). San Francisco, CA: Jossey-Bass.

Mellin, L. M. (1988). Responding to disordered eating in children and adolescents. *Nutrition News, 51,* 5–7.

Meltzoff, A. N. (1990). Foundations for developing a concept of self: The role of imitation in relating self to other and the value of social mirroring, social modeling, and self practice in infancy. In D. Cicchetti & M. Beeghly (Eds.), *The self in transition: Infancy to childhood* (pp. 139–164). Chicago: University of Chicago Press.

Meredith, W. H., Abbott, D. A., & Zheng, F. M. (1991). Self-concept and sociometric outcomes: A comparison of only children and sibling children from urban and rural areas in the People's Republic of China. *Journal of Psychology, 126,* 411–421.

Meredith, W. H., Wang, A., & Zheng, F. M. (1993). Determining constructs of self-perception for children in Chinese cultures. *School Psychology International, 14,* 371–380.

Messer, B., & Harter, S. (1989). *The Self-Perception Profile for Adults.* Unpublished manual, University of Denver, Denver, CO.

Miezdian, R. (1991). *Boys will be boys.* New York: Doubleday.

Miller, A. (1981). *The drama of the gifted child.* New York: Basic Books.

Miller, A. (1990). *Thou shalt not be aware.* New York: Meridan.

Miller, J. B. (1986). *Toward a new psychology of women* (2nd ed.). Boston: Beacon Press.

Miller, P. J., Potts, R., Fung, H., Hoogstra, L., & Mintz, J. (1990). Narrative practices and the social construction of self in childhood. *American Ethnologist, 17,* 292–311.

Mintz, L. B., & Betz, N. E. (1988). Prevalence and correlates of eating disordered behaviors among undergraduate women. *Journal of Counseling Psychology, 35,* 463–471.

Mischel, W. (1973). Toward a cognitive social learning reconceptualization of personality. *Psychological Review, 80,* 252–283.

Mizes, J. S. (1988). Personality characteristics of bulimic and non-eating-disordered female controls: A cognitive behavioral perspective. *International Journal of Eating Disorders, 7,* 541–550.

Monaco, N. M., & Gaier, E. L. (1992). Single sex versus coeducational environment and achievement in adolescent females. *Adolescence, 27,* 579–594.

Montemayor, R., & Eisen, M. (1977). The development of self-conceptions from childhood to adolescence. *Developmental Psychology, 13,* 314–319.

Moore, D. (1987). Parent–adolescent separation: The construction of adulthood by late adolescents. *Developmental Psychology, 23,* 298–307.

Moretti, M. M., & Higgins, E. T. (1990). The development of self-esteem vulner-abilities: Social and cognitive factors in developmental psychopathology. In R. J. Sternberg & J. Kolligian, Jr. (Eds.), *Competence considered* (pp. 286–314). New Haven, CT: Yale University Press.

Morrison, A. (1989). *Shame: The underside of narcissism.* Hillsdale, NJ: Analytic Press.

Mueller, N., & Silverman, N. (1990). Peer relations in maltreated children. In D. Cicchetti & V. Carlson (Eds.), *Child maltreatment: Theory and research on the causes and consequences of child abuse and neglect* (pp. 529–578). New York: Cambridge University Press.

Mullener, N., & Laird, J. D. (1971). Some developmental changes in the organiza-tion of self-evaluations. *Developmental Psychology, 5,* 233–236.

Munsch, J., Liang, S., & DeSecottier, L. (1996, April). *Natural mentors: Who they are and the roles they fill.* Poster presented at the biennial meeting of the Society for Research on Adolescence, Boston, MA.

Nadler, A., & Fischer, J. D. (1986) The role of threat to self-esteem and perceived control in recipient reaction to help: Theory development and empirical vali-dation. In L. Berkowitz (Ed.), *Advances in experiential social psychology* (Vol. 19, pp. 81–122). San Diego: Academic Press.

Nash, M., Hulsey, T., Sexton, M., Harralson, T., & Lambert, W. (1993). Long-term sequelae of childhood sexual abuse: Perceived family environment, psychopa-thology, and dissociation. *Journal of Consulting and Clinical Psychology, 61,* 276–283.

Navarre, E. L. (1987). Psychological maltreatment: The core component of child abuse. In M. R. Brassard, R. Germain, & S. N. Hart (Eds.), *Psychological mal-treatment of children and youth* (pp. 45–56). New York: Pergamon.

Neemann, J., & Harter, S. (1987). *The Self-Perception Profile for College Students.* Un-published manual, University of Denver, Denver, CO.

Neff, K. (1998). *Reasoning about rights and duties in the context of family life.* Unpub-lished manuscript, University of Denver, Denver, CO.

Neisser, U. (1991). Two perceptually given aspects of the self and their develop-ment. *Developmental Review, 11,* 197–209.

Nelson, K. (1986). *Event knowledge: Structure and function in development.* Hillsdale, NJ: Erlbaum.

Nelson, K. (Ed.). (1989). *Narratives from the crib.* Cambridge, MA: Harvard Univer-sity Press.

Nelson, K. (1990). Remembering, forgetting, and childhood amnesia. In R. Fivush & J. A. Hudson (Eds.), *Knowing and remembering in young children* (pp. 301–316). New York: Cambridge University Press.

Nelson, K. (1993). Events, narratives, memory: What develops? In C. A. Nelson (Ed.), *Memory and affect: Minnesota Symposia on Child Psychology* (Vol. 26, pp. 1–24). Hillsdale, NJ: Erlbaum.

Nemeroff, C. J., Stein, R. I., Diehl, N. S., & Smilack, K. M. (1994). From the Cleavers to the Clintons: Role choices and body orientation as reflected in magazine article content. *International Journal of Eating Disorders, 16,* 167–176.

Newberger, E. H. (1973). The myth of the battered child syndrome. In R. Bourne & E. H. Newberger (Eds.), *Critical perspectives on child abuse* (pp. 69–92). Lexington, MA: Lexington Books.

Ng, R. (1993, March). *The construction of true and false selves in adolescence.* Poster presented at the Society for Research in Child Development, New Orleans, LA.

Nicholls, J. G. (1990). What is ability and why are we mindful of it?: A developmental perspective. In R. J. Sternberg & J. Kolligian, Jr. (Eds.), *Competence considered* (pp. 11–40). New Haven, CT: Yale University Press.

Nikkari, D., & Harter, S. (1993). *The antecedents of behaviorally-presented self-esteem in young children.* Unpublished manuscript, University of Denver, Denver, CO.

Noam, G. G., & Borst, S. (Eds.). (1994). *Children, youth, and suicide: Developmental perspectives.* San Francisco: Jossey-Bass.

Nolen-Hoeksema, S. (1987). Sex differences in unipolar depression: Evidence and theory. *Psychological Bulletin, 101,* 259–282.

Nolen-Hoeksema, S. (1990). *Sex differences in depression.* Stanford, CA: Stanford University Press.

Nolen-Hoeksema, S., & Girgus, J. S. (1994). The emergence of gender differences in depression during adolescence. *Psychological Bulletin, 115,* 424–443.

Nolen-Hoeksema, S., Girgus, J. S., & Seligman, M. E. P. (1986). Learned helplessness in children: A longitudinal study of depression, achievement, and explanatory style. *Journal of Personality and Social Psychology, 51,* 435–442.

Nottelmann, E. D. (1987). Competence and self-esteem during the transition from childhood to adolescence. *Developmental Psychology, 23,* 441–450.

Oates, R. K., Forrest, D., & Peacock, A. (1985). Self-esteem of abused children. *Child Abuse and Neglect, 9,* 159–163.

Ogilvie, D. M., & Clark, M. D. (1992). The best and worst of it: Age and sex differences in self-discrepancy research. In R. P. Lipka & T. M. Brinthaupt (Eds.), *Self-perspectives across the life span* (pp. 186–222). Albany: State University of New York Press.

Olson, D. H. (1981). Family typologies: Bridging family research and family therapy. In E. E. Filsinger & R. A. Lewis (Eds.), *Assessing marriage: New behavioral approaches* (pp. 74–89). Beverly Hills, CA: Sage.

O'Malley, P., & Bachman, J. (1983). Self-esteem: Change and stability between ages 13 and 23. *Developmental Psychology, 19,* 257–268.

Oosterwegel, A., & Oppenheimer, L. (1993). *The self-system: Developmental changes between and within self-concepts.* Hillsdale, NJ: Erlbaum.

Orenstein, P. (1994). *School girls: Young women, self-esteem, and the confidence gap.* New York: Anchor Books, Doubleday.

Osgood, C. E., Suci, G. J., & Tannenbaum, P. H. (1971). *The measurement of meaning.* Urbana, IL: University of Chicago Press.

Overton, W. (1994). The arrow of time and the cycle of time: Concepts of change, cognition, and embodiment. *Psychological Inquiry, 5,* 215–237.

Oyserman, D., & Markus, H. R. (1993). The sociocultural self. In J. Suls (Ed.), *Psychological perspectives on the self* (Vol. 7, pp. 187–220). Hillsdale, NJ: Erlbaum.

Padin, M. A., Lerner, R. M., & Spiro, A. (1981). Stability of body attitudes and self-esteem in late adolescents. *Adolescence, 62,* 371-384.

Parsons, J., & Ruble, D. (1977). Developmental changes in attributions of descriptive concepts to persons. *Journal of Personality and Social Psychology, 48,* 1075-1079.

Pascual-Leone, J. (1988). Organismic processes for neo-Piagetian theories: A dialectical causal account of cognitive development. In A. Demetrious (Ed.), *The neo-Piagetian theories of cognitive development: Toward an integration* (pp. 25-65). Amsterdam: North Holland: Elsevier.

Patterson, C. J., Kupersmidt, J. B., & Griesler, P. C. (1990). Children's perceptions of self and of relationships with others as a function of sociometric status. *Child Development, 61,* 1335-1349.

Pedrabissi, L., & Santinello, M. (1992). II Self-Perception Profile for Children di Susan Harter. *Psicologia e Scuola, 61,* 3-14.

Pedrabissi, L., Santinello, M., & Scarpazza, V. (1988). Contributo all-adattamento italiano del Self-Perception Profile for Children di Susan Harter. *Bollettino di Psicolgia applicata, 185,* 19-26.

Pekrun, R. (1990). Social support, achievement evaluations, and self-concepts in adolescence. In L. Oppenheimer (Ed.), *The self-concept: European perspectives on its development, aspects, and applications* (pp. 107-119). Berlin, Heidelberg: Springer.

Pelham, B. W., & Swann, W. B., Jr. (1989). From self-conceptions to self-worth: On the sources and structure of global self-esteem. *Journal of Personality and Social Psychology, 57,* 672-680.

Pfeffer, C. R. (1986). *The suicidal child.* New York: Guilford Press.

Pfeffer, C. R. (1988). Risk factors associated with youth suicide. *Psychiatric Annals, 18,* 652-656.

Pfeffer, C. R., Lipkins, M. A., Plutchik, R., & Mirzruchi, M. (1988). Normal children at risk for suicidal behavior: A two-year follow-up study. *Journal of the American Academy of Child and Adolescent Psychiatry, 27,* 34-41.

Pfeffer, C. R., Zuckerman, S., Plutchik, R., & Mirzruchi, M. S. (1984). Suicidal behavior in normal school children: A comparison with child psychiatric in-patients. *Journal of the American Academy of Child Psychiatry, 23,* 416-423.

Phillips, D. A., & Zimmerman, M. (1990). The developmental course of perceived competence and incompetence among competent children. In R. J. Sternberg & J. Kolligian, Jr. (Eds.), *Competence considered* (pp. 41-66). New Haven, CT: Yale University Press.

Piaget, J. (1932). *The moral judgment of the child.* New York: Harcourt, Brace & World.

Piaget, J. (1960). *The psychology of intelligence.* Patterson, NJ: Littlefield-Adams.

Pierrehumbert, B., Plancherel, B., & Jankech-Caretta, C. (1987). Image de soi et perception des competences propres chez l'enfant. *Revue de Psycholgie Appliquée, 37,* 359-377.

Piers, E. V., & Harris, D. B. (1964). Age and other correlates of self-concept in children. *Journal of Educational Psychology, 55,* 91-95.

Pillemer, D. B., & White, S. H. (1989). Childhood events recalled by children and adults. In H. W. Reese (Ed.), *Advances in child development and behavior* (Vol. 21, pp. 297–340). San Diego: Academic Press.

Pintrich, P., & Blumenfeld, P. (1982, March). *Teacher and student behavior in different activity structures.* Paper presented at the annual meeting of the American Educational Research Association, New York, NY.

Pipher, M. (1994). *Reviving Ophelia: Saving the selves of adolescent girls.* New York: Ballantine.

Pipp, S. (1990). Sensorimotor and representational internal representational working models of self, other, and relationship: Mechanisms of connection and separation. In D. Cicchetti & M. Beeghly (Eds.), *The self in transition: Infancy to childhood* (pp. 243–264). Chicago: University of Chicago Press.

Pomerantz, S. C. (1979). Sex differences in the relative importance of self esteem, physical self-satisfaction, and identity in predicting adolescent satisfaction. *Journal of Youth and Adolescence, 8,* 51–61.

Pomerantz, E. V., & Ruble, D. N., Frey, K. S., & Greulich, F. (1995). Meeting goals and confronting conflict: Children's changing perceptions of social comparison. *Child Development, 66,* 723–738.

Pope, A. W., McHale, S. M., & Craighead, W. E. (1988). *Self-esteem enhancement with children and adolescents.* Boston, MA: Allyn & Bacon.

Potter-Efron, R. T. (1989). *Shame, guilt, and alcoholism: Treatment issues in clinical practice.* New York: Haworth Press.

Pratt, M. W., Pancer, M., Hunsberger, B., & Manchester, J. (1990). Reasoning about the self and relationships in maturity: An integrative complexity analysis of individual differences. *Journal of Personality and Social Psychology, 59,* 575–581.

Puig-Antich, J. (1982). Major depression and conduct disorder in prepuberty. *Journal of the American Academy of Child Psychiatry, 21,* 118–128.

Putnam, F. W. (1989). *Diagnosis and treatment of multiple personality disorder.* New York: Guilford Press.

Putnam, F. W. (1990). Disturbances of self in victims of childhood sexual abuse. In R. P. Kluft (Ed.), *Incest-related syndromes of adult psychopathology* (pp. 113–132). Washington, DC: American Psychiatric Press.

Putnam, F. W. (1991). Recent research on multiple personality disorder. *Psychiatric Clinics of North America, 14,* 489–502.

Putnam, F. W. (1993). Dissociation and disturbances of the self. In D. Cicchetti & S. Toth (Eds.), *Rochester Symposium on Developmental Psychopathology: Disorders and dysfunctions of the self* (Vol. 5, pp. 251–266). Rochester, NY: University of Rochester Press.

Pyszczynski, T., & Greenberg, J. (1986). Evidence for a depressive self-focusing style. *Journal of Research in Personality, 20,* 95–106.

Pyszczynski, T., & Greenberg, J. (1987). Self-regulatory perseveration and the depressive self-focusing style: A self-awareness theory of reactive depression. *Psychological Bulletin, 102,* 1–17.

Raciti, M. C., & Norcross, J. C. (1987). The EAT and EDI: Screening, interrelationships and psychometrics. *International Journal of Eating Disorders, 6,* 579–586.

Rand, C. S., & Kuldau, J. M. (1992). Epidemiology of bulimia and symptoms in a general population: Sex, age, race, and sociometric status. *International Journal of Eating Disorders, 11,* 37–44.

Reissland, N. (1985). The development of concepts of simultaneity in children's understanding of emotions. *Journal of Child Psychology and Psychiatry, 26,* 811–824.

Renick, M. J., & Harter, S. (1988). *The Self-Perception Profile for Learning Disabled Students.* Unpublished manual, University of Denver, Denver, CO.

Renick, M. J., & Harter, S. (1989). Impact of social comparisons on the developing self-perceptions of learning disabled students. *Journal of Educational Psychology, 81,* 631–638.

Renouf, A. G., & Harter, S. (1990). Low self-worth and anger as components of the depressive experience in young adolescents. *Development and Psychopathology, 2,* 293–310.

Rhee, U. (1993). Self-perceptions of competence and social support in Korean children. *Early Child Development and Care, 85,* 57–66.

Riesman, D. (1950). *The lonely crowd.* New Haven, CT: Yale University Press.

Riley, W. T., Treiber, F. A., & Woods, M. G. (1989). Anger and hostility in depression. *Journal of Nervous and Mental Disorders, 177,* 668–674.

Robinson, N. S. (1995). Evaluating the nature of perceived support and its relation to perceived self-worth in adolescents. *Journal of Research on Adolescence, 5,* 253–280.

Rogers, C. R. (1951). *Client-centered therapy.* Boston: Houghton Mifflin.

Rogers, C., & Dymond, R. (1954). *Psychotherapy and personality change.* Chicago: University of Chicago Press.

Rogoff, B. (1990). *Apprenticeship in thinking.* New York: Oxford University Press.

Rosales, I., & Zigler, E. F. (1989). Role taking and self-image disparity: A further test of cognitive-developmental thought. *Psychological Reports, 64,* 41–42.

Rosch, E. R. (1975). Cognitive representations of semantic categories. *Journal of Experimental Psychology, 104,* 192–233.

Rosen, G. M., & Ross, A. O. (1968). Relationship of body image to self-concept. *Journal of Consulting and Clinical Psychology, 32,* 100.

Rosenberg, M. (1979). *Conceiving the self.* New York: Basic Books.

Rosenberg, M. (1986). Self-concept from middle childhood through adolescence. In J. Suls & A. G. Greenwald (Eds.), *Psychological perspective on the self* (Vol. 3, pp. 107–135). Hillsdale, NJ: Erlbaum.

Rosenberg, S. (1988). Self and others: Studies in social personality and autobiography. In L. Berkowitz (Ed.), *Advances in experimental social psychology* (Vol. 21, pp. 56–96). New York: Academic Press.

Rosenberg, M., & Simmons, R. G. (1972). *Black and White self-esteem: The urban school child.* Washington, DC: American Sociological Association.

Rossman, B. B., & Rosenberg, M. S. (Eds.). (1998). *Multiple victimization of children.* New York: Haworth Press.

Rubin, K. H., Chen, X., & Hymel, S. (1993). Socioemotional characteristics of withdrawn and aggressive children. *Merrill-Palmer Quarterly, 39,* 518–534.

Rubin, K. H., Stewart, S. L., & Chen, X. (1995). Patterns of aggressive and withdrawn children. In M. Bornstein (Ed.), *Handbook of parenting* (Vol. 1, pp. 255–284). Hillsdale, NJ: Erlbaum.

Rubin, L. (1985). *Just friends: The role of friendship in our lives.* New York: Harper.

Ruble, D. N. (1988). Sex-role development. In M. H. Bornstein & M. E. Lamb (Eds.), *Developmental psychology: An advanced textbook* (2nd ed., pp. 411–460). Hillsdale, NJ: Erlbaum.

Ruble, D. N. (1998). Gender development. In W. Damon (Series Ed.) & N. Eisenberg (Vol. Ed.), *Handbook of child psychology: Vol. 3. Social, emotional and personality development* (5th ed., pp. 933–1016). New York: Wiley.

Ruble, D. N., & Dweck, C. (1995). Self-conceptions, person conception, and their development. In N. Eisenberg (Ed.), *Review of personality and social psychology: Development and social psychology: The interface* (Vol. 15, pp. 109–139). Thousand Oaks, CA: Sage.

Ruble, D. N., & Frey, K. S. (1991). Changing patterns of comparative behavior as skills are acquired: A functional model of self-evaluation. In J. Suls & T. A. Wills (Eds.), *Social comparison: Contemporary theory and research* (pp. 70–112). Hillsdale, NJ: Erlbaum.

Rudd, M. D. (1989). The prevalence of suicidal ideation among college students. *Suicide and Life-Threatening Behavior, 19,* 173–183.

Rutter, M. (1986). The developmental psychopathology of depression: Issues and perspectives. In M. Rutter, C. E. Izard, & P. B. Read (Eds.), *Depression in young people: Developmental and clinical perspectives* (pp. 3–32). New York: Guilford Press.

Rutter, M. (1987). Psychosocial resilience and protective mechanisms. *American Journal of Orthopsychiatry, 57,* 316–331.

Rutter, M. (1988). Epidemological approaches to developmental psychopathology. *Archives of General Psychiatry, 45,* 486–495.

Rutter, M. (1989). Isle of Wight revisited: Twenty-five years of child psychiatric epidemiology. *Journal of the American Academy of Child Adolescent Psychiatry, 28,* 633–653.

Rutter, M., Izard, C., & Read, P. (Eds.). (1985). *Depression in childhood: Developmental perspectives.* New York: Guilford Press.

Ryan, R., & Lynch, J. (1989). Emotional autonomy versus detachment: Revisiting the vicissitudes of adolescence and young adulthood. *Child Development, 60,* 340–356.

Ryckman, R. M., Robbins, M. A., Thornton, B., & Cantrell, P. (1982). Development and validation of a physical self-efficacy scale. *Journal of Personality and Social Psychology, 42,* 891–900.

Sadker, M., & Sadker, D. (1994). *Failing at fairness: How America's schools cheat girls.* New York: Scribner's.

Sakurai, S. (1983). Development of the Japanese version of Harter's Perceived Competence Scale for Children, *Japanese Journal of Educational Psychology, 31*, 245–249.

Salmons, P. H., Lewis, V. J., Rogers, P., Gatherer, A. J. H., & Booth, D. A. (1988). Body shape dissatisfaction in schoolchildren. *British Journal of Psychiatry, 15*, 27–31.

Sampson, E. E. (1988). The debate on individualism: Indigenous psychologies and their role in personal and societal functioning. *American Psychologist, 43*, 15–22.

Sander, L. (1975). Infant and caretaking environment: Investigation and conceptualization of adaptive behavior in a series of increasing complexity. In E. J. Anthony (Ed.), *Explorations in child psychiatry* (pp. 129–166). New York: Plenum.

Sandler, J., & Joffe, W. G. (1965). Notes on childhood depression. *International Journal of Psychoanalysis, 46*, 88–95.

Sarbin, T. R. (1962). A preface to a psychological analysis of the self. *Psychological Review, 59*, 11–22.

Savin-Williams, R. C., & Berndt, T. J. (1990). Friend and peer relations. In S. S. Feldman & G. Elliot (Eds.), *At the threshold: The developing adolescent* (pp. 277–307). Cambridge, MA: Harvard University Press.

Savin-Williams, R. C., & Demo, P. (1993). Situational and transitional determinants of adolescent self-feelings. *Journal of Personality and Social Psychology, 44*, 820–833.

Schneider-Rosen, K., Braunwald, K. G., Carlson, V., & Cicchetti, D. (1985). Current perspectives in attachment theory: Illustration from the study of maltreated infants. In I. Bretherton & E. Waters (Eds.), Growing points in attachment theory and research. *Monographs of the Society for Research in Child Development, 50*, 194–210.

Schneidman, E. S. (1991). The commonalities of suicide across the life span. In A. A. Leenaars (Ed.), *Life-span perspectives of suicide* (pp. 83–91). New York: Plenum.

Seligman, M. E. P. (1975). *Helplessness: On depression, development, and death.* San Francisco: Freeman.

Seligman, M. E. P. (1993). *What you can change and what you can't.* New York: Fawcett Columbine.

Seligman, M. E. P., & Peterson, C. (1986). A learned helplessness perspective on childhood depression: Theory and research. In M. Rutter, C. E. Izard, & P. B. Read (Eds.), *Depression in young people: Developmental and clinical perspectives* (pp. 223–249). New York: Guilford Press.

Selman, R. L. (1980). *The growth of interpersonal understanding.* New York: Academic Press.

Selman, R. L., & Schultz, L. H. (1990). *Making a friend in youth.* Chicago: University of Chicago Press.

Shaffer, D. (1974). Suicide in childhood and early adolescence. *Journal of Child Psychology and Psychiatry, 13*, 275–291.

Shaffer, D. (1985). Depression, mania, and suicidal acts. In M. Rutter & L. Hersov (Eds.), *Child and adolescent psychiatry: Modern approaches* (pp. 158–180). London: Blackwell.

Shaffer, D., & Fischer, P. (1981). The epidemiology of suicide in children and young adolescents. *Journal of American Academic Child Psychiatry, 20*, 545–565.

Shavelson, R. J., Hubner, J. J., & Stanton, G. C. (1976). Validation of construct interpretations. *Review of Educational Research, 46*, 407–441.

Shavelson, R. J., & Marsh, H. W. (1986). On the structure of self-concept. In R. Schwarzer (Ed.), *Anxiety and cognition* (pp. 305–330). Hillsdale, NJ: Erlbaum.

Shaver, P., & Rubenstein, C. (1983). Research potential of newspaper and magazine surveys. In H. T. Reis (Ed.), *Naturalistic approaches to studying social interaction* (pp. 133–149). San Francisco: Jossey-Bass.

Shaver, P. R., Wu, S., & Schwartz, J. C. (1992). Cross-cultural similarities and differences in emotion and its representation: A prototype approach. In M. S. Clark (Ed.), *Review of personality and social psychology* (Vol. 13, pp. 175–212). Newbury Park, CA: Sage.

Shell, R. M., & Eisenberg, N. (1992). A developmental model of recipients' reaction to aid. *Psychological Bulletin, 111*, 413–433.

Sherrill, C., Hinson, M., Gench, B., Kennedy, S. O., & Low, L. (1990). Self-concepts of disabled youth athletes. *Perceptual and Motor Skills, 70*, 1093–1098.

Shirk, S. R., & Eltz, M. (1998). Multiple victimization and the process and outcome of child psychotherapy. In B. B. R. Rossman & M. S. Rosenberg (Eds.), *Multiple victimization of children: Conceptual, developmental, research, and treatment issues* (pp. 233–252). New York: Haworth Press.

Shirk, S., & Harter, S. (1996). Treatment of low self-esteem. In M. A. Reinecke, F. M. Dattilio, & A. Freeman (Eds.), *Cognitive therapy with children and adolescents* (pp. 175–198). New York: Guilford Press.

Shirk, S. R., & Russell, R. L. (1996). *Change processes in child psychotherapy: Revitalizing treatment and research.* New York: Guilford Press.

Showers, C. (1995). The evaluative organization of self-knowledge: Origins, process, and implications for self-esteem. In M. H. Kernis (Ed.), *Efficacy, agency, and self-esteem* (pp. 101–122). New York: Plenum.

Shrauger, J. S., & Schoeneman, T. J. (1979). Symbolic interactionist view of self-concept: Through the looking glass darkly. *Psychological Bulletin, 86*, 549–573.

Shweder, R. A. (1991). *Thinking through cultures.* Cambridge, MA: Harvard University Press.

Shweder, R., & Bourne, E. (1982). Does the concept of person vary cross-culturally? In R. Shweder & R. LeVine (Eds.), *Culture theory: Essays on mind, self, and emotion* (pp. 158–199). New York: Cambridge University Press.

Shweder, R., & Miller, G. (1991). The social construction of the person. In R. Shweder (Ed.), *Thinking through cultures* (pp. 156–185). Cambridge, MA: Harvard University Press.

Siegler, R. S. (1991). *Children's thinking* (2nd ed.). Englewood Cliffs, NJ: Prentice-Hall.

Silberstein, L. R., Striegel-Moore, R. H., Timko, C., & Rodin, J. (1988). Behavioral and psychological implications of body dissatisfaction: Do men and women differ? *Sex Roles, 19*, 219–232.

Silverstein, B., Perdue, L., Peterson, B., & Kelly, E. (1986). The role of the mass media in promoting a thin standard of bodily attractiveness for women. *Sex Roles, 14,* 519–532.

Simmons, R. G., & Blyth, D. A. (1987). *Moving into adolescence: The impact of pubertal change and school context.* New York: Aldine de Gruyter.

Simmons, R. G., Blyth, D. A., Van Cleave, E. F., & Bush, D. (1979). Entry into early adolescence: The impact of school structure, puberty, and early dating on self-esteem. *American Sociological Review, 44,* 948–967.

Simmons, R. G., & Rosenberg, F. (1975). Sex, sex roles, and self-image. *Journal of Youth and Adolescence, 4,* 229–258.

Simmons, R. G., Rosenberg, F., & Rosenberg, M. (1973). Disturbances in the self-images at adolescence. *American Sociological Review, 38,* 553–568.

Simon, V. A., & Harter, S. (1998). *The role of self-focused attention in young adolescents' depressive reactions to negative self-evaluations.* Unpublished manuscript, University of Denver, Denver, CO.

Smith, K., & Crawford, S. (1986). Suicidal behavior among normal high school students. *Suicide and Life-Threatening Behavior, 16,* 313–325.

Smollar, J., & Youniss, J. (1985). Adolescent self-concept development. In R. L. Leahy (Ed.), *The development of self* (pp. 247–266). New York: Academic Press.

Snow, K. (1990). Building memories: The ontogeny of autobiography. In D. Cicchetti & M. Beeghly (Eds.), *The self in transition: Infancy to childhood* (pp. 213–242). Chicago: University of Chicago Press.

Snyder, D. K., & Smith, G. T. (1986). Classification of marital relationships: An empirical approach. *Journal of Marriage and the Family, 38,* 15–28.

Snyder, M. (1987). *Public appearances, private realities: The psychology of self-monitoring.* New York: Freeman.

Song, I. S., & Hattie, J. A. (1984). Home environment, self-concept, and academic achievement: A causal modeling approach. *Journal of Educational Psychology, 76,* 1269–1281.

Spence, J. T. (1985). Achievement American style: The rewards and costs of individualism. *American Psychologist, 40,* 1285–1295.

Spence, J. T., Helmreich, R., & Stapp, J. (1975). The Personal Attributes Questionnaire: A measure of sex role stereotypes and masculinity–femininity. *JSAS Catalog of Selected Documents in Psychology, 4,* 43–44.

Spencer, M. B. (1995). Old issues and new theorizing about African-American youth: A phenomenological variant of ecological systems theory. In R. L. Taylor (Ed.), *Black youth: Perspectives on their status in the United States* (pp. 37–70). Westport, CT: Praeger.

Spencer, M. B., & Markstrom-Adams, C. (1990). Identity processes among racial and ethnic minority children in America. *Child Development, 61,* 290–310.

Spencer, S., & Steele, C. M. (1995). *Under suspicion of inability: Stereotype vulnerability and women's math performance.* Unpublished manuscript, University of Michigan, Ann Arbor.

Spirato, A., Brown, L., Overholser, J., & Fritz, G. (1989). Attempted suicide in adolescence: A review and critique of the literature. *Clinical Psychology Review, 9,* 335–363.

Spirito, A., Stark, L. J., Cobiella, C., Drigan, R., Androkites, A., & Hewett, K. (1990). Social adjustment of children successfully treated for cancer. *Journal of Pediatric Psychology, 15,* 359–371.

Sroufe, L. A. (1990). An organizational perspective on the self. In D. Cicchetti & M. Beeghly (Eds.), *The self in transition: Infancy to childhood* (pp. 281–308). Chicago: University of Chicago Press.

Sroufe, L. A., & Fleeson, J. (1986). Attachment and the construction of relationships. In W. Hartup & Z. Rubin (Eds.), *Relationships and development* (pp. 51–71). New York: Cambridge University Press.

Sroufe, L. A., & Rutter, M. (1985). The domain of developmental psychopathology. *Child Development, 35,* 17–29.

Srull, T. K., & Wyer, R. S., Jr. (Eds.). (1993). *The mental representation of trait and autobiographical knowledge about the self: Vol. 5. Advances in social cognition.* Hillsdale, NJ: Erlbaum.

Stager, S. F., & Burke, P. J. (1982). A reexamination of body build stereotypes. *Journal of Research in Personality, 16,* 435–446.

Steele, C. M. (1988). The psychology of self-affirmation: Sustaining the integrity of the self. In L. Berkowitz (Ed.), *Advances in experimental social psychology* (Vol. 21, pp. 261–302). San Diego: Academic Press.

Stein, R. (1996). Physical self-concept. In B. A. Bracken (Ed.), *Handbook of self-concept* (pp. 374–394). New York: Wiley.

Steinberg, L. (1990). Interdependency in the family: Autonomy, conflict, and harmony in the parent–adolescent relationship. In S. Feldman & G. Elliot (Eds.), *At the threshold: The developing adolescent* (pp. 255–276). Cambridge, MA: Harvard University Press.

Steinberg, L., & Silverberg, S. B. (1986). The vicissitudes of autonomy in early adolescence. *Child Development, 57,* 841–851.

Stern, D. (1985). *The interpersonal world of the infant.* New York: Basic Books.

Stigler, J. W., Smith, S., & Mao, L. (1985). The self-perception of competence by Chinese children, *Child Development, 56,* 1259–1270.

Stipek, D. (1981). Children's perceptions of their own and their classmates' ability. *Journal of Educational Psychology, 73,* 404–410.

Stipek, D. (1983). A developmental analysis of pride and shame. *Human Development, 26,* 42–54.

Stipek, D. (1984). Young children's performance expectations: Logical analysis or wishful thinking? In J. Nicholls (Ed.), *Advances in motivation achievement* (Vol. 3, pp. 33–56). Greenwich, CT: JAI Press.

Stipek, D. (1995). The development of pride and shame in toddlers. In J. P. Tangney & K. W. Fischer (Eds.), *Self-conscious emotions: The psychology of shame, guilt, embarrassment, and pride* (pp. 237–252). New York: Guilford Press.

Stipek, D., Recchia, S., & McClintic, S. (1992). Self-evaluation in young children. *Monographs of the Society for Research in Child Development, 57,* 1–84.

Stiver, I. P., & Miller, J. B. (1988). *From depression to sadness in the psychotherapy of women* (Work in Progress No. 36). Wellesley, MA: Stone Center Working Paper Series.

Strauss, S. (1988). Sexual harassment in the school: Legal implications for principals. *National Association of Secondary School Principals Bulletin, 37*, 93–97.

Streigel-Moore, R. H., Silberstein, L. R., & Rodin, J. (1986). Toward an understanding of risk factors for bulimia. *American Psychologist, 41*, 246–263.

Strein, W. (1988). Classroom-based elementary school affective education programs: A critical review. *Psychology in the Schools, 25*, 288–296.

Stryker, S. (1987). Identity theory: Developments and extensions. In K. Yardley & T. Honess (Eds.), *Self and identity* (pp. 212–232). New York: Wiley.

Sullivan, H. S. (1953). *The interpersonal theory of psychiatry.* New York: Norton.

Suls, J., & Sanders, G. (1982). Self-evaluation via social comparison: A developmental analysis. In L. Wheeler (Ed.), *Review of personality and social psychology* (Vol. 3, pp. 67–89). Beverly Hills, CA: Sage.

Swann, W. B., Jr. (1985). Self-verification: Bringing social reality into harmony with the self. In J. Suls & A. G. Greenwald (Eds.), *Social psychological perspectives on the self* (Vol. 2, pp. 33–66). Hillsdale, NJ: Erlbaum.

Swann, W. B., Jr. (1987). Identity negotiation: Where two roads meet. *Journal of Personality and Social Psychology, 53*, 1038–1051.

Swann, W. B., Jr. (1996). *Self-traps.* New York: Freeman.

Talmi, A., & Harter, S. (1998). *The role of social support provided by parents and nonparental significant adults in the lives of young adolescents.* Unpublished manuscript, University of Denver, Denver, CO.

Tangney, J. P. (1995). Shame and guilt in interpersonal relationships. In J. P. Tangney & K. W. Fischer (Eds.), *Self-conscious emotions: The psychology of shame, guilt, embarrassment, and pride* (pp. 114–139). New York: Guilford Press.

Tangney, J. P., & Fischer, K. W. (Eds.). (1995). *Self-conscious emotions: The psychology of shame, guilt, embarrassment, and pride.* New York: Guilford Press.

Taylor, S. E. (1983). Adjustment to threatening events: A theory of cognitive adaptation. *American Psychologist, 38*, 1161–1173.

Taylor, S. E., & Brown, J. D. (1988). Illusion and well-being: A social psychological perspective on mental health. *Psychological Bulletin, 103*, 193–210.

Terr, L. (1990). *Too scared to cry.* New York: Basic Books.

Terr, L. (1991). Childhood traumas: An outline and overview. *American Journal of Psychiatry, 148*, 10–20.

Tesser, A. (1980). Self-esteem maintenance in family dynamics. *Journal of Personality and Social Psychology, 39*, 77–91.

Tesser, A. (1988). Toward a self-evaluation maintenance model of social behavior. In L. Berkowitz (Ed.), *Advances in experimental social psychology* (Vol. 21, pp. 181–227). New York: Academic Press.

Tesser, A., & Campbell, J. (1980). Self-definition: The impact of the relative performance and similarity of others. *Social Psychology Quarterly, 43*, 341–347.

Tesser, A., & Campbell, J. (1983). Self-definition and self-evaluation maintenance.

In J. Suls & A. G. Greenwald (Eds.), *Psychological perspectives on the self* (Vol. 2, pp. 1-32). Hillsdale, NJ: Erlbaum.

Tesser, A., & Cornell, D. (1991). On the confluence of self processes. *Journal of Experimental Social Psychology, 27,* 501-526.

Tessler, M. (1991). *Making memories together: The influence of mother–child joint encoding on the development of autobiographical memory style.* Unpublished doctoral dissertation, City University of New York Graduate Center, New York.

Thorne, A., & Michaelieu, Q. (1994, August). *Situating adolescent gender and self-esteem with personal memories.* Paper presented at the annual meeting of the American Psychological Association, Los Angeles, CA.

Tice, D. M. (1994). Pathways to internalization: When does overt behavior change the self-concept? In T. M. Brinthaupt & R. P. Lipka (Eds.), *Changing the self* (pp. 229-250). Albany: State University of New York Press.

Topol, P., & Reznikoff, M. (1982). Perceived peer and family relationships, hopelessness, and locus of control as factors in adolescent suicide attempts. *Suicide and Life-Threatening Behavior, 12,* 141-150.

Trent, L. M., Russell, G., & Cooney, G. (1994). Assessment of self-concept in early adolescence. *Australian Journal of Psychology, 46,* 21-28.

Triandis, H. C. (1989a). Cross-cultural studies of individualism and collectivism. In R. A. Diestbier & J. J. Berman (Eds.), *Nebraska Symposium on Motivation: Cross-cultural perspectives* (Vol. 37, pp. 232-259). Lincoln: University of Nebraska Press.

Triandis, H. C. (1989b). The self and social behavior in differing cultural contexts. *Psychological Review, 96,* 506-520.

Trilling, L. (1971). *Sincerity and authenticity.* Cambridge, MA: Harvard University Press.

Trungpa, C. (1976). *The myth of freedom.* Berkeley, CA: Shambhalla Books.

Tulku, T. (1978). *Skillful means.* Berkeley, CA: Dharma Publishing.

Tulving, E. (1972). Episodic and semantic memory. In E. Tulving & W. Donaldson (Eds.), *Organization of memory* (pp. 382-403). New York: Academic Press.

Tulving, E. (1983). *Elements of episodic memory.* New York: Oxford University Press.

Turiel, E., & Wainryb, C. (in press). Social reasoning and the varieties of social experiences in cultural contexts. In H. W. Reese (Ed.), *Advances in child development and behavior* (Vol. 9). New York: Academic Press.

Vallacher, R. R. (1980). An introduction to self-theory. In D. M. Wegner & R. R. Vallacher (Eds.), *The self in social psychology* (pp. 3-30). New York: Oxford University Press.

Vanderheyden, D. A., Fekken, G. C., & Boland, F. J. (1988). Critical variables associated with bingeing and bulimia in a university population: A factor analytic study. *International Journal of Eating Disorders, 7,* 321-329.

van der Kolk, B. A. (1987). *Psychological trauma.* Washington, DC: American Psychiatric Association Press.

van der Werff, J. J. (1985). *Identity problems: Self-conceptions in psychology.* Muiderberg, The Netherlands: Dick Coutinho.

van Dongen-Melman, J. E. W. M., Koot, H. M., & Verhulst, F. C. (1993). Cross-cultural validation of Harter's Self-Perception Profile in a Dutch sample. *Educational and Psychological Measurement, 53,* 739–753.

van Rossum, J. H. A., & Vermeer, A. (1994). Harter's vragenlijst naar vaargenomen competentie: Een Nederlandstalige versie. *Ped. T., 19,* 9–30.

Wallbott, H. G., & Scherer, K. R. (1995). Cultural determinants in experiencing shame and guilt. In J. P. Tangney & K. W. Fischer (Eds.), *Self-conscious emotions: The psychology of shame, guilt, embarrassment, and pride* (pp. 465–487). New York: Guilford Press.

Waters, P. L. (1993, March). *Consistency in relationship styles across three contexts: Intimate partners, coworkers and supervisors.* Poster presentation at the Biennial Meeting of the Society for Research in Child Development, New Orleans, LA.

Waters, P. L., & Gonzales, R. (1995, March). *Level of voice among young adolescent males and females.* Paper presented at the meeting of the Society for Research in Child Development, Indianapolis, IN.

Waters, P. L., & Harter, S. (1998). *Backlast attitudes against the women's movement as a function of relationship style with one's intimate partner.* Unpublished manuscript, University of Denver, Denver, CO.

Watson, M. (1990). Aspects of self development as reflected in children's role playing. In D. Cicchetti & M. Beeghly (Eds.), *The self in transition: Infancy to childhood* (pp. 281–307). Chicago: University of Chicago Press.

Watson, M. W., & Fischer, K. (1993). Structural change in children's understanding of family roles and divorce. In R. R. Cocking & K. A. Renninger (Eds.), *The development and meaning of psychological distance* (pp. 123–144). Hillsdale, NJ: Erlbaum.

Webb, N. M., & Kenderski, C. M. (1985). Gender differences in small group interaction and achievement in high-achieving and low-achieving classrooms. In L. C. Wilkinson & C. B. Marret (Eds.), *Gender-related differences in classroom interaction* (pp. 209–226). New York: Academic Press.

Weiner, B. (1985). An attributional theory of achievement motivation and emotion. *Psychological Review, 92,* 271–282.

Weiner, B. (1986). *An attributional theory of motivation and emotions.* New York: Springer.

Weis, L., & Fine, M. (1993). *Beyond silenced voices.* Albany: SUNY University of New York Press.

Westen, D. (1993). The impact of sexual abuse on self structure. In D. Cicchetti & S. Toth (Eds.), *Rochester Symposium on Developmental Psychopathology: Disorders and dysfunctions of the self* (Vol. 5, pp. 223–250). Rochester, NY: University of Rochester Press.

Wexler, D. B. (1991). *The adolescent self: Strategies for self-management, self-soothing, and self-esteem.* New York: Norton.

White, K., Speisman, J., & Costos, D. (1983). Young adults and their parents: Individuation to mutuality. In H. D. Grotevant & C. R. Cooper (Eds.), *New directions for child development: Adolescent development in the family* (pp. 61–76). San Francisco: Jossey-Bass.

White, R. (1959). Motivation reconsidered: The concept of competence. *Psychological Review, 66,* 297–333.

Wicklund, R. (1975). Objective self-awareness. In L. Berkowitz (Ed.), *Advances in experimental social psychology* (Vol. 8, pp. 233–275). New York: Academic Press.

Wicklund, R. A., & Frey, D. (1980). Self-awareness theory: When the self makes a difference. In D. M. Wegner & R. R. Vallacher (Eds.), *The self in social psychology* (pp. 31–54). New York: Oxford University Press.

Wigfield, A., Eccles, J. S., MacIver, D., Reuman, D. A., & Midgley, C. (1991). Transitions during early adolescence: Changes in children's domain-specific self-perceptions and general self-esteem across the transition to junior high school. *Developmental Psychology, 27,* 552–565.

Wigfield, A., Eccles, J. S., & Pintrich, P. R. (1996). Development between the ages of 11 and 25. In D. C. Berliner, & R. C. Calfee (Eds.), *Handbook of educational psychology* (pp. 148–185). New York: Simon & Schuster/Macmillan.

Wilkinson, L., Lindow, J., & Chiang, C. (1985). Sex differences and sex segregation in students' small-group communication. In L. Wilkinson & C. Marett (Eds.), *Gender influences in classroom interaction* (pp. 185–207). Orlando, FL: Academic Press.

Williamson, D. A., Netemeyer, R. G., Jackman, L. P., Anderson, D. A., Funsch, C. L., & Rabalais, J. Y. (1995). Structural equation modeling of risk factors for the development of the eating disorder symptoms in female athletes. *International Journal of Eating Disorders, 17,* 387–393.

Winnicott, D. W. (1958). *From paediatrics to psychoanalysis.* London: Hogarth Press.

Winnicott, D. W. (1965). *The maturational processes and the facilitating environment.* New York: International Universities Press.

Wiseman, C. V., Gray, J. J., Mosimann, J. E., & Ahrens, A. H. (1992). Cultural expectations of thinness in women: An update. *International Journal of Eating Disorders, 11,* 85–89.

Withers, L. E., & Kaplan, D. W. (1987). Adolescents who attempt suicide: A retrospective clinical chart review of hospitalized patients. *Professional Psychology: Research and Practice, 18,* 341–393.

Wolf, D. P. (1990). Being of several minds: Voices and version of the self in early childhood. In D. Cicchetti & M. Beeghly (Eds.), *The self in transition: Infancy to childhood* (pp. 183–212). Chicago: University of Chicago Press.

Wolfe, D. (1989). *Child abuse.* Newbury Park, CA: Sage.

Wood, J. V. (1989). Theory and research concerning social comparisons of personal attributes. *Psychological Bulletin, 106,* 231–248.

Wundt, W. (1907). *Outlines of psychology.* New York: Stechert.

Wyer, R. S., & Srull, T. K. (1989). *Memory and cognition in its social context.* Hillsdale, NJ: Erlbaum.

Wylie, R. C. (1979). *The self concept: Theory and research on selected topics* (Vol. 2). Lincoln: University of Nebraska Press.

Wylie, R. C. (1989). *Measures of self-concept.* Lincoln: University of Nebraska Press.

Youngblade, L., & Belsky, J. (1990). The social and emotional consequences of child maltreatment. In R. Ammerman & M. Herssen (Eds.), *Children at risk: An evaluation of factors contributing to child abuse and neglect* (pp. 109–146). New York: Plenum.

Zahn-Waxler, C., Cole, P., & Barrett, K. C. (1991). Guilt and empathy: Sex differences and implications for the development of depression. In K. Dodge & J. Garber (Eds.), *Emotional regulation and dysregulation* (pp. 242–272). New York: Cambridge University Press.

Zahn-Waxler, C., Radke-Yarrow, M., & King, R. A. (1979). Childrearing and children's prosocial initiations toward victims of distress. *Child Development, 50,* 319–330.

Zahn-Waxler, C., & Robinson, J. (1995). Empathy and guilt: Early origins of feelings of responsibility. In J. P. Tangney & K. W. Fischer (Eds.), *Self-conscious emotions: The psychology of shame, guilt, embarrassment, and pride* (pp. 143–173). New York: Guilford Press.

Zajonc, R. B. (1984). On the primacy of affect. *American Psychologist, 39,* 117–123.

Zastrow, C. (1994). Conceptualizing and changing the self from a rational therapy perspective. In T. M. Brinthaupt & R. P. Lipka (Eds.), *Changing the self* (pp. 175–120). Albany: State University of New York Press.

Zumpf, C. L., & Harter, S. (1989, April). *Mirror, mirror on the wall: The relationship between appearance and self-worth in adolescent males and females.* Paper presented at the annual meeting for the Society for Research in Child Development, Kansas City, MO.

Index

(Page numbers in italics refer to figures or tables)